This book is to be returned on or before
the last date stamped below.

IMMUNOLOGY, BIOCHEMISTRY, AND BIOTECHNOLOGY

SERIES EDITORS:

Praveen Tyle
Sandoz Research Institute
Sandoz Pharmaceutical Corporation
P.O. Box 83288
10401 Highway 6
Lincoln, NE 68501 USA

Bhanu P. Ram
Idetek, Inc.
1057 Sneath Lane
San Bruno, CA 94066 USA

IMMUNOLOGY, BIOCHEMISTRY, AND BIOTECHNOLOGY

Immunology: Clinical, Fundamental, and Therapeutic Aspects

IMMUNOLOGY, BIOCHEMISTRY, AND BIOTECHNOLOGY

Immunology: Clinical, Fundamental, and Therapeutic Aspects

EDITORS:

Bhanu P. Ram
Idetek, Inc.

Mary C. Harris
Children's Hospital of Philadelphia

Praveen Tyle
Sandoz Pharmaceuticals Corporation

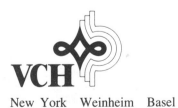

VCH

New York Weinheim Basel Cambridge

Bhanu P. Ram
Idetek, Inc.
1057 Sneath Lane
San Bruno, CA 94066 USA

Mary C. Harris
Department of Pediatrics
University of Pennsylvania
    School of Medicine
The Children's Hospital of Philadelphia
34th Street and Civic Center Boulevard
Philadelphia, PA 19104 USA

Praveen Tyle
Sandoz Research Institute
Sandoz Pharmaceutical Corp.
P.O. Box 83288
10401 Highway 6
Lincoln, NE 68501 USA

Library of Congress Cataloging-in-Publication Data

Immunology : clinical, fundamental, and therapeutic aspects / editors,
    Bhanu P. Ram, Mary C. Harris, Praveen Tyle.
        p.   cm. — (Immunology, biochemistry, and biotechnology)
    Includes bibliographical references.
    ISBN 0-89573-763-9
    1. Immunology.   I. Ram, Bhanu P., 1951–   .
II. Harris, Mary C.   III. Tyle, Praveen, 1960–   .   IV. Series.
    [DNLM: 1. Immunity.   QW 504 I36384]
QR181.I4283   1990
616.07'9—dc20
DNLM/DLC
for Library of Congress   89-24846
                                                                                                                            CIP

British Library Cataloguing in Publication Data
Immunology.
    1. Immunology
    I. Ram, Bhanu P.   II. Harris, Mary C.   III. Tyle, Pravcen
    IIII. Series
    574.2'9

    ISBN 0-527-27854-0

Printed in the United States of America.
ISBN 0-89573-763-9 VCH Publishers
ISBN 3-527-27854-0 VCH Verlagsgesellschaft

Printing History:
10 9 8 7 6 5 4 3 2 1

Published jointly by:

VCH Publishers, Inc.
220 East 23rd Street
Suite 909
New York, New York 10010

VCH Verlagsgesellschaft mbH
P.O. Box 10 11 61
D-6940 Weinheim
Federal Republic of Germany

VCH Publishers (UK) Ltd.
8 Wellington Court
Cambridge CB1 1HW
United Kingdom

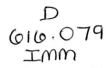

Contributors

MARK R. ALBERTINI, Departments of Human Oncology, Pediatrics, and Genetics, University of Wisconsin, Madison, WI 53792 USA

WILLIAM BENJAMIN, Roche Research Center, Hoffmann-LaRoche, Inc., Nutley, NJ 07110 USA

MILAN BUC, Faculty of Medicine, Comenius University, Bratislava, Czechoslovakia

RICHARD CHIZZONITE, Roche Research Center, Hoffmann-LaRoche, Inc., Nutley, NJ 07110 USA

SHARAD D. DEODHAR, Department of Immunopathology, Cleveland Clinic Foundation, Cleveland, OH 44195-5131 USA

OSCAR L. FRICK, HSW 1404A, School of Medicine, University of California, San Francisco, CA 94143 USA

L. PATRICK GAGE, Roche Research Center, Hoffmann-LaRoche, Inc., Nutley, NJ 07110 USA

MARVIN R. GAROVOY, Immunogenetics and Transplantation Laboratory, University of California Medical Center, San Francisco, CA 94143 USA

MAURICE GATELY, Roche Research Center, Hoffmann-LaRoche, Inc., Nutley, NJ 07110 USA

BRADFORD GRAVES, Roche Research Center, Hoffmann-LaRoche, Inc., Nutley, NJ 07110 USA

JOHN HAKIMI, Roche Research Center, Hoffmann-LaRoche, Inc., Nutley, NJ 07110 USA

MARY C. HARRIS, Department of Pediatrics, University of Pennsylvania School of

Medicine, The Children's Hospital of Philadelphia, 34th Street and Civic Center Boulevard, Philadelphia, PA 19104 USA

Věra Hříbalová, Institute of Hygiene and Epidemiology, Prague, Czechoslovakia

Grace Ju, Roche Research Center, Hoffmann-LaRoche, Inc., Nutley, NJ 07110 USA

Naynesh R. Kamani, Division of Allergy-Immunology, University of Pennsylvania School of Medicine, The Children's Hospital of Philadelphia, 34th Street and Civic Center Boulevard, Philadelphia, PA 19104 USA

Joseph Kaplan, Children's Hospital of Michigan, 3901 Beaubien Boulevard, Detroit, MI 48201 USA

Evžen Kasafírek, Research Institute for Pharmacy and Biochemistry, Prague, Czechoslovakia

Patricia Kilian, Roche Research Center, Hoffmann-LaRoche, Inc., Nutley, NJ 07110 USA

Vladimír Lackovič, Virological Institute, Slovak Academy of Sciences, Bratislava, Czechoslovakia

Michael E. Lambert, Department of Immunology, Scripps Clinic and Research Foundation, 10666 North Torrey Pines Road, La Jolla, CA 92037 USA

Daniel Levitt, Roche Research Center, Hoffmann-LaRoche, Inc., Nutley, NJ 07110 USA

Olivia Martinez, Immunogenetics and Transplantation Laboratory, University of California Medical Center, San Francisco, CA 94943 USA

Kathleen Miller, Lawrence Berkeley Laboratory, University of California at Berkeley, Building 74, One Cyclotron Road, Berkeley, CA 94720 USA

Dušan Mlynarčík, Univerzita Komenskeho Nositelka Radu Republiky, Katedra biochemie a mikrobiologie, 832 32 Bratislava, Kalinciakova 8, Czechoslovakia

Jan Pekárek, Czechoslovakia Institute of Sera and Vaccines, Prague, Czechoslovakia

Bhanu P. Ram, Idetek, Inc., 1057 Sneath Lane, San Bruno, CA 94066 USA

Ross Rocklin, Fisons Corporation, Two Preston Court, Bedford, MA 01730 USA

Jozef Rovenský, State Institute for Control of Drugs, Bratislava, Czechoslovakia

Paul M. Sondel, Departments of Human Oncology, Pediatrics, and Genetics, K4/448 UWCSC, 600 Highland Avenue, University of Wisconsin, Madison, WI 53792 USA

Rakesh Srivastava, Department of Immunology, Scripps Clinic and Research Foundation, 10666 North Torrey Pines Road, La Jolla, CA 92037 USA

Gary Truitt, Roche Research Center, Hoffmann-LaRoche, Inc., Nutley, NJ 07110 USA

Yvonne Tsien, Roche Research Center, Hoffmann-LaRoche, Inc., Nutley, NJ 07110 USA

Praveen Tyle, Sandoz Research Institute, Sandoz Pharmaceuticals Corporation, P.O. Box 83288, 10401 Highway 6, Lincoln, NE 68501 USA

Edward W. Voss, Jr., Department of Microbiology, 131 Burrill Hall, 407 South Goodwin, University of Illinois, Urbana, IL 61801 USA

Robert W. Wilmott, Wayne State University School of Medicine, 3901 Beaubien Boulevard, Detroit, MI 48201 USA

Mervin S. Yoder, Indiana University Medical Center, Indianapolis, IN 46223 USA

Chester M. Zmijewski, University of Pennsylvania Medical Center, 3400 Spruce Street, Philadelphia, PA 19104-4283 USA

Preface

Diagnostics and therapeutic immunology has expanded tremendously in recent years. T. S. Eliot once said, "Where is the knowledge we have lost in information?" Many books (elementary and advanced) have been published on immunological sciences trying to keep pace with the voluminous information available in this area that necessitated various subdivisions in immunology—immunogenetics, clinical immunology, etc. The present book discusses the clinical, fundamental, and therapeutic effects of immunology. Each chapter begins with the basic terminologies, and their explanations, then takes the reader to a much higher level of complexity so that he can appreciate some of the latest achievements of this decade. Thus, the book is useful for people who are beginning to understand immunology yet advanced enough for researchers who are venturing to find new niches in research.

The book begins with fundamentals of immunology and proceeds to explore the subject at increasing levels of detail. The first section delves into the present "state of the art" knowledge of the immune system and immunoglobulins, and its development over the years. Crystallographic structure of immunoglobulin is presented in Chapter 3, which contains the latest findings on this topic. This basic foundation, interwoven with use of immunology in biology (immunobiology), is detailed in the second section. The third section presents the immunological mechanisms that protect human beings against infectious disease and cancer. In addition, this section covers immune deficiency diseases. The fourth section presents drugs of immune origin, especially derived interleukins and immunoregulatory drugs. This area is still in its infancy but the next decade will see the tremendous potential offered by such drugs. This section is included to encourage researchers to develop drugs that are compatible with the immune systems.

The book is designed to give a glance at various aspects of immunology impacting upon the field of biomedicine, both from the basic and clinical view point, and should be of interest to biologists, biochemists, pharmaceutical scientists, immunologists, and biotechnologists, both in industry and academia. The book is directed to students as well as advanced researchers who might be exploring areas away from the beaten path in immunology. It may also be used as a textbook for advance study in immunology.

We would like to thank Christina Martin and Ed Immergut for their editorial help and Sue Kendrick for word processing various aspects of this volume.

Bhanu P. Ram
Mary C. Harris
Praveen Tyle

Contents

BASIC IMMUNOLOGICAL CONSIDERATIONS

CHAPTER 1

Immunology: Yesterday, Today, and Tomorrow

Mary Catherine Harris

Department of Pediatrics, The Children's Hospital of Philadelphia, 34th Street and Civic Center Boulevard, Philadelphia, PA 19104 USA

Bhanu P. Ram

Idetek, Inc., 1057 Sneath Lane, San Bruno, CA 94066 USA

Praveen Tyle

Sandoz Research Institute, Sandoz Pharmaceuticals Corporation, P.O. Box 83288, 10401 Highway 6, Lincoln, NE 68501 USA

Introduction

The field of immunology has expanded tremendously in recent years because of the unprecedented development of new concepts in answer to fundamental scientific questions and the introduction of powerful technologies that have both diagnostic and therapeutic impact. In previous years, immunology was considered part of microbiology, and research in the field investigated problems related to the diagnosis and treatment of infectious diseases. Following significant scientific advances, however, immunology developed into its own science, apart from those of microbiology, pathology, biochemistry, and molecular biology, which nursed its original development. Recently, moreover, with its ever expanding research applications and technologies, the field of immunology has provided important information of use to physicians and scientists in many disciplines, including neonatology, nephrology, genetics, medicine, and surgery. Immunology is currently at the forefront of the medical sciences and has become a most exciting, challenging, and promising field!

The term "immune" derives from the Latin *immunis,* which means "free or exempt from taxes or expenses". In the most classical sense, then, immunology, or the study of the immune system, is concerned with the mechanisms or processes that protect the host from damage caused by invading microorganisms. Moreover, the immune system functions to maintain homeostasis between the internal body milieu and the external environment. Under normal conditions, the immune system effectively defends the host against foreign substances, such as pathogenic microbial agents, as well as native cells that have undergone neoplastic transformation. Defective functioning of the immune system results in disease. It is now well recognized that not all immune responses are helpful to the host. For example, the interaction of the immune system and the environment may produce injury to target cells, termed hypersensitivity or allergy. Likewise, target cells may be directly damaged via autoimmune mechanisms. When immunologic surveillance fails, the manifestations may be those of malignant disease. Bellanti,[1] therefore, has characterized the three functions of the immune system as defense, homeostasis, and surveillance.

Thus, the field of immunology includes contributions from both basic and clinical research investigations. The current text, therefore, has been developed to include contributions from workers in the spheres of both basic and clinical sciences. The first two sections of this text, "Basic Immunological Considerations" and "Immunobiology," reflect contributions from basic scientists, whereas Sections III and IV, "Clinical Immunology" and "Drugs of Immune Origin," review the application of basic immunological principles to clinical problems and drug development.

Brief History

The origin of immunology lies buried in the past and is derived primarily from the study of resistance to infection. It was known from centuries that individuals acquired immunity against a particular disease, eg, smallpox, following recovery from the disease. The first effective immunization was performed by Edward Jenner, an English Physician (1749–1823), who observed that persons who got well after infection with cowpox were protected against smallpox. The enhancement and further development of preventative immunization almost a century later was made possible by Louis Pasteur, who coined the term "vaccine" (from *vacca*: L, cow) in honor of Jenner's contribution. Pasteur's research led to the development of germ theory. He developed techniques to grow microorganisms in vitro. The organisms (living, heat killed, and attenuated) were used as vaccines for the disease they caused. It was observed by Pasteur that old cultures (attenuated) of fowl cholera organism, when inoculated into fowl, produced no disease, although the fowls were found to be resistant to subsequent infection with the organism and were strongly immune.

Humoral Immunity

Robert Koch (1843–1910), while attempting to develop a vaccine for tuberculosis, observed the phenomenon known today as delayed hypersensitivity or cell-mediated immunity. Fodor in 1886 observed a direct action of an immune serum on microbes during the course of his studies on anthrax bacilli. Behring and Kitasato (1890) demonstrated the neutralizing antitoxic activity of sera from animals immunized with diphtheria or tetanus toxin. They injected the serum from animals and demonstrated that normal animals became resistant to the disease. Thus, they concluded that blood (serum) of resistant animals contained a substance, antitoxin, that could neutralize the toxic effect of bacteria.

Rudolf Kraus (1897) demonstrated that a bacterial filtrate became clouded with a precipitate when mixed with serum from immune animals. The immune serum (antiserum) thus contained precipitins. At the same time it was also discovered that an antiserum reacted not only with bacterial products but also with the bacteria themselves. Pfifer observed that certain antisera dissolved bacterial cells (lysis). Gruber and Durham reported that certain other antisera glued bacteria together (agglutination). These reactions as well as others (opsonins, reagins, conglutinins) occurred because of the presence of substances in the serum that were later termed "antibodies." Substances stimulating the appearance of antibodies were then designated "antigens." Yet another serum factor involved in the immune reaction, which was distinctly different from antibodies, was discovered by Hans Buchner in 1893. Confirming Buchner's observation, Bordet observed that goat antiserum to vibro cholerae lysed bacteria when fresh, but when the serum has been heated at 58°C for 1 h, it lost its lysing activity. However, this lysing activity of the serum was regained when some fresh serum from nonimmunized guinea pig was added to the heated serum. It was concluded that goat serum contained two kinds of substances: (1) specific thermostable antibodies, and (2) heat-liable alexin, which was later renamed complement.

Antibodies

Initially, it was believed by microbiologists that antibodies could be produced only against microorganisms. However, it became clear that antibodies could be produced virtually against any molecule—big or small. In addition, the antibodies were found to be very specific in that they reacted with the substance they were produced against.

Later it became apparent that antibodies were proteins. Lloyd D Felton and GH Bailey were the first to isolate the pure antibody generated against pure polysaccharide from pneumococcal bacteria. Fractionation of the serum in ammonium sulfate gave a precipitate and a soluble portion, which were termed, respectively, "globulin" (thought to be related to hemoglobin) and "albumin" (resembling egg white). It was not until the development of an electrophoresis apparatus by Arne W Tiselius that the serum proteins were separated under electric current, yielding peaks with globulin activity. Globulins with antibody activity were designated "immunoglobulins" by JF Heremans.

What makes antibodies manage to distinguish so many antigens with great specificity? This was explained by Paul Ehrlich in 1900 by his theory of stereoscopic complementarity of two kinds of molecule. The antibody molecule is shaped to fit a particular antigen, and only that antigen, like a key and lock.

Karl Landsteiner and his collaborators explained the antigenicity of small molecules. He later termed these molecules "haptens." By conjugating haptens to proteins, he studied the immune response of such conjugates. He concluded that haptens had to be attached to a carrier (protein) to elicit antibody response. The contribution of chemistry to immunology led Svante Arrhenius in 1907 to suggest the name "immunochemistry," denoting a combination of the two, which is accepted today.

Cellular Immunity

At around the turn of the century, there emerged two different points of view of immunology, from which two lines of thought later developed: (1) the humoral theory of immunity, that is mediated by soluble substance (antibodies) present in body fluids, and (2) the cellular theory of immunity, whose emphasis is the biologic effects of intact cells involved in the host's response to foreignness. The Russian zoologist Elie Metchnikoff was the founder of the cellular theory of immunity. His theory held that the body's scavanger cells, the phagocytes, were the primary detectors of foreign material as well as its primary defense system. Now, it is established that both cellular and humoral factors are involved in understanding the principles underlying the immunologic processes that result in tissue injury.

The realization that cellular and humoral immunity are governed by different organs has led some immunologists to speculate that there are two different kinds of lymphocytes—one processed by the bursa and involved primarily in the humoral immunity, and the other processed by the thymus and involved primarily in cellular immunity. William A Ford, Malcolm AS Moore, and some other investigators observed that there were indeed two pathways of lymphocyte development. One passes through the thymus and leads to thymus-derived lymphocytes or T cells, and the other passes through the bursa, leading to bursa-derived lymphocytes, or B cells. Thus, removal of thymus not only inhibits cellular immunity but depresses antibody response by preventing helper T cells (T_H) from maturing.

Recent Periods in Immunology

Discovery of B and T cells made a big impact on immunological understanding. The increasing importance of blood grouping in medicine led to a search for more blood groups in humans and animals. This made geneticists aware of the possibilities that immunological methods had to offer for the study of inheritance. This led to the development of a new branch of immunology, termed "immunogenetics" by M Robert Irwin in 1936. Slowly other new branches of immunology started emerging. An overview of related fields is presented in Figure 1-1.

Present Concepts in Immunology

Two fundamental aspects of immunology persist today; to wit, (1) immunologic phenomena are considered "defense mechanisms" and (2) the organism, under normal conditions, does not react against its own constituents.

In his presidential address to the American Association of Immunologists, William Paul[2] has characterized two centuries in the development of immunology. The first period, from 1880 to the present, marked the century of immunological

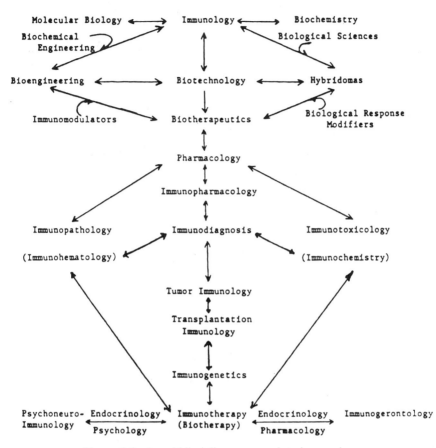

Figure 1-1. A multidisciplinary approach to immunology.
(Courtesy Professor Albert Awad of Ohio Northern University.)

specificity. The second century of immunology, beginning in the 1980s, is proposed to be the century of immunological regulation and the physiology of the immune system. The new era of molecular immunoregulation has already dawned, as evidenced by the proliferation of research and published material in this area. Important concepts include the recognition that antibody production requires the cooperation of helper T and B cells as well as current understanding of the functions of helper and suppressor cells and idiotype–anti-idiotype interactions. In addition, soluble products of the immune system, including cytokines, interleukens, and hematopoietic growth factors, are important regulators of the immune system and may ultimately suggest new pharmacologic mechanisms for the treatment of disease. With regard to the physiology of the immune system, current knowledge is accumulating to elucidate basic biochemical mechanisms of cell function, and to establish cooperative cellular and molecular interactions as the basis for the transmission of information between cells. This network of communicating cells involves a molecular language that controls the development and function of other cells to maintain the integrity of the host within the environment. Further insight is also being gained into genetic information, molecular surface components, and developmental cellular processes. Many of these concepts are presented in detail in the various chapters of this book.

The first section of this book reviews basic immunological considerations. Although presenting a general overview of the immune system, Chapter 2 details recent advances in the area of cellular immunology. The concept of immune regulation is presented as well as some current approaches in immunotherapy. During the past two decades, rapid progress has been made in understanding the structure and formation of antibodies. The information theory of antibody synthesis holds that it is the antigen that dictates the specific structure of the antibody. This theory has been abandoned in favor of genetic theory proposed by Haurowitz in 1970, which holds that the information for synthesis of all possible configurations of antibodies exists in the genome and that specific receptors on immunocompetent cells are normally present, as foreseen by Ehrlich. Chapters 3 and 4 of this book present some of the latest developments in this area, including the crystallographic structures of antibodies. The major histocompatibility complex (MHC) is a chromosomal region consisting of genes that are intimately involved in both cellular and humoral immunity, as well as disease states. The MHC molecules, therefore, provide an additional level of immunological specificity; the structure, expression, and function of class-I genes are detailed in Chapter 5. Antigen–antibody interactions, occurring in both primary and secondary stages, may have either beneficial or deleterious effects on the host, depending on tertiary biological manifestations (Chapter 6). Overall, these first chapters review many principles of structure, function, specificity, and regulation of the immune system.

The next two sections of this book present concepts in immunobiology and clinical immunology and are closely related. Both the cellular components and expression of cell-mediated immunity are included in Chapter 7, along with a discussion of clinical disease states and pharmacologic mediation. The chapter on hypersensitivity (Chapter 8) details the immunologic reactions that have adverse consequences for the host, as summarized earlier. Likewise, the section on tumor immunology (Chapter 10) presents evidence in states where the immunologic balance or surveillance has been evaded in the situation of malignancy. Additional subsections review the host response to the tumor and address novel approaches and current modalities for tumor immunotherapy. These modalities combine standard therapies with immunotherapy, in the hopes of enhancing survival for additional cancer patients. Again, in a similar fashion, autoimmune diseases (Chapter 14) represent a perturbation in the immunological balance, whereby the target cells of the host are injured directly. Additional chapters describe the immunobiology of transplantation (Chapter 9) and the regulation of the immune response to infectious agents (Chapters 11 and 12). The emergence of the AIDS epidemic and daily increasing number of HIV infections is a matter of extreme importance to both clinicians and basic scientists. Chapter 13 presents immunodeficiency diseases, but as well details current information on the acquired immunodeficiency syndrome.

The last section of the book (Chapters 15–18) describes current advances in the soluble mediators, such as the lymphokines and interleukens, which play a critical role in immunoregulation. Perhaps, this next century of immunology will develop around concepts of interacting cells and mediators and will ultimately suggest immunomodulatory therapies for the successful eradication of disease.

Future Prospects

Present and future trends within the field of immunology are again bridging the gap between the basic sciences and clinical medicine. Various new immunologic techniques are becoming available, such as the use of monospecific antisera and T cell subset enumeration and flow cytometry, which are useful in the diagnosis of disease. For example, application of antibodies in the field of diagnostics and medicine has revolutioned the various fields of medical sciences. Progress is so rapid that by the time this book is published there will be some new methods and use. One of the areas that fetched the Nobel prize to Kohler and Milstein is the generation of hybridomas that produce monoclonal antibodies. Monoclonal antibodies are more popular now than conventional antisera because they can be produced in unlimited amounts. Also, clones can be selected to produce monoclonal antibodies tailored to a particular need. For a long time, it was possible to produce only murine monoclonal antibodies, but with the refinement of technique and new knowledge human–human hybridomas are being constructed. Production of chimeric antibodies through genetic manipulation was another breakthrough of the late 1980s.

These antibodies have been used in diagnostics to develop state-of-the-art immunoassays to detect antigens at extremely low levels. In many cases, sensitivity of immunoassay surpasses the sensitivity achieved by conventional organic methods, such as high-performance liquid chromatography. The best use of the antibodies is to develop tests for household or physicians office. By the turn of the century, tests for some of the common ailments such as diabetes are expected to be found in public places, such as restrooms, like a weight machine. Antibodies are being used to develop biosensors that respond like a pH meter.

Newer treatment modalities have also been proposed and are likely to be further explored in the not too distant future. Antibodies, especially monoclonals, are being used as therapeutic agents to cure cancer. This area appears to be so promising that some new biotechnology companies are producing monoclonals tailored to the need of the cancer patient. These monoclonals are then used to deliver toxic substances to destroy the tumor cells while sparing the healthy ones. In addition, there is likely to be an increasing rate of success with organ transplantation, and immunodeficiency disease may become correctable with immunotherapy. Perhaps, the future may also allow the manipulation of the immune response, which will prove valuable as therapy for patients with AIDS. Preventative as well as therapeutic strategies should evolve from the constant interface between clinical medicine and the fundamental laboratory. These advances are hoped to allow a greater maintenance of health, reduction of disease, and ultimately prolongation of life in the not too distant future.

Conclusions

It is beyond the scope of this book to enumerate all recent developments in immunology that have impacted on the biomedical field, but a glance at various chapters of the book may give some of the most important contributions of the recent past. However, there are many unanswered questions as there are unanswered issues, and the more we know, the more questions we have. Perhaps, we have to be content with Robert Frost's line: "The woods are lovely, dark and deep. But I have promises to keep". It appears that we have just started understanding immunology!

References

1. Bellanti JA. Introduction to immunology. In Bellanti JA, Kadlec JV, eds. *Immunology III*, Philadelphia: WB Saunders Company; 1985:1–15.

2. Paul WE. *J Immunol.* 1987;139:1–6.

CHAPTER 2

The Immune System: An Overview

Kathleen L. Miller

Division of Cell and Molecular Biology, Lawrence Berkeley Laboratory, University of California at Berkeley, Berkeley, CA 94720 USA

Introduction

The immune system functions through a complex network of interactions between cells and their products. These interactions govern the ability of the cells of the immune system to recognize and respond specifically to foreign substances (antigens). Antigen-specific immune responses are mediated by two types of lymphocytes; T lymphocytes (thymus dependent), which mediate cellular immunity, and B lymphocytes (bone marrow derived), which mediate humoral immunity via the production of antibody (immunoglobulin). In addition, nonspecific effector mechanisms can amplify these antigen-specific functions. The ability to recognize self and nonself (foreign) is central to the immune system, and the events that produce a specific immune response are regulated by cell-surface molecules that can distinguish between diverse foreign substances (nonself) and self.

This chapter provides an overview of the general characteristics of the immune system; specificity, recognition of self/nonself, and memory. The cells and molecules that are involved in various types of immune responses are also reviewed. Particular emphasis is placed on recent advances in the area of basic cellular immunology. Present thinking on how cells and their products interact to regulate the immune response is addressed. In addition, current approaches in immunotherapy are discussed. Fascinating and highly complex, the immune system offers many challenges to those seeking to manipulate its various components selectively.

Characteristics of the Immune System

Specific immune responses can be induced by an almost limitless variety of foreign substances (antigen). Contact with antigen alters the immune system and imparts a heightened responsiveness or "memory" so that when it comes in contact again with the same antigen, the response is more rapid and intense. The immune system is characterized by its specificity, the ability to distinguish self from nonself, and memory. Hallmarks of the immune system, these criteria are used to characterize a particular response as being due to a specific immunological response.

Specificity

The specificity of the immune response resides in antigen-specific receptors present on the surface of B and T lymphocytes. These receptors, surface immunoglobulin on B cells and the immunoglobulin-like receptor on T cells, recognize and specifically bind to determinants on foreign molecules (antigens). "Specific" means that the antigen reacts in a selective fashion with its corresponding receptor and not with a multitude of other antigen receptors present on other cells.

Self-Recognition

In addition to discriminating between a variety of foreign molecules, the immune system must also have the ability to discriminate between foreign (nonself) and self. The inability to discriminate and therefore to limit the immune response to nonself may result in damage to self tissues. The distinction between foreign (nonself) and self is made by a specific-recognition system that involves cell surface molecules encoded by genes of the major histocompatibility complex (MHC). The MHC encodes, in part, for cell surface proteins that are expressed on essentially all cells in the body. These proteins, the major transplantation or histocompatibility antigens, are responsible for provoking the immunological rejection of tissue grafts. However, their actual biological function is to control the ability of T lymphocytes to recognize self and respond to foreign (nonself) antigens.

Memory

Upon initial exposure to antigen (primary response) there is a lag phase before the immune system responds, for example, with the production of antibody that can specifically bind the antigen (see Figure 2-1). During this primary response, memory cells capable of responding to the same antigen are generated, in addition to cells that secrete specific antibody.[1] The immune system is altered and, since memory cells can persist for prolonged periods, it retains specific memory for that antigen. Upon a second encounter with the same antigen (secondary response), the immune system responds more rapidly and with higher antibody levels (see Figure 2-1). The secondary response differs from the primary response because of the presence of antigen-specific memory cells. The memory of foreignness and the ability to mobilize a rapid response upon reexposure to antigen can provide long-lasting immunity, resistance to disease. The stimulation of long-lasting and effective immunity is the goal of vaccine strategies.

Components of the Immune System

The immune system contains a number of components, including antigen, lymphoid organs and tissues, the MHC, lymphoid cells and their products, immunoglobulin,

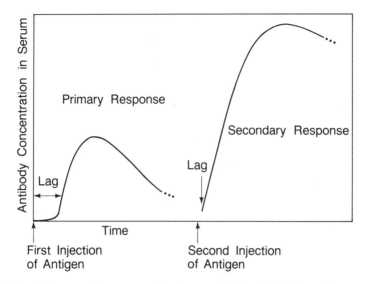

Figure 2-1. Antigen-specific serum antibody concentrations following a first exposure to antigen (primary response) and second exposure to the same antigen (secondary response). Note that the antibody response is more rapid and more intense on second exposure to antigen.

and cytokines. Antigens (foreign substances) are responsible for the induction of specific immunological responses. Lymphoid organs and tissues provide the sites for the development of lymphoid cells and for the generation of immune responses. The cells of the immune system include antigen-specific T and B lymphocytes and nonspecific accessory cells that play a role in immune responses through their ability to process antigen, to secrete soluble factors, and to mediate effector mechanisms. The ability of the immune system to recognize antigen as foreign (nonself) is controlled by gene products of the MHC. In addition, cellular interactions, immunoglobulin, and cytokines regulate the development and outcome of immune responses.

Antigen

A variety of macromolecules can behave as antigens, including most proteins, many polysaccharides, lipoproteins, and nucleoproteins. An antigen has two properties: immunogenicity, the capacity to stimulate the production of specific antibody, and antigenicity, the ability to specifically bind with antibody.[2,3] Immunogenicity is not an inherent property of a macromolecule. The putative immunogen must be recognized as foreign (nonself) and must be able to be presented effectively to the immune system. For instance, small low molecular weight determinants, known as haptens, although capable of binding to antibodies, cannot themselves induce their production.

Although it is conventional to refer to foreign substances as antigens, what is recognized by antigen receptors on lymphocytes and immunoglobulin is not the entire molecule but particular antigenic determinants (epitopes) on the molecule. For example, a single protein molecule may possess a variety of epitopes that can each be recognized by a unique clone of lymphocytes.

Some molecules are able to stimulate T and B cells nonspecifically. These molecules are usually of high molecular weight and contain multiple repeating units. They stimulate a large number of T- and/or B-cell clones, other than those with specific receptors for the antigen, and are therefore known as polyclonal activators. In contrast, antigens stimulate only one or a few specific clones. Antigens that can directly activate B cells to proliferate, without the apparent need for T-cell help, are often referred to as T-independent antigens. A number of substances of bacterial or plant origin have been found to possess this property. Concanavalin A (Con A) and phytohemagglutinin (PHA) are plant lectins that nonspecifically stimulate T cells to proliferate and have been termed mitogens (mitosis promoting agents).[4] Another plant lectin, pokeweed mitogen (PWM), is a potent stimulator of B cells. In addition, lipopolysaccharides (LPS) from gram-negative bacteria and extracts of *Staphylococcus aureus* Cowan strain (SAC) are also potent B-cell mitogens. The level of response of T and B cells to such mitogens is frequently used as a method to monitor, nonspecifically, the functional capacity of these lymphocyte populations.

The route of administration, dose, adjuvants, previous antigenic exposure to the same or crossing reacting antigens, antigen form (soluble or aggregated), and presence of other antigens can all affect the immunogenicity and type of immune response that is induced to a particular immunogen. Adjuvants are substances that enhance the immunogenicity of immunogens and can themselves be immunogenic. Inorganic gels, such as aluminum hydroxide and water–oil emulsions, act by increasing the persistance of antigen and serve as a depot for antigen. The addition of living or dead mycobacteria to water–oil emulsions, complete Freund's adjuvant (CFA), activates macrophages and T cells and increases their effectiveness. Chronic inflammation at the site of injection, however, prevents the use of CFA in humans. Purified cell wall products of mycobacteria, such as muramyl dipeptide, have also proved effective.

Agents, such as adjuvants, that can potentiate the immune response are of great interest and are often referred to as biological response modifiers (BRMs) or immunomodulatory agents.[5,6] Bacterial endotoxin (LPS) is one of the most potent immunomodulators known; however, it also has associated toxic effects. Subunit vaccines are often poorly immunogenic. As a result, safe and effective adjuvants for use in humans are sorely needed. The search is on for new products that can be used to stimulate enduring immunity through an adjuvant effect.

Lymphoid Organs and Tissue

Primary lymphoid organs generate lymphoid cells with specific immunological potential, whereas secondary lymphoid organs serve as sites for the generation of immune responses, that is, the activation by antigen of the proliferation and differentiation of lymphocytes. The primary lymphoid organs are the bone marrow and the thymus and the secondary lymphoid organs include the spleen, lymph nodes, tonsils, and gut- and mucosae-associated lymphoid tissue. Lymphocytes derive their name from the fact that they are abundant in the lymphatic system, a network of vessels that drain fluid (lymph) from the tissues. Lymphocytes have been shown to recirculate from blood to lymph to blood.[7] Most of the recirculating lymphocytes are long-lived T cells; B cells also recirculate but to a lesser extent. As they circulate lymphocytes pass through the spleen and lymph nodes. These organs are highly efficient at trapping and presenting antigen to the cells of the immune system.[3] Lymphocytes can also enter into the tissues via the lymph.

During their differentiation from stem cells, lymphocytes proceed through a series of differentiation events that generate a variety of T- and B-cell clones, each of which expresses a unique antigenic specificity. For B cells, these events take place in the fetal lymphoid tissue and in the adult bone marrow. For T cells, these events are initiated in the same primary lymphoid organs but are concluded in the thymus.

The thymus plays a central role in the development of functional mature T cells and in the specificity of the immune system. Stem cells migrate into the thymus and undergo both differentiation and selection. Through mechanisms that have yet to be fully delineated, T cells are "educated" to be able to recognize antigen in the context of self-MHC-encoded cell-surface molecules; eg, they are "MHC restricted."[8] A major paradox of the immune system, the education of T cells involves the selection for and the development of tolerance to self-MHC. Within the thymus, T cells bearing antigen receptors with no or high affinity for self-MHC are postulated to be eliminated.[9,10]

According to the clonal selection theory of Burnet,[11] lymphocytes become committed to the restricted expression of surface antigen receptors prior to exposure to antigen. Selection of these precommitted antigen-specific lymphocytes by antigen leads to their proliferation and clonal expansion. Following antigen activation, the cells of a particular B-cell clone continue to produce antibody with the same antigen binding site, although the class or isotype of the antibody may be switched under the regulatory influence of T cells.[12] The concept of a cell clone is complicated by the fact that not all its members, which arise from one antigen-specific lymphocyte, are identical. A B-cell clone can contain cells in different states of differentiation. For example, a clone of B cells, specific for a particular antigen, may contain cells that are antibody-secreting B cells (plasma cells) and memory B cells. How a clone develops and its composition of different cell types is determined by a number of regulatory mechanisms.

Cells of the Immune System

The immunological specificity of the immune system is based upon the antigen-specific receptors of T and B lymphocytes. These receptors are the surface immunoglobulin on B cells[13,14] and the immunoglobulin-like receptor on T cells.[15-18] In addition, other cell types play a nonspecific role in the processing and presentation of antigen to lymphocytes and mediate a variety of effector functions. These cells are often collectively referred to as accessory cells. For example, macrophages play a central role in the immune system through their ability to present antigen to lymphocytes and to produce soluble mediators that regulate the immune response.[19,20]

The cells of the immune system are now classified using an array of antibodies that recognize antigenic determinants on a number of their cell-surface molecules. These molecules, whose biological function often is unknown, serve as cell markers for various differentiation states and for functional subpopulations. They are also used to characterize lymphoid malignancies.[21] The use of monoclonal antibody (Mab) to identify cell-surface structures has greatly facilitated studies of cell differentiation and cellular interactions.

Human lymphocytes are currently defined according to a "clusters of differentiation (CD) system."[22,23] A large array of Mab are available that react with the same or different epitopes on a particular cell-surface molecule. Clusters of differentiation represent a clustering of those antibodies that recognize the same cell-surface molecule. For the mouse, in some cases, the Ly (lymphocyte antigen) designation has been retained.[24]

B Lymphocytes

The standard marker for B cells is their membrane or surface immunoglobulin (sIg).[13,14] Other surface antigens, such as CD19 and CD20, are also found on B cells (see Table 2-1). B cells are heterogeneous in their surface molecule expression, their state of maturation, and their ability to function in antibody responses.[25–27] However, unlike T cells, the presence of distinct B-cell lineages remains unresolved. Distinct B-cell lineages are thought to arise from the bone marrow, one representing precursors of antibody-producing B cells and the other representing precursors of memory B cells.[26,27] No doubt there are distinct B-cell subpopulations; however, their existence is not yet fully documented or widely accepted.

T Lymphocytes

The standard marker for murine T lymphocytes is the Thy 1 antigen (thymocyte antigen), CD2 for human T lymphocytes[24] (Table 2-1). More recently, the CD3 surface molecule has been employed as a marker for mature T lymphocytes. The T lymphocytes have been classified into subpopulations based upon the expression of different cell-surface molecules known as CD4 and CD8.[28–30] The CD4+ and CD8+ T-cell subsets are functionally distinct and the regulatory mechanisms that maintain this disparity have not yet been delineated (Table 2-1). The CD4+ T cells exert helper-inducer activity (T_H) for the differentiation of B cells and T cells. They also mediate certain immune-inflammatory responses, such as delayed-type hypersensitivity (T_{DTH} or T_{INF}). The CD8+ T cells mediate the direct killing of target cells, cytotoxic lymphocytes (T_{CTL}), and mediate suppressor functions, T suppressor cells (T_S). The relationship between phenotype and function has not been absolute for the CD4+ and CD8+ T cells. For example, a subpopulation of CD4+

Table 2-1. Cells of the Immune System

		Some Surface Markers	
Cell Type	Function	Mouse	Human
ANTIGEN SPECIFIC			
B lymphocyte	Production of immunoglobulin	sIg	sIg
		Lyb4	CD19, CD20
T lymphocyte		Thy 1	CD2
		CD3	CD3
T helper (T_H)	Provides help to antigen-stimulated B cells and to other T cells	L3T4 (CD4)	CD4
T delayed hypersensitivity (T_{DTH} or T_{INF})	Activates macrophages and mediates killing of intracellular organisms and delayed-type hypersensitivity	L3T4 (CD4)	CD4
T cytotoxic lymphocyte (T_{CTL})	Lysis of target cells (MHC restricted)	Ly2 (CD8)	CD8
T suppressor (T_S)	Blocks induction and/or action of T-helper cells	Ly2 (CD8)	CD8
NONSPECIFIC			
Monocyte-macrophage	Antigen processing, secretion of IL-1	Mac-1,2,3 CD11	CD11 CD14

Source: based on Holmes KL, Morse HC, *Immunol Today*. 1988;9:345.

T cells has been shown to function as cytotoxic T cells, whereas some CD8[+] T cells have been shown to provide help to B cells.[28]

Studies of cloned mouse T-cell lines have revealed two major functional phenotypes of CD4[+] T helper cells.[31−33] At this time there are no surface markers to distinguish these two murine T cell subpopulations, which are currently defined by differences in their patterns of cytokine synthesis and functional properties. These subpopulations, referred to as T_H1 and T_H2, appear to play distinct roles in protective immunity and to have different activation pathways. The T_H1 cells are thought to predominate in cell-mediated immunity to intracellular pathogens, whereas the T_H2 cells are thought to predominate in humoral immunity to extracellular pathogens. Similar subpopulations, OX-22[+] and OX-22[−], have been observed for rat T cells.[34] Attempts to demonstrate similar subpopulations of human T cell clones, either by monoclonal antibody or by clonal analysis of lymphokine production, have not met with success. Human T-cell clones appear to have the potential to exert multiple functions upon stimulation and to retain a degree of pluripotency.[35] Differences in the nature of the stimulus (antigen, mitogen, Mab to CD3) and the length of time maintained in culture in producing T clones may account for this, or there may not be a human equivalent to the functional dichotomy observed with rodent T cells.

The CD4[+] T cell subpopulation in humans has been subdivided by the expression of surface antigens recognized by Mab 2H4 (CD45RA) and 4B4 (CD45RO) (UCHL1).[36] The CD4[+] 2H4[+] subset has been shown to function as inducers of CD8[+] T suppressor cells and the CD4[+] 4B4[+] T-cell subset to provide help to B cells for antibody production. Depending upon the type of activation, T cells have the potential to mediate a variety of functions, such as help, suppression, and cytotoxicity. Through the release of soluble mediators, T lymphocytes also play a pivotal role in regulating the immune system.

Antigen-Presenting Cells

Complex antigens appear to require "processing" and presentation by macrophages to become immunogenic.[19,37] Usually T-helper cells are not directly activated by foreign molecules. Rather they have evolved to recognize antigen, on the surface of certain antigen-presenting cells (APC), in association with self-MHC-encoded molecules.[8,38] It has been postulated that antigen processing serves to select for the epitope on the antigen molecule that has an affinity for the MHC-encoded molecule. Antigen presentation typically requires antigen processing, a sequence of events that includes internalization of antigen, denaturation or digestion of antigen into fragments, and its return to the surface in the context of MHC-encoded molecules.

Antigen-presenting cells (APC) other than the classical macrophages can also function in the presentation of antigen.[37,39-42] B cells, Langerhans cells of the skin, dendritic cells of the lymphoid organs, and the vascular endothelia have all been shown to present antigen. Not all APCs are equivalent. For example, some APCs, such as macrophages, also secrete soluble factors, such as interleukin-1 (IL-1), that serve to activate T lymphocytes.[19,20] It is not clear whether all APCs must provide such additional signals for the activation of T_H cells. Differences in the level of expression of MHC-encoded molecules by APC and in the abilities to process antigen and to produce soluble factors in diverse anatomic compartments may serve to modulate the immune response. The process by which antigens are endocytosed, modified, and returned to the cell surface in an immunogenic form is an area of intense investigation.

Immunoglobulin

Antibodies are specialized protein molecules (immunoglobulin) that specifically bind to their target molecule antigen. Immunoglobulin molecules are composed of two identical light chains (either κ or λ) and two identical heavy chains (μ, γ, δ, α or ϵ) that are held together by disulfide bonds (Figure 2-2). Each chain has an amino-terminal variable (V) region and a carboxy-terminal constant (C) region.[2] The V and C regions are encoded by separate germline genes, which are rearranged and joined during lymphocyte development.[43] The heavy-chain C region defines the class (isotype) of the immunoglobulin molecule. There are five major classes of immunoglobulin (Ig): IgA, IgD, IgE, IgG, and IgM. The IgG class is subdivided into four subclasses IgG_1, IgG_2, IgG_3, and IgG_4 (Table 2-2).

Antibodies serve two specific functions: specific binding to antigenic determinants and participation in effector functions. These two functions are carried out by

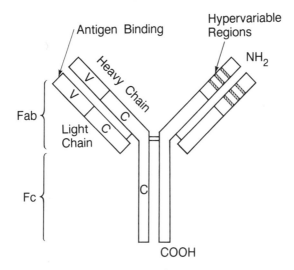

Figure 2-2. Representation of an immunoglobulin molecule. The molecule is composed of two identical heavy chains (H) and two identical light chains (L) linked by disulfide bonds. Both the H and L chains contain variable (V) regions, hypervariable regions, and constant (C) regions. Digestion of the molecule with papain yields the Fab fragment, which contains the antigen binding sites, and the Fc fragment, which determines the biological activities of the molecule.

different domains of the antibody molecule, known as the Fab (antigen binding fragment) and the Fc region[44] (Figure 2-2). Antigen combines with antibody in an antigen binding site that is formed, mainly, by the hypervariable regions of the V region of heavy and light chains. The cavity formed by the antibody–antigen binding site is complementary to a specific epitope on the antigen molecule.[2] The constant region, which determines the isotype of the immunoglobulin molecule, is responsible for a variety of effector functions, such as[45] the fixation of complement, binding to receptors on cells for the Fc region of immunoglobulin (FcR),[46] and passage across the placenta (Table 2-2).

Immunoglobulin M is the major surface immunoglobulin on early B cells and it is the first antibody produced by antigen-activated B cells during a primary immune response. It is present in the serum as a pentamer joined together by a J chain, a protein molecule that does not share homology with immunoglobulin.[47] Immunoglobulin G is the most abundant immunoglobulin in the serum and the only immunoglobulin to cross the placenta in humans. Immunoglobulin D, a major surface immunoglobulin of early B cells, appears to function in a regulatory capacity, but its biological significance is not known.[48] Immunoglobulin A is the principle immunoglobulin of mucous secretions, and B cells producing it are particularly abundant around mucin glands of the intestinal, respiratory, and genitourinary mucosae. It plays a role in protecting mucosal surfaces from pathogens. Its secretion across the epithelium is dependent upon the addition of a protein molecule

Table 2-2. Some Properties of Human Immunoglobulin Classes

Property	IgM	IgG$_1$	IgG$_2$	IgG$_3$	IgG$_4$	IgA$_1$	IgA$_2$	IgD	IgE
Molecular weight ($\times 10^{-3}$)	900	150	150	150	150	150–600	150–600	185	190
Basic number of 4-chain subunits	5[a]	1	1	1	1	1, 2[b]	1, 2[b]	1	1
Average conc. in serum (mg/mL)	1	8	4	1	0.4	3.5	0.4	0.03	0.0001
% Total immunoglobulin	6	80	80	80	80	13	13	1	0.002
Principle surface Ig on B cells	+	–	–	–	–	–	–	+	–
Complement fixation	++	++	+	++	–	–	–	?	–
Binds to mast cells	–	–	–	–	–	–	–	–	+
Binds to macrophage	–	++	+	++	±	–	–	–	–
Transmitted across the placenta	+	±	+	+	–	–	–	–	–
Predominate in mucous secretions	–	–	–	–	–	+	+	–	–

Source: adapted from Eisen HN. *Immunology.* New York: Harper & Row; 1980.

[a]Pentamer held together with J chain (Koshland ME. *Adv Immunol.* 1974;20:41).

[b]Polymeric forms in external secretions contain a J chain and a secretory component (Cebra J. *Adv Exp Med Biol.* 1974;45:23).

known as the "secretory piece."[49] In the secretions IgA is present as dimers, trimers, etc., joined by a J chain. Immunoglobulin E is the principle skin-sensitizing (reaginic) immunoglobulin in humans. It binds to mast cells, basophils, and eosinophils via their cell-surface receptors for the Fc portion of the IgE molecule (Fc_ER).[50] IgE mediates certain allergic responses in humans. It is present in elevated levels in the serum of "atopic" individuals and during infections with certain helminth parasites.

Antibodies display a remarkably diverse range of antigen binding specificities. From a relatively small number (a few hundred) of genes the mammalian immune system has been estimated to be capable of expressing as many as 10^{10} different antibody specificities. Antibody diversity arises from a number of sources, including associations of different heavy and light chains, gene rearrangements in the B cell line, and the recognition of several epitopes by some antibodies.[51,52] To code for immunoglobulin molecules there are separate variable (V), joining (J), diversity (D), and constant (C) gene segments.[53] During the development of B cells the gene segments are rearranged into a complete gene.[43] An array of germline (V) region genes, which code for distinct amino acid sequences, combine with various D and J segments to give rise to a diverse primary immunoglobulin repertoire. Somatic mutation in the V region then generates immunoglobulin of higher affinity for antigen.[54] The rearrangement of V gene families and H and L genes during the ontogeny of B cells is not random and appears to be a programmed process.[55]

The earliest B-cell precursors have only cytoplasmic μ heavy chains. When a light chain is synthesized entire immunoglobulin molecules are expressed on the membrane ($sIgM^+$) and the cells are then able to recognize and respond to antigen.[25,52] The selective activation of B cells with sIg by a particular antigen is followed by proliferation (clonal expansion) and immunoglobulin gene rearrangement coupled with further maturation (isotype switching). Upon antigen activation the phenotypic changes that occur in B cells include shifts in the phenotype of surface and secreted immunoglobulin progressing from IgM^+ to IgM^+ IgD^+ to IgM^+ IgD^-. Mature B cells may retain sIgM or sIgD or acquire sIgA, sIgG, sIgE. The mechanisms regulating the isotype switch involve both T-helper cells and soluble factors and are still not fully understood.[56] In addition to antibody-secreting plasma cells, other cells become memory B cells.

After immunization in vivo or in vitro, B cells can be immortalized as hybridoma lines by cell fusion with immortal B cell lines.[57] These hybridoma lines make monoclonal antibody. Since these monoclonal antibodies are the product of a single B-cell clone they are homogeneous, and each particular Mab has a single defined antigen specificity and only one heavy- and one light-chain isotype. In contrast, polyclonal serum antibody populations are heterogeneous and composed of multiple individual immunoglobulins representing the products of multiple individual B-cell clones, each with a distinct antigen binding specificity and one of potentially five heavy-chain and two light-chain isotypes.

Curiously, a number of lymphocyte cell-surface molecules have been shown to possess immunoglobulin-like domains and to share sequence homology, suggesting a common evolutionary origin. The members of this "immunoglobulin-gene super-family" include the T-cell surface molecules CD3, CD4, and CD8; the T-cell antigen receptor; and MHC-encoded molecules. Based upon this observation, immunoglobulins are thought to have evolved from cell-surface molecules that played a role in basic cell-surface recognition.[58]

Cytokines

A variety of soluble factors are made by the cells of the immune system. These molecules play an essential role in the induction and regulation of immune responses. Products of lymphocytes, largely T-cell derived, are called lymphokines while products of monocytes or macrophages are called monokines. In addition, some mediators that are made by and act upon leukocytes are called interleukins (IL). Collectively they are all considered cytokines. It is now recognized that many of these factors are not made exclusively by and do not act exclusively on cells of the immune system. In fact, they are part of a puzzling and complex network that serves to link the immune system with the other systems in the body including the inflammatory and hemopoietic systems. It is now accepted that a particular cytokine can have multiple biological activities, act synergistically with other cytokines, or inhibit the action of other cytokines depending upon the target tissue and its state of differentiation. Different stages in the lymphocyte proliferative cascade require different factors to act as activation factors, growth factors, and differentiation factors. The cytokine network controlling the cells of the immune system is highly complex and not fully understood. However, several general properties of cytokines have been documented, based primarily on in vitro observations (Table 2-3).

Interleukin-1 (IL-1) plays a dual role as a mediator of immune cell interactions and as a major mediator of the inflammatory response.[59,60] There are two distinct molecules, IL-1α and IL-1β, which share about 40% homology and appear to bind to the same cell receptor. Interleukin-1 is produced by a variety of cells and has a broad range of biological activities in both lymphoid and nonlymphoid tissues. Released by activated macrophages it plays a role in the activation of T cells. It induces the production of IL-2 by T cells and the expression of interleukin-2 receptors (IL-2R) on T cells. Whether all T cells require such activation by IL-1 is not clear. Interleukin-2 is thought to be essential to the clonal expansion of T cells,[61] a property that has been exploited to produce and maintain T-cell clones and hybridomas in vitro. Originally thought to act only on T cells, IL-1 and IL-2 may also have regulatory effects on B cells.

Cytokines are also essential to the growth and differentiation of B cells. At least six cytokines, IL-1, IL-2, IL-4, IL-5, IL-6, and interferon-γ (IFN-γ), have been shown to influence antigen-stimulated B cells.[56,62,63] Some of them, IL-4 and IL-5, have been recently shown to play a role in the preferential induction of particular immunoglobulin isotypes by T_H cells. In addition cytokines stimulate nonspecific

Table 2-3. Soluble Mediators of the Immune System

Factor	Functions
IL-1α, IL-1β	Stimulates T-cell differentiation; costimulates B cells, endogenous pyrogen, hemopoietin-1
IL-2	Stimulates growth of T cells; costimulates B-cell differentiation (T-cell growth factor, TCGF)
IL-3	Multipotential hemopoietic growth factor; stimulates mast cell growth
IL-4	Costimulates B-cell proliferation; stimulates limited T-cell growth; enhances IgE and IgG$_1$ production; stimulates Ia expression (B-cell stimulatory factor-1, BCSF-1)
IL-5	Costimulates B-cell growth; enhances IgA production; enhances eosinophil differentiation (B-cell growth factor-2, BCGF-2)
IL-6	Costimulates B- and T-cell growth, Interferon β$_2$ (B-cell differentiation factor, BCDF)
IL-7	Stimulates growth of early B cells (Lymphopoietin 1)
IFN-γ	Inhibits viral replication; activates NK cells and macrophages; induces expression of Ia; inhibits action of IL-4 on B cells

Source: adapted from Mossman TR, Coffman RL. *Immunol Today*. 1987;8:223.

accessory cells. For example, IL-3 and IL-4 have been shown to induce the differentiation of mast cells and IL-5 to induce the differentiation of eosinophils.

Other cytokines may also regulate immune responses. Transforming growth factor β (TGFβ) has been shown to be a potent inhibitor of both T- and B-cell proliferation in vitro.[64,65] Since many of the observations on the action of cytokines have been in vitro, the in vivo role played by these cytokines is still an area of active research.[66] The unraveling of how these cytokines regulate the cellular interactions of the immune system and how to use this knowledge to manipulate the immune system is one of the more exciting areas of immunology today.

The Major Histocompatibility Complex (MHC)

Central to the immune system is the ability to recognize foreign substances as nonself and to make an appropriate immune response. The MHC, a cluster of genes, codes for cell-surface molecules essential for the recognition of one cell of the immune system by another, for the recognition of foreign substances, and for regulation of immune responses.[67,68] The MHC of humans, on chromosome 6, is known as the human leukocyte antigen (HLA) complex. In the mouse the MHC, on chromosome 17, is known as the histocompatibility-2 (H-2) complex.

All vertebrates possess one MHC, containing three major classes of genes. In addition, there are many minor histocompatibility regions. Class-I genes code for the major histocompatibility or transplantation antigens. These cell-surface proteins are expressed on essentially all cells in the body and provoke the immunological rejection of tissue grafts. They were discovered as a result of transplantation stud-ies. Generally, grafts of tissue are rapidly rejected when donor and recipient are mismatched at the MHC. Class-I molecules are coded by loci A, B, and C of the human HLA complex and loci K and D of the mouse H-2 complex. The MHC is highly polymorphic, with each locus having 20–50 alleles. This is why it is so difficult to find histocompatible donors when performing organ transplants. Class-I molecules are composed of two chains, a heavy chain and β_2-macroglobulin, that are noncovalently associated on the cell surface.

Class-II genes code for cell-surface molecules known as immune-response-asso-ciated (Ia) molecules that regulate the ability of lymphocytes to respond to antigen. They were discovered when the ability of different inbred strains of mice to make or not make antibody to simple peptides was shown to be determined by gene products of a region of the MHC.[38,69] This region is known as the immune-response (Ir) region. Class-II molecules are coded by loci DP, DQ, and DR in humans and loci I-A and I-E in the mouse.[70] Class-II molecules are heterodimers composed of an α and a β chain, which are noncovalently associated. Unlike class-I molecules, class-II (Ia) molecules are not expressed on all cells. They are found on only a few cells in the body, primarily of the reticuloendothelial system. These include macrophages, Langerhans cells of the skin, and dendritic cells of lymphoid organs. They are also expressed on B cells. All these cells are associated with being effective APC.[39,42] In addition, the expression of Ia molecules on cells is not constitutive and subject to both positive and negative regulation. Class-III genes encode for a variety of protein molecules, including proteins of the complement (C') system. Recently the genes coding for tumor necrosis factor α and β (TNF) have also been shown to be in the MHC region. Both C' and TNF have been shown to play regulatory roles in the immune system.

One of the most significant findings in immunology is the demonstration that CD4$^+$ T-helper cells appear to recognize antigen in association with class-II (Ia) molecules, whereas CD8$^+$ T cytotoxic cells appear to recognize antigen in associa-tion with class-I molecules.[38,69] It has been proposed that by limiting the expression of Ia to certain cells and regulating its expression T_H cells are less likely to recog-nize antigens on cells that do not bear class-II molecules, eg, most cells in the body. How the expression of Ia molecules is regulated by lymphocyte products such as IFN-γ and IL-4 is not known.[71]

T- and B-Cell Antigen Recognition

T cells differ from B cells in their recognition of antigen. It has been generally held that B cells recognize conformational determinants on native proteins, whereas T cells recognize relatively short sequences of peptides that result from the processing of native molecules by APC. However, the general rule of linear peptide presenta-tion is not obeyed by all T cells.[72] Unlike B cells, T cells do not appear to recognize protein antigens in their native conformation but require that they be processed by antigen processing cells via an endosomal- or lysosomal-mediated mechanism to expose a peptide fragment or a domain that contains the T-cell antigenic determinant (epitope).[37] In addition, T cells have been shown to recognize antigen in association with cell-surface molecules encoded by the MHC.[38,73] This requirement is referred to as "MHC restriction."

These differences in antigen recognition by T and B lymphocytes reside in the nature of their antigen-specific receptors. In the case of B cells the receptor is membrane immunoglobulin[13,14] and in the case of T cells the receptor is a complex of immunoglobulin-like molecules that are capable of recognizing both antigen and self-MHC-encoded molecules.[15,18] Two types of T-cell receptor (TCR), TCRαβ and TCRγδ, have been demonstrated on distinct T-cell subpopulations.[74] On the surface of T cells, the TCR is thought to interact with invariant molecular complexes, including CD3, CD4, and CD8. How these molecules interact and signal the T cell is largely speculative.

B-Cell Antigen Recognition

B cells recognize antigen via the antigen-binding sites of membrane-bound immunoglobulin. The antigen binding site is largely made up of the hypervariable segments of the V regions of both the light and heavy chains. Framework amino acid residues appear to interact to hold the antigen-binding site in place.[2] Despite knowledge about the structure of the antigen binding site and the nature of its interaction with antigen, there is still debate as to how B cells recognize and bind to antigen. It is still not clear what makes an effective B-cell epitope or whether there are conformational changes in the antibody when antigen is bound. x-Ray crystallographic studies of Fab fragment–antigen complexes, currently in progress, are being used to provide a better understanding of the interactions between antibody and antigen.[75]

MHC Restriction of T Cells

The MHC restriction of T cells was observed in early studies of the ability of cytotoxic T cells to kill virally infected target cells.[73] Mice of the H-2^k inbred strain were injected with sublethal doses of lymphocytic choriomeningitis (LCM) virus to induce cytotoxic T cells specific for LCM-infected target cells. Lymphocytic choriomeningitis-specific T cells from the H-2^k strain of mice were able to kill LCM-infected target cells only if the infected target cells were of the same H-2 strain (Figure 2-3). Cytotoxic T cells from the LCM-immunized H-2^k strain mice would not lyse LCM-infected H-2^b target cells. The cytotoxic T cells were recognizing not only viral antigens on the surface of infected cells but also MHC-encoded proteins. It is now known that CD8$^+$ cytotoxic T cells recognize antigen, on the cell surface, in association with class-I MHC-encoded molecules. Such MHC restriction also extends to the collaborative interactions of CD4$^+$ T$_H$ cells with B cells and antigen-processing cells. The CD4$^+$ T$_H$ cells recognize antigen in association with class-II Ia molecules on the surface of APC. Apparently, T cells have evolved to recognize antigen in association with MHC-encoded molecules. Processed antigen can bind to class-I or class-II MHC molecules and different antigen-processing pathways may be involved.[76]

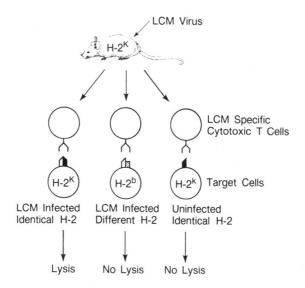

Figure 2-3 MHC restriction of T-cell recognition in cytotoxic T-cell killing of virally infected target cells. T cells from H-2ᵏ strain, LCM-virus-immunized mice are able to kill target cells infected with LCM virus only if the infected target cells are of the same H-2 strain, H-2ᵏ. Based upon Zinkernagel RM, Doherty PC. *Adv Immunol.* 1979; 27:51; and Goodenow RS, et al., *Science.* 1985; 230:777.

Studies of the epitopes that are recognized by T cells have suggested that the immunodominant peptides for T cells are those that can assume the three-dimensional structure of an amphipathic helix in which uncharged hydrophobic amino acids serve as T-cell recognition sites,[77] a structure that appears well suited to binding to MHC proteins. Currently, interactions with purified MHC molecules and immunogenic peptides are being used to determine what makes an effective T-cell epitope.[78]

T-Cell Antigen Receptor (TCR)

As discussed earlier, it is generally accepted that CD4$^+$ T$_H$ cells recognize antigen associated with class-II MHC-encoded molecules, while CD8$^+$ T cytotoxic cells recognize antigen associated with class-I MHC-encoded molecules. Antigen-specific MHC complex restricted recognition of antigen by CD4$^+$ and CD8$^+$ T cells is mediated by the T-cell receptor (TCR).[15-18] The TCR recognizes two ligands simultaneously, antigen and proteins encoded for by genes of the MHC locus. The TCR is a disulfide-linked heterodimer composed of an α chain and a β chain. The genes coding for the TCR have been shown to be composed of several gene segments, variable (V), diversity (D), and joining (J), that rearrange during development to form genes. This process generates unique receptors for each T cell. There are similarities with the antigen receptor (immunoglobulin) of B cells. Both construct combining sites through the use of heterodimers and both use VDJ transloca-

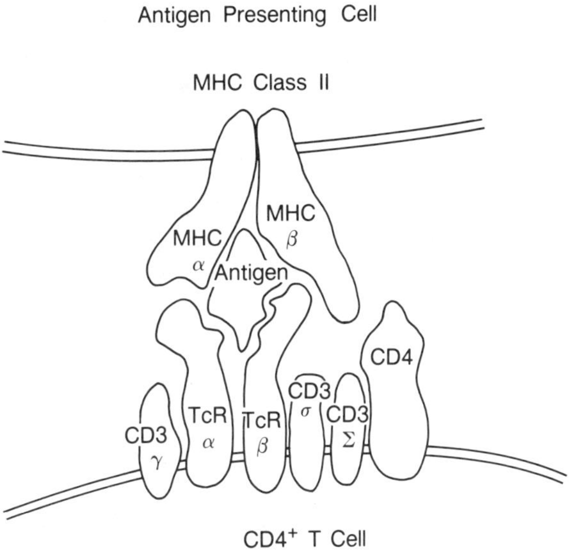

Antigen Presenting Cell

MHC Class II

CD4+ T Cell

Figure 2-4. The T-cell antigen–receptor (TCR)–CD3 complex on a CD4+ T-helper cell and the MHC-encoded class II molecule on an antigen-presenting cell. The two chains (α and β) of the TCR and the three chains (γ, σ, and Σ) of the CD3 molecule are illustrated. The TCR–CD3 complex on T cells interacts with antigen in association with MHC-encoded molecules on the antigen-presenting cell. Based upon Traunecher A, et al., *Immunol Today.* 1989; 10:29.

tions to assemble the gene for transcription. The genes for the TCR, unlike immunoglobulin genes, do not appear to undergo somatic mutation and there appears to be no T-cell counterpart to B-cell isotype switching.

The antigenic repertoire of T cells is postulated to arise from germline genes for the α and β chain of the TCR, removal of self-reactive T-cell clones during the induction of tolerance to self-antigens in the thymus, and positive selection of cells bearing receptors biased for recognition of antigen in association with self-MHC molecules.[8–10] Immunological tolerance is defined as the impairment of the ability to respond to an antigen, resulting from previous exposure to it.[79] Largely a mysterious process, clonal deletion of self-responding TCRαβ+ T cells is thought to occur via interactions of CD4+ CD8+ thymocytes with Ia+ dendritic cells of the thymus.[9]

On the T-cell surface the TCRαβ is noncovalently associated with the CD3 multichain complex. This complex consists of at least five proteins including the invariant γ, σ, and Σ chains (Figure 2-4). The TCRαβ–CD3 complex serves as the antigen receptor on T cells. The CD3 complex, present on all T cells, is thought to stabilize the binding of antigen, in the context of MHC, by T cells and to provide a transducing signal when the TCRαβ binds antigen. The invariant CD4 and CD8 accessory molecules present on the cell surface of distinct T-cell subpopulations are also thought to deliver positive signals during T-cell antigen activation.[80] Class-II recognition is thought to be the consequence of the binding of invariant sites on the class-II MHC encoded proteins by the CD4 molecule, which is thought to act as the signaling component of the TCR–class-II MHC complex. The CD8 molecule may act in a similar fashion by physically associating with the TCRαβ during recognition of antigen and class-I MHC-encoded proteins.

A second TCR, TCRγδ, is found on CD4[-], CD8[-] T cells and is composed of a γ and a δ chain.[74] The TCRγδ[+] T cells appear to represent a separate lineage of T cells. They have been found to be the dominant T-cell population in the epidermis of the skin and have been postulated to mediate immune surveillance of the epithelia.[81,82]

T- and B-Cell Interactions

The immune response to antigen requires the interaction or collaboration of cells within the immune system. For the production of antibody by B cells, T_H cells collaborate with B cells and provide antigen-specific help via cellular interactions and the release of cytokines. In some instances, the participation of nonspecific accessory cells, such as macrophages, is also required. These cells function by processing and presenting antigen and, in some cases, by releasing cytokines. The helper inducer cells also collaborate with other T cells to generate the effector cells of cell-mediated immunity, such as T_{CTL} and T_{DTH}, from T-cell precursors. The early events of T- and B-cell collaboration are still not fully understood. Increasing evidence that B cells are effective antigen-presenting cells and the discovery of distinct T_H subpopulations is changing our concept of how these cells interact via a network of cytokines.

Hapten–Carrier Effect

The antibody response to antigen requires the cooperation between B cells and helper T cells specific for the same antigen molecule. Early studies showed that the secondary antibody response to small chemically defined determinants (haptens) was influenced by the "carrier" molecule to which it was chemically coupled.[83-85] For example, when mice were primed with hapten (dinitrophenyl, DNP) coupled to the carrier bovine serum albumin (BSA) a second injection of DNP–BSA several weeks later gave a vigorous secondary anti-DNP response (Figure 2-5a). However, if the second injection was made with hapten (DNP) coupled to another carrier molecule, ovalbumin (OVA), the secondary anti-DNP response was minimal. Further studies, in which antigen-primed T and B cells were adoptively transferred into irradiated mice, showed that in addition to hapten-specific B cells, T cells that recognized the carrier molecule were also required for the production of hapten-specific antibody.[86] The "hapten–carrier" effect was explained by an "associative-recognition" model of T- and B-cell interaction.[83-87] In this model, T cells recognize antigenic determinants on the carrier molecule and provide help via cytokines to B cells that recognize haptenic determinants on the same antigen molecule (Figure 2-5b). The T-helper cell and the B cell interact via an "antigen

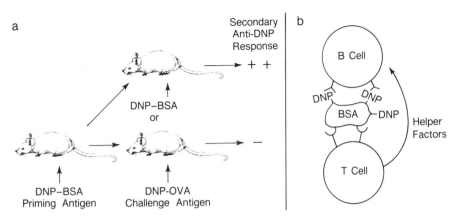

Figure 2-5. (a) The hapten–carrier effect. A secondary antibody response to hapten, such as dinitrophenyl (DNP), is only obtained when mice have been previously primed with both the hapten (DNP) and the same carrier, such as bovine serum albumin (BSA), to which it is linked. If mice primed with DNP–BSA are later challenged with hapten (DNP) linked to another carrier, ovalbumin (OVA), there is no secondary anti-DNP response. (b) B cells specific for haptenic determinants on the antigen interact with T cells specific for carrier determinants on the same antigen. T cells provide a second signal to B cells via the release of soluble factors.

bridge," which stabilizes the interaction and serves to focus the release of cytokines.[88] The result is the activation of B cells to produce anti-hapten antibody. The prevailing view for B-cell activation is the "two signal theory of lymphocyte activation,"[87] the initial event being the interaction of antigen with surface immunoglobulin, which results in the crosslinking of immunoglobulin antigen receptors. Subsequent clonal expansion of antigen-stimulated B cells and their differentiation into cells that secrete antibody is induced by secondary signals provided by T-helper cells.

Models of T- and B-Cell Interaction

In addition to antigen-specific T and B lymphocytes, nonspecific antigen-presenting cells (APC) have also been shown to be required for antibody production by B cells.[20,89–91] T-helper cells are thought to provide help via two distinct mechanisms: cell interactions, which require MHC-restricted collaboration, and cytokine-mediated help. The MHC restriction of this interaction implies that the T cell recognizes antigen on the surface of antigen-presenting cells in the context of MHC-encoded molecules. As discussed earlier, in the majority of cases antigen presentation also requires antigen processing, a sequence of events that includes internalization of antigen, denaturation or digestion of antigen into fragments, and its return to the surface in the context of MHC-encoded molecules.

In the generally accepted model of T- and B-cell interaction, antigen-presenting cells (classically macrophages) process antigen and present it to T-helper cells in the context of class-II MHC molecules. The TCRαβ recognizes antigen in the context

CELL MEDIATED IMMUNITY

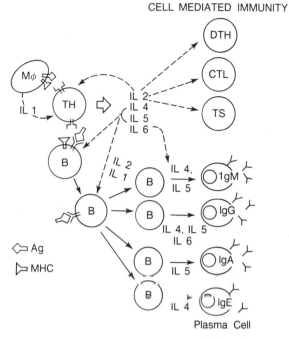

Plasma Cell

HUMORAL IMMUNITY

Figure 2-6. Generalized scheme to illustrate the postulated sequence of events leading to the activation, proliferation, and differentiation of B cells into antibody-secreting plasma cells (humoral immunity) and the induction of T-cell-mediated responses; cytotoxic T cells (CTL), delayed-type hypersensitivity (DTH), and T-suppressor cells (T_s) (cellular immunity). Cytokines are produced by activated helper T cells (TH) in response to macrophage (MΘ) and/or B-cell presentation of antigen (Ag) in the context of MHC-encoded molecules (MHC). These cytokines regulate the proliferation and differentiation of cells in the network. Based upon Abbas AK. *Immunol Today.* 1988; 9:89; and Miyajima A, et al. *Fed Proc Am Soc Exp Biol.* 1988; 2:2462.

of Ia molecules aided by accessory molecules, such as CD3 and CD4. In addition, the T cell receives a second signal, IL-1, from the antigen-presenting macrophage (Figures 2-4 and 2-6). The activated T_H cell produces IL-2 and expresses receptors for IL-2 (IL-2R), which results in the clonal expansion of the antigen-specific T-cell clone. The T cell, in turn, presents antigen to B cells specific for haptenic groups on the antigen. The activated T cells also produce cytokines, such as IL-4, IL-5, and IL-6, which serve to expand the B cells clonally and anti-hapten antibody is produced.

Recent observations have led to a reinterpretation of this model. These include the observation that B cells may be efficient APC to MHC class-II restricted T cells,[37,40-42] the definition of subsets of T_H cells (at least in rodents),[31-33] and the in vitro effects of recombinant cytokines on T and B cells.[59-64] The concept of T cells as active regulatory cells and B cells as passively regulated cells has been reevaluated. B cells have been shown to be very effective at antigen processing and presentation to. T cells through their immunoglobulin antigen receptors. Antigen presentation by B cells is particularly useful when antigen is present in low concentration as antibody can facilitate the uptake of antigen.

In another model of T- and B-cell interaction, the B cell, specific for hapten, is thought to capture antigen and after processing it, to present a portion of the carrier molecule to the T cell (Figure 2-6). The T cells are then stimulated to secrete cytokines that induce B-cell growth and differentiation. It is still unclear at what stage in its activation pathway the normal B cell can present antigen to obtain help.

Thus the primary response to antigen can be initiated in essentially two ways: (1) The T helper cell can interact with antigen on B cells and the T cell then provides helper signals to the B cell for proliferation and differentiation. (2) The T-helper cell interacts with antigen on nonspecific APCs and, in turn, presents antigen to the B cells and provides helper signals to the B cell. Antigen-activated T helper-inducer cells also provide a helper function, via IL-2 production, to other T cells for the generation of T cytotoxic cells, T suppressor cells, and the T cells that mediate delayed-type hypersensitivity and killing of intracellular pathogens (Figure 2-6).

Effector Mechanisms of the Immune System

The immune system is thought to have evolved to protect against foreign pathogens and to limit neoplastic disease. Resistance to infection may be natural or acquired as the result of a specific immune response. The mechanisms involved in natural immunity are largely those responsible for reacting in a nonspecific way to tissue damage with the production of an inflammatory response. Specific immune responses, mediated by T and B lymphocytes, serve to amplify and focus these preexisting natural mechanisms. A variety of effector mechanisms, involving both antibody and cells, are employed by the immune system to protect the body from foreign pathogens[92,93] (see Table 2-4).

Table 2-4. Mechanisms of Protective Immunity

Effector Mechanism	Effector Cells and Molecules
ANTIBODY DEPENDENT	
Neutralization, inhibition of invasion	Antibody
Complement fixation and cytolysis	Antibody (complement fixing) and complement
Phagocytosis	Antibody (opsonizing) and phagocytic cells, such as macrophages (enhanced with complement fixation)
Antibody-dependent cell-mediated cytotoxicity (ADCC)	Antibody and variety of cells, including neutrophils, eosinophils, and mast cells
CELL MEDIATED	
Cell-mediated lysis	MHC-restricted T cells or non-MHC-restricted NK cells
Macrophage activation	T cells and macrophage
Secretory mucosal response	T cells, goblet cells, and inflammatory cells, such as mast cells

Source: adapted from Mitchell GF. *Immunology*. 1979;38:209.

Antibody Mediated

Binding of antibody alone can be sufficient to prevent the penetration of tissue by microorganisms and to neutralize the action of toxins. For the majority of microorganisms, however, help is required for antibody effectively to remove the invading organisms. After combining with antigen, antibody can recruit, via the Fc region of the molecule, a variety of defense systems such as phagocytosis, cell-mediated killing, and the fixation of complement.[45] Receptors for the Fc portion of the immunoglobulin molecule (FcR) are found on a variety of cells, including lymphocytes, monocyte-macrophages, neutrophils, and mast cells.[46] Binding to the Fc portion of the antibody complexed with antigen stimulates phagocytic cells, such as macrophages, to engulf the organism. Intracellular killing of phagocytized organisms may then occur via lysosomal enzymes or the production of toxic reactive oxygen substances.[19,20,94]

Complement (C') plays a major role in the effector mechanisms of the immune system.[94,95] It mediates a diverse range of biologic activities depending upon its mode of activation. Complement is actually 14 or more serum proteins that are normally present in an inactive form. Upon activation they act in an ordered cascade. Complement may be activated via the classical pathway in which the binding of the $C1_q$ protein to antigen antibody complexes activates the C' cascade. Complement may also be activated via an alternative pathway, which does not require the presence of antibody. In this case the C_3 protein is activated by the surface of some cells or microorganisms. The activation of C' generates a group of molecules that can mediate chemotaxis, adherence of antigen–antibody complexes to neutrophils and macrophages, phagocytosis, and cytolysis. Lymphocytes, neutrophils, monocytes, and other cells have been shown to possess receptors for the activated components of C_3.[96]

Cell Mediated

Other effector mechanisms seem to have evolved to deal with larger multicellular parasites.[97–99] Cells such as macrophages, eosinophils, basophils, and mast cells possess FcR and can bind to antibody and/or complement bound to the surface of pathogens. As a result they are stimulated to degranulate and/or secrete cytokines. This mechanism is known as antibody-dependent cell-mediated cytotoxicity (ADCC). Upon activation eosinophils, neutrophils, and mast cells release a variety of pharmacologically active substances that can damage the target organisms.

Some cells are also capable of killing target cells without the presence of antibody. There appears to be no consensus as to the mechanisms and molecules involved in this type of cell killing. Antigen-specific cytotoxic CD8 + T cells (T_{CTL}) bind to antigen on specific target cells and, through mechanisms that are not yet clear, can directly kill target cells.[100–102] The cytokine tumor necrosis factor β (TNFβ), also known as lymphotoxin, a lytic pore-forming protein (PFP)/perforin, T-cell proteinases, or the initiation of autolysis have all been proposed as possible mechanisms.[101,102] Upon activation by T cells (CD4 +) macrophages can act nonspecifically to kill pathogens and certain tumor cells.[103] This mechanism appears to reflect a distinct stage of macrophage activation from that required for ADCC.[104] Activated macrophages release a variety of substances, among them tumor necrosis factor α (TNFα), which has been shown to kill certain tumor cell lines in vitro and certain transplanted tumors in vivo.[105] Other cell types, such as natural killer cells (NK), have also been shown to kill tumor cells directly.[106,107] These large granular lymphocytes (LGLs) are thought to be a subpopulation of immature T cells (CD3$^-$). Unlike classical CD8$^+$ cytotoxic T cells, NK cells are not MHC restricted in their killing of target cells. Present in nonimmunized hosts they require activation by IFN or IL-2 and are thought to kill target cells via the secretion of TNF.

In addition to the mechanisms discussed above, the immune system has evolved specialized effector mechanisms, often unique, for particular nonlymphoid organs and tissues. For instance the presence of IgA antibody in the secretions of the mucosal surfaces, and lymphocytes that can infiltrate the epithelial lining of the small intestine.[108]

Regulation of the Immune Response

The immune system is regulated by highly complex interactions between cells and their products. A variety of mechanisms have been proposed to explain how the immune system regulates itself. These include idiotype–anti-idiotype networks, antibody-mediated feedback inhibition, soluble surface receptors, cytokines, and T suppressor cells. How these interact to direct the immune response along a particular course—cellular versus humoral, help versus suppression, IgE versus IgG production—is not yet fully understood. Based, in some cases, largely on in vitro observations, the role of these mechanisms in vivo and their molecular basis are far from clear. Understanding the processes that regulate the immune system will aid in the development of strategies to suppress or stimulate particular immune responses.

Idiotype Networks

In addition to antigen-driven regulation, regulatory mechanisms are postulated to discriminate between lymphocytes, enhancing some and inhibiting others, via idiotypes expressed on the antigen binding sites of their surface immunoglobulin (B cells) or surface TCR (T cells). Antibody molecules can themselves serve as antigens. The antigenic part of the variable region of antibody is known as its idiotype.[109] An idiotype is made up of a set of epitopes (idiotopes) displayed by the variable region of the immunoglobulin molecule. Most, but not all, idiotopes are within the antigen-binding site. Idiotypes represent the individually distinctive antigenic determinants of a single immunoglobulin molecule or shared determinants of a small number of immunoglobulins.

An animal is thought to possess in its immunological repertoire antigen binding sites that can recognize any idiotope appearing in the species and therefore can regulate its level of expression. Antigen receptors have specificity not only for antigen (epitopes) but also for antigenic determinants on other antigen binding sites (idiotopes) and an idiotypic specificity in which it itself acts as an antigen. For instance, the introduction of antigen X stimulates production of anti-X antibodies. These anti-X antibodies and B cells that make them share the same idiotype. The anti-X antibodies, in turn, stimulate the production of antibody to their particular idiotype, anti-anti-X. The anti-anti-X (anti-idiotype) may resemble the original antigen X, as both have an affinity for anti-X. The anti-anti-X antibodies can recognize anti-X on the surface of other B cells and regulate their response to antigen. Anti-idiotype antibodies binding to the antigen binding site of cells can substitute for antigen; they mimic antigen and are thought to provide an "internal image" of the antigen. The result can be stimulation or inhibition of the cell. For example, the injection of antibody against an idiotype into an animal can suppress lymphocytes that have antigen receptors with that idiotype.[110]

According to Jerne,[111] each idiotype occurring on an antibody molecule or cell-surface antigen receptor molecule is recognized with different degrees of precision by antigen combining sites which occur on other antibody molecules or receptors in the same immune system. Each antigen binding site recognizes a set of idiotypes occurring within the system. The immune system is thus a network of antibody molecules and antigen receptor molecules that recognize and are recognized by other antibody molecules and lymphocytes. This network is postulated to be a functional network and an essential regulatory mechanism of the immune system.[111-113] The production of anti-idiotype antibody has been shown to be a normal component of the immune response; however, the extent of the control that the idiotypic network exerts on immune function remains to be determined.

Antibody (Fc)-Mediated Regulation

Immunoglobulin molecules can participate in the regulation of the immune response via idiotypic networks, a function of the V region of the molecule and in regulatory functions involving the isotypic determinants of the Fc region of the molecule. Antibody–antigen complexes can exert antigen-specific feedback inhibition.[114-116] By binding to the FcR and the immunoglobulin antigen receptor on B cells and co-crosslinking them, they exert an inhibitory effect on B-cell differentiation. Recently, IL-4 has been shown to overcome Fc-dependent suppression by antibody.[116] Interleukin-4 is thought to induce the loss of immune complexes bound to the FcR, perhaps by inducing turnover of the FcR. Antibody–antigen complexes may also enhance the response by binding to the surface of antigen-presenting cells through their FcR and enhancing antigen presentation.[91] The binding of C' to antigen–antibody complexes is also thought to exert regulatory effects depending upon whether the activated C' components are soluble or complexed to antigen–antibody complexes.[117-118]

A family of proteins exists that share the property of binding to the Fc region of immunoglobulin, including FcR and immunoglobulin binding factors (IBFs).[119-124] In addition to the receptor for IgE (Fc_ER), three distinct classes of FcR for IgG, with distinct isotype specificity, are currently being characterized. As well as mediating a number of effector functions, FcRs, have been shown recently to play a role in the regulation of specific immunoglobulin isotypes, either on the cell surface or as soluble IBFs. The regulation of IgE production by IBFs with an affinity for the Fc portion of the IgE molecule (IgE–IBF) has been the most well studied.[120-123] Immunoglobulin E-specific IBFs have been shown to enhance or suppress IgE production depending upon the degree of glycosylation.[122] They are antigenically related to Fc_ER (CD23) and are thought to be a (25-kd) proteolytic fragment of the 45-kd Fc_ER. In addition, there is now considerable evidence that the regulation of IgE production by IL-4 is mediated by the increased release of soluble Fc_ER. However, the precise effects of IL-4 on IgE production remain to be determined.

Immunoglobulin binding factors are structurally heterogeneous, and some possess class-II MHC determinants; however, their action is not MHC restricted.[119-124] They may directly suppress B-cell clones with the matching isotype via interaction with sIg or FcR of B cells. Because both T, in some cases, and B cells have been shown to possess FcR, they are both capable of regulating and being regulated by the release of IBFs.

Cytokines

The availability of purified cytokines has greatly accelerated studies of their role in the regulation of immune function. In addition, the demonstration of $CD4^+$ T_H subsets with apparent differences in their patterns of cytokine production has led to interesting proposals as to how cytokines regulate the immune response to antigen. Both T_H1 and T_H2 can help B cells to produce antibody; however, the nature of the help appears to be qualitatively different.[31-33,71] The T_H1 cells produce IL-2, IFN-γ, and TNFβ, whereas T_H2 cells produce IL-4 and IL-5 (Table 2-5). The four lymphokines that define the differences in T_H1 and T_H2 subpopulations, IL-2, IL-4, IL-5, and IFN-γ, have potent effects on in vitro immune responses[56,62,63,71,125-127]

Table 2-5. Types of Mouse T-Helper Cells

Property	$T_H 1$	$T_H 2$
CYTOKINE SYNTHESIS		
IL-2	+	−
IFN-γ	+	−
Lymphotoxin (TNFβ)	+	−
IL-4	−	+
IL-5	−	+
IL-3	+	+
FUNCTIONS		
B-cell help	+	++
IgE help	−	+
Cytotoxicity	+	−
Delayed-type hypersensitivity	+	−

Source: Adapted from Mossman TR, Coffman RL. *Immunol Today*. 1987;8:223.

(see Table 2-3). For instance, IL-4 enhances the production of IgE and IgG_1 by stimulated B cells, whereas IFN-γ blocks this enhancement. Interferon-γ induces IgM, IgG_3, and IgG_2 production in the same LPS-stimulated B cells. Thus IFN-γ and IL-4 appear to act by antagonizing each other's action.[125]

Extrapolating from these differences, T_H2 T cells in vivo can be expected to provide help selectively for IgE and IgG_1 (via IL-4) and IgA production (via IL-5), whereas T_H1 T cells can be expected to suppress the production of IgE and IgG_1 (via IFN-γ), despite their ability to provide help for other isotypes. In addition to enhancement of IgE production, T_H2 could promote mast-cell growth (via IL-3 and IL-4) and eosinophil growth (via IL-5) and therefore promote IgE-mediated allergic reactions. The T_H1 cells would then be expected to suppress IgE-mediated inflammation and to mediate delayed-type hypersensitivity. Preferential activation of T_H1 or T_H2 subpopulations by particular antigen–adjuvant or antigen–APC combinations would result in the preferential induction of cellular or humoral immune responses and/or isotypes of antibody. The multiple effects that have been associated with cytokines suggest that the physiology and regulation of the immune system is extremely complex. Illuminating the precise nature of their actions will no doubt occupy immunologists for some time.

T-Suppressor Cells

T-suppressor (T_S) cells are potent modulators of the immune response and are thought to play a major role in modulating and terminating excessive immune responses.[128] Although it is generally accepted that T_S cells belong to the CD8$^+$ T-cell subset there is no consensus on what they do and how they act.[87,91,128–132] They appear to be heterogeneous in their actions. They may be antigen specific, idiotype specific, or isotype specific. They may act on T or B cells, and they can "arm" nonspecific accessory cells with soluble factors. A number of mechanisms have been proposed to explain how they act, including idiotype–anti-idiotype interactions and soluble suppressor factors.

Studies in the mouse have revealed that the antigen-specific suppression of the immune response by T_S involves a complex cascade of cellular interactions that are mediated by antigen-specific antigen-binding molecules.[128–132] This cascade is initiated by the T_S inducer cell and its antigen-specific product, T-cell suppressor inducer factor (T_SiF). This factor induces the generation of T_S effector cells (Ly 2$^+$) (CD8$^+$) from precursor T cells. The T_SiF is composed of at least two non-covalently linked molecules, an antigen-binding molecule and an antigen-non-specific accessory molecule.[133] A single-chain T_SiF has also been described.[134] By combining with different antigen-specific molecules the antigen-nonspecific component produces T_SiFs of different antigenic specificities. To add to the complexity, the two molecules composing the T_SiF appear to be the products of two distinct T cells. It has been suggested that the antigen-binding molecule of the T_SiF is a soluble form of the TCR$\alpha\beta$.[131] The nature of the nonspecific accessory molecule is not known. It bears the I-J determinant, which has been linked to the class-II MHC region, and is thought to be an inducible determinant on a T-cell surface molecule found on both T_H and T_S cells.[135] Antigen-specific T_S cells are thought to act by blocking the action and/or induction of T_H cells through mechanisms that have yet to be fully understood.

The T_S cells are also postulated to function in both idiotype- and isotype-specific suppression of B cells.[130] Through idiotype–anti-idiotype interactions T_S cells are proposed to directly suppress antigen-specific B and T cells. In addition, T cells may mediate isotype-specific suppressor effects at the B-cell level through the release of IBF derived from their FcR. The in vivo role of T_S cells in regulating immune function is still poorly understood; nevertheless, they do appear to play a major role in the regulation of the immune response by T cells.

Soluble Cell-Surface Molecules

In addition to the regulation of the immune system by immunoglobulin and cyto-kines, cell-surface molecules of lymphocytes also appear to have immunomodulato-ry effects. As discussed earlier, FcRs released from the cell surface as IBFs have regulatory effects on the production of specific immunoglobulin isotypes, such as IgE, by B cells. In addition, a portion of the TCR is thought to contribute to the T_SiF complex responsible for the induction of antigen-specific T_S cells, which act on other T cells.

Cell-surface molecules, such as CD8 and IL-2R, released upon activation of T cells, are found in the circulation and are currently being used to monitor the level of T-cell activation in the body during disease or following treatment.[136–138] Cir-culating IL-2R has been shown to increase during infection. The soluble IL-2R may compete with cell-bound IL-2R for IL-2 and down regulate the immune response. This mechanism has been proposed to explain, in part, the immunosuppression associated with malaria infection.[138] An interesting possibility, the importance of these soluble cell-surface molecules in the regulation of the immune system, has yet to be determined.

Hypersensitivity and Autoimmunity

In some cases the secondary immune response to foreign substances becomes over-zealous and tissue damage results. Both antibody- and cell-mediated mechanisms can be involved. In addition, the immune response can be directed against self-antigens, autoimmunity. These two phenomena may overlap. For instance, the immune response to antigens on foreign pathogens may result in damage to normal tissues in the body that share cross-reacting antigens. Therapeutic strategies for intervention require a better understanding of how these processes evolve.

Hypersensitivity

Under certain circumstances the response to a second exposure to antigen is associ-ated with exaggerated reactions that may result in tissue damage. Some of these "hypersensitivity" reactions occur immediately upon antigen exposure, whereas

Table 2-6. Hypersensitivies

Type	Mechanisms	Examples
IMMEDIATE (ANTIBODY MEDIATED)		
I Anaphylaxis	Antigen binds to IgE antibody bound to mast cells or basophils, which release vasoactive amines	Anaphylactic shock, hayfever, hives, asthma (some forms)
II ADCC	Antibody-dependent cell-mediated cytotoxicity, antibody to autologous (self) cells and complement-dependent lysis and/or degranulation of neutrophils or other cells	Autoantibodies to some self-antigens, Rh disease
III Immune complexes	Antigen and antibody complexes fix complement and infiltrating neutrophils release lysosomal enzymes	Arthus reaction; serum sickness Immune complex disease
DELAYED (CELL-MEDIATED)		
IV Delayed-type hypersensitivity	Antigen-activated T cells release lymphokines, which activate nonspecific effector macrophages	Tuberculin reaction

others are delayed in development. Hypersensitivities were originally categorized by Coombs and Gell into types I, II, III, and IV (Table 2-6).[139] Types I–III are primarily antibody mediated (passively transferred with serum), whereas type IV is mediated by cells (adoptively transferred with cells). Hypersensitivity is synonymous with allergy and is defined as an altered state, induced by antigen, in which subsequent exposure to antigen results in pathological reactions. Antigens involved in allergic reactions are often called allergens or sensitizers. Although hypersensitivity reactions have been divided into two general types, immediate (antibody mediated) and delayed (cell mediated), a particular allergic reaction is more likely a complex interplay between both. Certain types of immediate responses form an important component for the development of type III and IV interactions by altering the permeability of the vascular endothelia and facilitating the accumulation of effector cells.

In serum sickness and the Arthus reaction, soluble antigen–antibody complexes (formed in antigen excess) initiate focal vascular lesions as a result of the fixation of C' by immune complexes. The fixation of complement by localized immune complexes results in the infiltration of neutrophils and the release of lysosomal enzymes, causing tissue damage.[94,95] Anaphylaxis is the result of the acute release of pharmacologically active substances by mast cells, eosinophils, and–or basophils.[140–142] The principle skin-fixing or reaginic antibody in humans is IgE,[50] which is bound to the surface of these cells via their Fc_ER. Upon binding of specific antigen by the cell-bound IgE, the cells are signaled to degranulate and release a variety of soluble factors, such as histamine, prostaglandins, and leukotrienes, that mediate tissue damage. Normally IgE is present at low levels, but certain "atopic" individuals produce excessive levels in response to certain antigens (allergens). Immunoglobin E is also found in elevated levels during infection with certain helminth parasites. In delayed-type hypersensitivity antigen-activated T_{DTH} cells release cytokines, which activate nonspecific effector cells and cause tissue damage. Tissue injury results from the T-cell-dependent tissue infiltration of activated lymphocytes, mononuclear cells, and neutrophils.[103,143]

Autoimmunity

The destruction of "altered self" cells is a normal activity of T cells. Self-reactive T cells are thought to be deleted during development in the thymus if they encounter a self-peptide complexed with an MHC molecule.[8-10] Such complexes exist in the body all the time. Yet under certain circumstances self-reactive immune responses are generated and can result in significant pathology. Autoimmune diseases are thought to be due to the effects of autoantibody, fixation of C′ to immune complexes, and nonspecific or specific effector cells. Autoantibodies have been implicated in a number of diseases, including myasthenia gravis, systemic lupus erythematosus (SLE), and rheumatoid arthritis.[144] Occasionally self-reactivity can be traced to a lack of tolerance to tissue antigens, such as the eye, brain, and testis, normally sequestered from contact with lymphocytes or to nonspecific lymphocyte activation; however, often the cause is not known.[145] Autoimmunity may result when antibody formed against foreign substances attacks normal cells that have these antigens attached to their cell surfaces. Autoantibodies do not appear to be the result of genetic abnormalities in germline genes or in the generation of the immunologic repertoire.[146] However, certain autoimmune diseases have been found to be associated with specific HLA antigens. Autoimmunity is often secondary to infection or to the use of drugs and may represent a normal part of the disposal of damaged and/or altered material and the failure to regulate the immune response. Postinfection autoimmunity may result from molecular mimicry (a chance sharing of antigens by host and pathogen), changes in endogenous antigens (viral alterations of cell surfaces), or disturbances in host immunoregulation. Several mechanisms have been suggested that act to control self-reactive cells and maintain tolerance to self-antigens. These include clonal deletion, active suppression by T_S cells, and "veto" cells.[9,10,79,128,147] Veto cells are lymphoid cells with the apparent ability to prevent the generation of cytotoxic T cells to self-MHC antigens.[147] The use of immunotherapy to control hypersensitivity and autoimmunity will require a better understanding of how these processes evolve.

Immunotherapy

The major goals of immunotherapy are the control of specific immunosuppression and the control of immunoenhancement. Present emphasis in immunosuppression is to ablate certain populations of immune cells without a crippling loss of immune function. Currently, traditional pharmacologic principles are being applied to creating agents that will allow us to attain these goals. Monoclonal antibody technology, purified recombinant cytokines, T-cell cloning techniques, and new in vivo animal models have made these goals more obtainable.

Animal Models

Severe combined immunodeficiency (SCID) mice, lacking detectable B and T cells or lymphocyte functions, are being used as an in vivo animal model to study the human immune system.[148] The SCID–human chimeric mouse provides a model that allows direct analysis of the human immune system.[149] In addition, transgenic mice have also proved useful in vivo models for the study of the immune system and its components.[150,151]

Monoclonal Antibody

Monoclonal antibodies are currently being evaluated as therapeutic agents for a variety of diseases. For example, anti-idiotype antibody directed against the idiotypic determinants of the surface immunoglobulin on B-cell lymphomas and leukemias is being evaluated.[152] Monoclonal antibody to the CD3 complex of T cells has been shown to have both immunopotentiating and immunosuppressive effects in vivo, depending upon the dose.[153] The production of human Mab to specific tumor-associated antigens is being tried, using the patient's own lymphocytes. Monoclonal antibodies are also being used to target drugs, toxins, and radioisotopes.[154–157] They are being used in combination with cytokines, such as IFN, in the treatment of cancer. Hybrid Mab molecules, specific for both tumor antigens and the TCR, are also being evaluated.[158] In addition, the use of antibodies (idiotypes) produced during infection as surrogate antigens for vaccines has met with some success in animal models.[159–161]

There are current limitations to the effectiveness of Mab. Target cells can endocytose antigen and antibody complexes and modulate their cell-surface antigen. In addition, efficient production of human Mab has lagged behind that of rodent Mab. Mouse Mab, however, is potentially immunogenic in humans, resulting in the production of antibodies that accelerate blood clearance and block binding to antigen. The paucity of high-affinity human Mab has led to an attempt to develop chimeric Mab.[162–163] These include the chemical coupling of mouse Fab to human Fc, genetic engineering of divalent mouse V region–human C region constructs, and genetic constructs that place only the mouse hypervariable region in the human V region. The ability to generate Mab with a defined antigen specificity and with effector functions selected for particular clinical requirements is of current interest.

Cytokines

Cytokines are becoming increasingly available for use in vivo.[66,164] As potent immunomodulators they can be used as natural adjuvants to potentiate immune responses during immunization and to improve defects in immune function. They can also be employed to suppress immune function. For instance, IL-2, a potent stimulator of T cells, is being used[61,165] to improve the potency of vaccines and in the treatment of cancer. There is a great deal of interest in agents that can modulate IL-2 production and IL-2 action via IL-2R. The finding that IL-2R is expressed solely by antigen-activated T cells has led to the possibility of using agents that inhibit IL-2R action for therapeutic immunosuppression to improve survival of allografts and new therapies for autoimmune diseases.[166] The use of anti-IL-2R is based upon the fact that T cells involved in autoimmune diseases are in a state of activation (IL-2R$^+$) in contrast to resting cells (IL-2R$^-$). Glucocorticoids or cyclosporine suppress the immune system through the selective inhibition of IL-2 production while having little influence on IL-2R expression.[167] Monoclonal antibody reactive to the IL-2R have been shown specifically to prevent cardiac allograft rejection, and to suppress the development of autoimmunity and delayed-type hypersensitivity in mice.[167–169] In addition, bacterial toxin–IL-2 conjugates can suppress antigen-specific responses.[170] Neutralizing Mab may be replaced with other antagonists, when they are available, such as competitive ligands for the receptor.

Other cytokines are also being evaluated for their immunomodulating potential. For instance, TGFβ is a potent inhibitor of the proliferation of both T and B cells.[64,65] Tumor necrosis factor α (TNFα), a product of activated macrophages, causes necrosis of certain transplanted tumors and is being evaluated, along with IFN, in the treatment of human cancer.[105] Potent chemical messengers, cytokines can also mediate pathological sequelae, and some of the symptoms of human disease, such as autoimmunity and the anemia of chronic disease, may be mediated, in part, by the overproduction of cytokines. High levels of cytokines can be found in the fluid of rheumatoid joints and TNFα is a potent inhibitor of red blood cell production.[59,60,171] Control of cytokine production would alleviate symptoms. For instance, anti-IFN is being used to inhibit inflammatory responses associated with acute vascular thrombosis and to promote the survival of skin transplants.[172,173] Still in its infancy, the potential use of cytokines as therapeutic agents looks very promising.

Adoptive Cellular Immunity

Adoptive cellular immunity also has great potential. Specific T cells could provide resistance to infection and neoplastic disease and reconstitute immunodeficiencies.[174,175] Specific T_S cells may alleviate allergic states and autoimmunity. Lymphocytes cytotoxic for autologous tumors can be generated in vitro from a patient's own lymphocytes. A number of activation procedures, including stimulation with tumor cells, allogeneic peripheral blood leukocytes, and IL-2, have been used. Leukocytes from blood and spleen activated by IL-2 become cytotoxic for tumor cells in vitro and regress solid tumors in vivo.[176] These lymphokine-activated killer (LAK) cells are heterogeneous but have been shown to be primarily an activity of NK cells.[177] Cell cloning techniques are currently being applied to further refine the development of killer T cell clones and to provide antigen-specific T-cell clones.

Tumor infiltrating lymphocytes, isolated from resected human cancers, are being used and may be more effective than LAK. Small numbers of cloned T cells, "T-cell vaccination," have also been used in an attempt to stimulate anti-T-clonotype (anti-idiotype) T cells for the treatment of autoimmunity.[178]

A variety of the components of the immune system are available as potential immunotherapeutic agents, including monoclonal antibodies, cytokines, and specific T-cell clones. They can also be used in combination with drugs and immunomodulating agents. There is no doubt that they will be a part of future immunotherapeutics and strategies to manipulate the immune response.

Summary

Our understanding of how the immune system specifically recognizes foreign substances and responds with the production of specific antibody and/or specific effector T cells has been increased in recent years by several advances. These include the characterization and molecular cloning of the TCR and MHC-encoded molecules, the availability of purified recombinant cytokines, and the delineation of functionally distinct subpopulations of T cells.

Thymus dependent (T) and bone marrow derived (B) lymphocytes share a number of similarities: Their antigen receptors are composed of heterodimers; the genetic mechanisms responsible for the construction of the antigen binding sites on their antigen receptors involve VDJ joining and the generation of a similar degree of diversity; they both require two signals for their activation, which results in their clonal expansion and the generation of memory cells; and they are both regulated by networks of cytokines, anti-idiotype interactions, and suppressor cells. There are also differences in T and B cells. Unlike B cells, T cells have evolved to recognize antigen in the context of self-MHC molecules. In addition, T cells appear to require antigen to be processed, while B cells appear to recognize antigen in its native state. These dissimilarities arise from the differences in their antigen receptors, immunoglobulin in the case of B cells and the immunoglobulin-like TCR of T cells. For instance, the interaction of TCR with antigen appears to require the contribution of other T-cell-surface molecules, such as CD3, CD4, and CD8. These molecules may serve to stabilize the interaction with antigen and/or MHC-encoded molecules and to transduce signals across the membrane. The self-/nonself-discriminatory powers, selected for in the thymus, make T cells the sentinels of the immune system.

The immune system employs a number of effector mechanisms to protect the body from foreign pathogens. These include both antibody-mediated mechanisms, such as C' fixation and ADCC, and cell-mediated ones, such as cytotoxic T cells and activation of macrophages. The induction and mediation of these immune responses is regulated by complex cellular interactions and a variety of mechanisms are thought to be involved, including idiotype–anti-idiotype interactions, antibody-mediated suppression, and T_S cells. Their precise role, however, remains unclear. Autoimmunity and allergy can result when there is a failure in regulation of an immune response. Rationales for therapeutic intervention will depend upon an increased understanding of how the components of the immune system interact.

The Future

A number of rapidly evolving areas in immunology should deepen our understanding of the immune system. These include the role of cytokines in cell signaling and immune regulation, T-cell recognition of antigen, antigen processing and presentation, characterization of T- and B-cell subpopulations, and the biochemistry of cell signaling mechanisms. A number of questions remain unanswered, for example, the role played by accessory molecules, such as CD3, CD4, and CD8, in transmembrane signaling of T cells; what makes an effective T- or B-cell epitope; the mechanisms by which APCs transport antigen to and from the membrane; the early events of T- and B-cell collaboration; and the role played by various cytokines in vivo. Unraveling the mysteries of the highly complex immune system will no doubt occupy those wishing to understand and manipulate it for years to come.

Acknowledgments

The author wishes to thank Dr Michele Jungery, Ms Marcia Wood, and Ms Birgitta Kullgren for their helpful discussions and editorial comments during the preparation of this manuscript. This work was supported in part by the Office of Health and Environmental Research, U.S. Department of Energy, under contract DE-AC03-76SF00098, and by Lawrence Berkeley Laboratory Director's Program Development Funds #3669.01.

References

1. Paul WE, Siskind GW, Benacerraf B, Ovary Z. *J Immunol,* 1967;99:760.

2. Kabat EA, Mayer MM. *Structural Concepts in Immunology and the Immune Response Immunochemistry.* New York: Holt, Rinehart and Winston Inc; 1961.

3. Nossal GJV, Ada GL. *Antigens, Lymphoid Cells and the Immune Response.* New York: Academic Press Inc; 1971.

4. Oppenheim JJ, Rosenstreich DL. *Mitogens in Immunobiology.* New York: Academic Press Inc; 1976.

5. Fenichel RL, Chirigos MA. *Immune Modulation Agents and Their Mechanisms.* New York: Marcel Dekker Inc; 1984.

6. Masihi KN, Lange W. *Immunomodulation and Nonspecific Host Defense Mechanisms Against Microbial Infections.* New York: Pergamon Press; 1988.

7. Gowans J, McGregor D. *Prog Allergy.* 1965;9:1.

8. Katz DH. *Fed Proc Am Soc Exp Biol.* 1979;38:2065.

9. Singer A. *J Immunol.* 1988;140:2481.

10. Marrack P, Kappler J. *Immunol Today.* 1988;9:309.

11. Burnet FM. *Self and Nonself.* Cambridge: Cambridge University Press; 1969.

12. Pernis B, Chiappino G, Kelus A, Gell PGH. *J Exp Med.* 1965;122:678.

13. Vitetta ES, Uhr JW. *Science.* 1975;189:964.

14. Marchalonis JJ. *Science.* 1975;190:20.

15. Kronenberg M, Siu G, Hood LE, Shasti N. *Annu Rev Immunol.* 1986;4:529.

16. Allison JP, Lanier LL. *Annu Rev Immunol.* 1987;5:503.

17. Reinherz E. *Nature (London).* 1987;325:660.

18. Marrack P, Kappler J. *Sci Am.* 1986;254:36.

19. Unanue ER, Allen PM. *Science*. 1987;236:551.

20. Nathan CF. *J Clin Invest*. 1979;2:319.

21. Greaves MF. *Science*. 1986;234:697.

22. Reinherz E, Haynes BF, Nadler LM, Bernstein ID, eds. *Leukocyte Typing*. New York: Springer Verlag; 1986.

23. Holmes KL, Morse HC. *Immunol Today*. 1988;9:345.

24. Boyse EA, Miyezarral M, Aoki T, Old LJ. *Proc R Soc Biol*. 1968;178:175.

25. Melchers F, Anderson J. *Annu Rev Immunol*. 1986;4:13.

26. Hayakawa K, Herzenberg LA. *J Exp Med*. 1985;161:1554.

27. Linton PJ, Gilmore GL, Klinman NR. In Witte O, Howard M, Klinman NR, eds. *B Cell Development: UCLA Symposia on Molecular and Cellular Biology*. New York: Alan R Liss; 1989; 139.

28. Swain SL. *Immunol Rev*. 1983;74:129.

29. Beverly PC. *Immunol Lett*. 1987;14:263.

30. Sprent J, Webb SR. *Adv Immunol*. 1987;41:39.

31. Kurt-Jones EA, Hamberg S, O'Hara J, Paul WE, Abbas AA. *J Exp Med*. 1987;219:166.

32. Mossmann TR, Cherwinski H, Bond MW, Giedller MA, Coffmann RL. *J Immunol*. 1986;136:2348.

33. Bottomly K. *Immunol Today*. 1988;9:268.

34. Arthur RP, Mason D. *J Exp Med*. 1986;163:774.

35. Patel SS, Duby AD, Thiele DL, Lipsky PE. *J Immunol*. 1988;141:3726.

36. Meuer SC, Schlossman SF, Reinherz EL. *Proc Natl Acad Sci (USA)*. 1982;79:4395.

37. Pernis B. In Silverstein S, Vogel H, eds. *Antigen Processing and Presentation*. New York: Academic Press; 1988.

38. Katz DH. *Pharmacol Rev*. 1982;32:51.

39. Lipsky PE, Kettman J. *Immunol Today*. 1982;3:209.

40. Rock KL, Benacerraf B, Abbas AK. *J Exp Med*. 1984;160:1102.

41. Janeway CA, Ron C, Katz ME. *J Immunol*. 1987;138:1051.

42. Ashwell JD. *J Immunol*. 1988;140:3697.

43. Hozumi N, Tonegawa S. *Proc Soc Acad Sci*. 1976;73:3628.

44. Porter RR. *Biochemistry*. 1959;73:119.

45. Morgan EL, Weigle WO. *Adv Immunol*. 1987;40:61.

46. Basten A, Warner NL, Mandel T. *J Exp Med*. 1976;135:627.

47. Koshland ME. *Adv Immunol*. 1974;20:41.

48. Thorebecke GJ, Leslie GA, eds. *Immunoglobulin D: Structure and Function*. New York: New York Academy of Science; 1982.

49. Cebra J. *Adv Exp Med Biol*. 1974;45:23.

50. Metzger H, Kinet JP. *Fed Proc Am Soc Exp Biol*. 1988;2:3.

51. Leder P. *Sci Am*. 1982;246:104.

52. Alt F. *Science*. 1987;238:1079.

53. Early P, Huang H, Davis M, Calame K, Hood L. *Cell*. 1980;19:981.

54. Tonegawa S. *Nature (London)*. 1983;302:575.

55. Yancopoulos GD, Desiderio SV, Paskind M. *Nature* (London). 1984;311:727.

56. Howard M, Paul WE. *Annu Rev Immunol*. 1983;1:307.

57. Kohler G, Milstein C. *Nature (London).* 1975;256:495.

58. Hood L, Kronenberg M, Hunkapiller T. *Cell.* 1985;40:225.

59. Dinarello CA, Mier JW. *Annu Rev Immunol.* 1986;37:173.

60. Oppenheim JJ, Kovacs EJ, Matsushima K, Durum DK. *Immunol Today.* 1986;7:45.

61. Smith K. *Adv Immunol.* 1988;42:165.

62. Pike BL, Alderson MR, Nossal GJV. *Immunol Rev.* 1987;99:119.

63. Miyajima A, Miyatake S, Schreurs J, De Vries J, Arai N, Yokota T, Arai KI. *Fed Proc Am Soc Exp Biol.* 1988;2:2462.

64. Ellingsworth LR, Akayama D, Segarini P, Dasch J, Carrillo P, Waegell W. *Cell Immunol.* 1988;114:31.

65. Sporn MB, Roberts AB, Wakefield LM, Assoian RK. *Science.* 1986;233:532.

66. Fauci AS, Rosenberg SA, Sherwin SA, Dinarello CA, Longe DL, Lane HC. *Ann Int Med.* 1987;106:421.

67. Dorf M, ed. *The Role of the Major Histocompatibility Complex in Immunobiology.* New York: Garland/STM Press; 1985.

68. Klein J. *Natural History of the Major Histocompatibility Complex.* New York: J. Wiley & Sons; 1986.

69. Benacerraf B, McDevitt HO. *Science.* 1972;175:273.

70. Steinmetz M, Minard S, Horvath S, McNicholas J, Frelinger J, Wake C, Long E, Mach B, Hood L. *Nature (London).* 1982;300:35.

71. Mossman TR, Coffman RL. *Immunol Today.* 1988;8:223.

72. Bixler GS, Abassi MZ. *Biotechnology.* 1985;3:47.

73. Zingernagel RM, Doherty PC. *Adv Immunol.* 1979;27:51.

74. Brenner MB, McLean J, Dialynes DP. *Nature (London).* 1986;322:145.

75. Sutton B. *J Immunol.* 1988;Suppl.1:31.

76. Morrison LA, Luckacher AE, Bracialie VL. *J Exp Med.* 1986;163:903.

77. Berzofsky JA. *Science.* 1985;229:932.

78. Babbit BP, Allen PM, Matseueda G. Nature (London). 1985;317:359.

79. Weigle WO. *Adv Immunol.* 1973;16:61.

80. Schrezenmeir H, Fleischer B. *J Immunol.* 1988;141:398.

81. Konig F, Stingl G, Yokoyama WM. *Science.* 1987;236:837.

82. Janeway CA, Jones B, Hayday A. *Immunol Today.* 1988;9:73.

83. Siskind G, Paul WE, Benacerraf B. *J Exp Med.* 1966;123:673.

84. Rajewsky K, Schirrmacher V, Nase S, Jerne NK. *J Exp Med.* 1969;129:1131.

85. Mitchison NA. *Eur J Immunol.* 1971;1:18.

86. Miller JFA, Mitchell GF. *J Exp Med.* 1968;128:801.

87. Greaves MF, Owen JJT, Raff MC. *T and B Lymphocytes.* Amsterdam: Excertpa Medica; 1974.

88. Sanders VM, Snyder JM, Uhr JW, Vitetta ES. *J Immunol.* 1986;137:2395.

89. Mosier DB, Coppleson LW. *Proc Nat Acad Sci* (USA). 1988;61:542.

90. Miller JAPF, Basten A, Sprent J, Cheers C. *Cell Immunol.* 1971;2:469.

91. Feldman M, Basten A, Boylston A, Erb P, Gorczynski R, Greaves M, Hogg N, Kilburn D, Kontianinen C, Parker D, Pepys M, Schrader J. *Prog Immunol.* 1974;II,Vol.3:65.

92. Mitchell GF. *Immunology.* 1979;38:209.

93. Oppenheim JJ, Jacob D, eds. *Leukocytes and Host Defense*. New York: Alan Liss; 1986.

94. Austen FK. *J Immunol*. 1978;121:793.

95. Porter RR, Reid KBM. *Nature (London)*. 1978;26:699.

96. Loy WH, Nussenzweig V. *J Exp Med*. 1968;128:991.

97. Capron A. *Immunol Rev*. 1982;61:41.

98. McLaren D, Terry R. *Parasite Immunol*. 1982;4:129.

99. Payne CM, Linde A, Kibler R. *J Cell Sci*. 1985;77:27.

100. Cerattini JC, Brunner KT. *Adv Immunol*. 1974;18:67.

101. Chang TW, Eisen HN. *J Immunol*. 1980;124:1028.

102. Ding J, Young E, Cohn ZA. *Adv Immunol*. 1988;41:268.

103. Mackaness GB. *J Infect Dis*. 1971;123:439.

104. Ralph P, Nakowiz I. *Cancer Res*. 1981;41:3546.

105. Beutler B, Cerami A. *Adv Immunol*. 1988;42:213.

106. Herberman RB, ed. *NK Cells and Other Natural Effector Cells*. New York: Academic Press; 1982.

107. Hercend T, Schmidt RE. *Immunol Today*. 1988;9:291.

108. Hanson LA, Svanborg-Eden C, eds. Mucosal Immunobiology. *Monograph in Allergy*. 1987;24:1.

109. Oudin J. *Ann Inst Pasteur*. 1974;8:1.

110. Hippen JE, Nisonoff A. *Adv Immunol*. 1971;13:57

111. Jerne NK. *Ann Immunol (Inst Pasteur)*. 1974;125C:373.

112. Iverson GM, Dresser DW. *Nature*. 1970;227:274.

113. Bona CA. *Regulatory Idiotypes*. New York: John Wiley & Sons; 1987.

114. Sinclair NRS. *Pharmacol Ther*. 1979;4:355.

115. Sindau NR, Panoskaltsis A. *Immunol Today*. 1987;8:76.

116. O'Garra A, Rigley KP, Holman M, McLaughlin JB, Klaus GB. *Proc Natl Acad Sci (USA)*. 1987;84:6254.

117. Pepys MB. *Trans Rev*. 1976;32:93.

118. Melchers F, Erdei A, Schulz T, Dierich MP. *Nature (London)*. 1985;317:264.

119. Fridman W, Golstein P. *Cell Immunol*. 1974;11:442.

120. Neuport Santes C, Dueron M, Teillard J, Blank U, Fridman W. *Int Immunol*. 1986;1:237.

121. Ishizaka K. *Annu Rev Immunol*. 1984;2:159.

122. Gordon J, Guy GR. *Immunol Today*. 1987;8:339.

123. Metzger H. *Adv Immunol*. 1988;43:277.

124. Lynch RG. *Adv Immunol*. 1987;40:135.

125. Snapper CM, Paul WE. *Science*. 1987;236:944.

126. Paul WE. *Fed Proc Am Soc Exp Biol*. 1987;1:456.

127. Harriman GR, Strober W. *J Immunol*. 1987;139:3553.

128. Gershon RK, Cohen P, Hencin R, Liebhaber SA. *J Exp Med*. 1972;108:586.

129. Eardley DE. *Fed Proc Am Soc Exp Biol*. 1980;39:3114.

130. Lynch RG, Milburn GL. *Fed Proc Am Soc Exp Biol*. 1983;42:688.

131. Green DR, Flood PM, Gershon RK. *Annu Rev Immunol*. 1983;1:439.

132. Asherson GL, Zembala M. *Annu Rev Immunol*. 1986;4:37.

133. Yamauchi K, Chao N, Murphy DB, Gershon RK. *J Exp Med*. 1982;155:655.

134. Webb DR, Kapp JA, Pierce CW. *Annu Rev Immunol.* 1983;1:423.

135. Tada T, Asano Y, Nakayama T, Fujisama I. In David CS, ed. *H-2 Antigens, Genes, Molecules, Function.* New York: Plenum Press; 1987:435.

136. Fujimoto J. *J Exp Med.* 1983;159:752.

137. Male D, Lelchuk M, Curry S, Pryce S, Playfair JHL. *Immunology.* 1985;56:119.

138. Ho M, Webster K, Green B, Looareesuwan S, Kongchareon S, White NJ. *J Immunol.* 1988;141:2755.

139. Gell PGH, Coombs PRA. *Clinical Aspects of Immunology.* Oxford: Blackwell Scientific Publications; 1968.

140. Bach MK. *Annu Rev Microbiol.* 1982;36:371.

141. Gleich GJ, Adolphson CR. *Adv Immunol.* 1986;39:124.

142. Ford-Hutchison AW. *Fed Proc Am Soc Exp Biol.* 1985;44:1214.

143. Granger GA. *Am J Pathol.* 1970;54:469.

144. Waksman B. *Medicine.* 1963;41:93.

145. Streilein JW, Wegmann TG. *Immunol Today.* 1987;8:362.

146. Theofilopoulos AN, Dixon FJ. *Adv Immunol.* 1985;37:269.

147. Miller RG. *Nature (London).* 1980;287:544.

148. Bosma GC, Custer RP, Bosma J. *Nature (London).* 1983;301:527.

149. McCune JM, Namikawa R, Kaneshima H, Shultz LD, Lieberman M, Weissman L. *Science.* 1988;241:1632.

150. Taurog JD, Lowen L, Forman J, Hamner RE. *J Immunol.* 1988;141:4020.

151. Miller JFAP. *Immunol Today.* 1989;10:53.

152. Miller RA, Maloney DG, Waunke R. *New Engl J Med.* 1982;306:517.

153. Ellenhorn E, Hirsch R, Schreiber J, Bluestone A. *Science.* 1988;242:569.

154. Vitetta ES, Krolick KA, Miyama-Inaba M, Cushley W, Uhr JW. *Science.* 1983;219:644.

155. Basham TY, Kaminski MS, Kitamura K, Levy R, Merigan TC. *J Immunol.* 1987;137:3019.

156. Klausner A. *Biotechnology.* 1986;4:185.

157. Ram BP, Tyle P. *Pharmacol Res.* 1987;4:181.

158. Jung G, Muller-Eberhard HJ. *Immunol Today.* 1988;9:256.

159. Sacks D, Esser KM, Sher A. *J Exp Med.* 1981;155:1108.

160. Kohler H, Bona C, eds. *Idiotypic Vaccines.* New York: Academic Press; 1986.

161. Hiernaux JR. *Infect Immunol.* 1988;56:1407.

162. Morrison SL. *Science.* 1985;229:123.

163. Reichmann L, Clark M, Waldmann H, Winter G. *Nature (London).* 1988;332:323.

164. Balkwill F. *Cytkokines in Cancer Therapy.* Oxford: Oxford University Press; (1989).

165. Smith KA. *Science.* 1988;240:1169.

166. Cantrell DA, Smith KA. *Science.* 1984;224:198.

167. Gillis S, Crabtree GR, Smith KA. *J Immunol.* 1979;123:1624.

168. Banerjee S, Wei BY, Hillman K, Lerthra CS, David CS. *J Immunol.* 1988;141:11508.

169. Kelley VE, Naor T, Gaulton GN, Strom TB. *J Immunol.* 1988;140:59.

170. Ogata M, Lorbertoum-Galski H, Fitzgerald D, Pastan I. *J Immunol.* 1988;141:4224.

171. Roodman GD. *Blood Cells.* 1987;13:171.

172. Billiau A. *Immunol Today*. 1988;9:37.

173. Jacob C, VanderMeer PH, McDevitt HO. *J Exp Med*. 1987;166:798.

174. Greenberg PD. In Gale RP, Truitt RL, Buorton MM, eds., *Cellular Immunotherapy of Cancer*. New York: Alan R. Liss; 1988.

175. Anichim A, Fossata G, Parmiani G. *Immunol Today*. 1987;8:385.

176. Rosenberg S. *J Natl Cancer Inst*. 1985;75:595.

177. Herberman RB. *Immunol Today*. 1987;8:178.

178. Cohen IR, Weiner HL. *Immunol Today*. 1988;9:332.

CHAPTER 3

Antibody and Immunoglobulin: Structure and Function

Edward W. Voss, Jr.

Department of Microbiology, 131 Burrill Hall, 407 South Goodwin, University of Illinois, Urbana, IL 61801 USA

Introduction and Background

Historically, research defining the antibody (Ab) molecule at the macromolecular structure–function level has lagged behind other protein systems (eg, enzymes, polypeptide hormones, and small proteins with prosthetic groups such as myoglobin). The delay can be attributed in part to time-consuming temporal progressions from the polyclonal → myeloma → hybridoma stages. Since Porter's classical antibody structure studies,[1] significant progress has been made in the general understanding of the nature and functional scope of protein structure. Recent years have witnessed a formulation and conceptualization of protein tertiary structure and increased understanding of domain structure, including functional and dynamical consequences, and a genetic basis in the exon/intron gene mosaic. With availability of homogeneous immunoglobulin (Ig) reagents (myelomas and hybridomas) comparative primary structure determinations led to the multigene origin of immunoglobulins based on distinguishable variable- and constant-region expression products. However, homogeneous immunoglobulins have not crystallized efficiently, delaying procurement of comprehensive three-dimensional information. Amzel and Poljak[2,3] provided the original three-dimensional understanding of the structure of complexes involving antigen binding fragments (Fab) of myeloma immunoglobulins bound to small ligands. Although these initial studies were important they established neither the range of precise shapes and sizes of antibody combining sites nor the nature and extent of antigen-induced effects on the antibody macromolecule.

Future advancements in antibody structure–function analyses will depend on development and characterization of appropriate and chemically defined epitope systems as a prelude to systematic studies. Simple and complex immunogens usually induce heterogeneous immune responses in a variety of hosts. However, some biochemically distinct antigens elicit restricted responses characterized by relatively low-affinity interactions with homologous antigen and consisting of families of antibodies that are structurally and immunologically related. Such restricted immune responses have been described for phosphorylcholine, dextran, arsonate, (4-hydroxy-3-nitrophenyl) acetyl (NP),[4] and poly($Glu_{60}Ala_{30}Tyr_{10}$).[5,6] Analyses of restricted responses have also shown that diversification of antibodies encoded by germline genes results from several mechanisms, possibly all working in concert.[7] However, the proposed functional correlates of these processes (ie, specificity, affinity maturation, etc) are not well understood but provide the foundation upon which structure–function principles of antibodies will be formulated. For example, it is not known if mechanisms responsible for generation of antibody diversification also result in affinity maturation.[8] Certain aspects of this question are important. First, what is the ontogeny and structural basis of high-affinity antibodies? Are such molecules derived from low-affinity antibodies by mechanisms generally involved in antibody diversification or are they encoded within germline repertoires? Second, what is the contribution of different immunoglobulin gene products within an unrestricted response to diversity and affinity maturation by association? While studies of restricted responses have elucidated many aspects of antibody diversification, regulation, and genetics, they have not fully clarified these questions because of inherent limitations.

Immune responses exhibiting significant diversity and affinity maturation provide potential for more complete elucidation of structure–function relationships. In this regard, hapten systems, such as the fluorescein epitope,[9,10] have become attractive models.

Another such system is the 2-phenyl-5-oxazolone (Ox1) response. An important series of studies[11–13] involving mRNA sequencing of antibodies produced in response to the oxazolone epitope, have elucidated certain structural and genetic mechanisms of affinity maturation within this restricted response. Sequencing of hybridoma antibodies isolated following primary (day 7 or 14) or secondary immunizations indicated the following: (1) the response after 7 days was restricted and 11 of 15 clones expressed heavy and light chains encoded by two germline genes; (2) by day 14, six of 11 used similar but not identical sequences, indicating somatic mutational processes; and (3) during the secondary response, only 4 of 22 clones used genes identified in the early response and the substitutions were correlated with an increased affinity for hapten. It is readily apparent that model systems, such as the anti-oxazolone response, provide diverse immunological reagents suitable for methodical structure–function studies. However, model systems should also include a thorough characterization of the resulting antibody active sites as the anti-fluorescein response. For example, monoclonal anti-fluorescein antibodies have been obtained through hybridoma methodology covering the range of 10^4 M^{-1} to approximately 10^{11} M^{-1}. Monoclonal and polyclonal anti-fluorescein active sites of various affinities have been characterized using such parameters as fluorescence quenching of ligand; intrinsic fluorescence quenching of tryptophan residues within or near the antibody-active site; ligand binding association and dissociation rate kinetics; spectral shift of bound ligand (active site polarity); iodide quenching for accessibility of bound fluorescyl ligand; thermodynamic properties, including high-pressure studies,[14] heavy- and light-chain reassociation, and intermixing studies; deuterium oxide perturbation of hydrogen bonding within the active site; fluorescence lifetime measurements and their distribution to determine conformational states; and fine specificity to ascertain degree and extent of immunological cross reactivity.[9] Comprehensive active site characterizations are important in eventually understanding functional aspects of primary, secondary, tertiary, and quaternary structural information. Extensive active site characterizations and integration of appropriate structural information lead to the expanded term "structure–function–mechanism."

Protein antigens such as the lysozyme–antilysozyme system have proved important as shown in crystallization studies of immune complexes.[15] However, the lysozyme system has not afforded extensive diversity and a continuum of crystallizable reagents for comparative studies. Similar studies have been performed with structural analyses of neuraminidase–anti-neuraminidase (Fab) crystallized immune complexes. An important structure–function model system based on the use of murine IgM anti-IgG monoclonal autoantibodies (rheumatoid factors) has also been developed.[16]

Thus, various model systems are being established in which a series of characterized antibodies to the same epitope will provide important comparative information from which the rules governing structure–function relationships in antibodies will evolve.

Immunoglobulin Structure: Fundamental Properties and Principles

Identifying and emphasizing important historical steps fundamental in the eventual elucidation of structure–function relationships associated with antibody molecules requires judgements and perceptions that differ with each investigator. However, the hallmark studies by Porter[1] and colleagues in the late 1950s—which determined that rabbit antibodies (150 kd) incubated with the proteolytic enzyme papain cleaved the macromolecule into two components of similar size, but with different structural and functional properties—must be considered indispensable to the story that evolved during the convening 30 years. Overwhelmingly, the literature that has advanced the structure–function understanding of antibody molecules depends on Porter's studies[17] as an experimental reference point.

The two nearly equivalent sized (50-kd) papain-derived Ig fragments were termed Fab and Fc upon ion-exchange chromatographic resolution (Figure 3-1). Stoichiometrically, a ratio of two Fab fragments to one Fc was obtained per digested antibody molecule. Critical to Porter's experiments and their interpretation was the determination that quantitatively the three fragments accounted for almost total recovery of digested protein. Quantitative recovery inferred resistance to further proteolysis by papain and suggested three globular structures held together by short exposed peptides.[17] Functionally, both Fab fragments retained native antigen binding properties of the parental molecule, while the Fc fragment possessed structural features responsible for immunoglobulin effector functions. Subsequent to Ab proteolysis studies, it was determined that sequential incubations of immunoglobulins with thiol-reducing and -dispersing agents (urea, acid, or detergent) resulted in

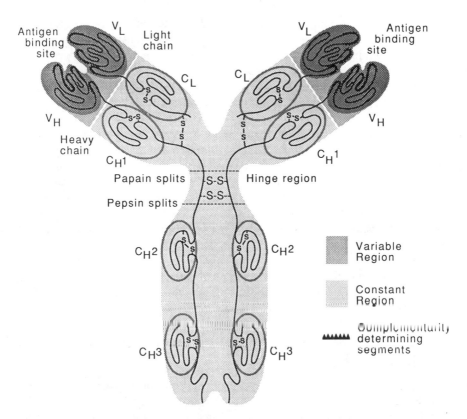

Figure 3-1. Basic four-chain immunoglobulin model. Heavy- (H) and light- (L) chain designations are noted as subscripts. Variable (V) and constant (C) regions and domains are represented in a tertiary structural configuration featuring the immunoglobulin folds. Intrachain and interchain disulfide (—S—S—) bonds are noted except in the variable domains, because of the complexity of the drawing. (Figure reproduced from Ref 147 by permission.)

selective reduction of covalent disulfide bonds and molecular dissociation into two pairs of polypeptide chains of unequal size.[18,19] The largest protein (50–75 kd) was termed the heavy chain (H), and the smaller polypeptide (22–23 kd) the light chain (L) (Figure 3-1). Collectively, these studies not only formed the basis for eventual refined structure–function studies but also provided the foundation for continuing advances in the understanding of immunoglobulin genes, their rearrangement and immunological diversity. Analyses of the overlapping structural products derived from proteolytic digestion and thiol reduction-dispersing agent experiments led to the first linear model of the immunoglobulin molecule (Figure 3-1).[18-20]

Importantly, it was shown that the antibody molecule was also susceptible to digestion with other proteolytic enzymes, such as pepsin and trypsin under appropriate conditions.[21] Unlike papain digestion the Fc was selectively degraded with pepsin and trypsin. However, an important final product termed F(ab)₂ remained intact. This fragment represented two Fab fragments joined covalently through an

H–H interchain disulfide bond. Bivalent F(ab)$_2$ fragments retained the intrinsic antigen binding properties as well as secondary reactions such as immunoprecipitation and agglutination. Univalent Fab fragments are derived from F(ab)$_2$ fragments through mild thiol reduction. Structure–function studies have continuously deemed it important to obtain and analyze substructural reagents to systematically define and elucidate Ig properties.

Although significant advances continue toward a more thorough understanding of the primary, secondary, tertiary, and quarternary structures of antibodies, the initial linear model has remained an accurate approximation of the essential features of Ig structure (Figure 3-1). Immunoglobulins are glycoproteins composed of a basic monomeric structure of four polypeptide chains composed of pairs of H and L chains. The four polypeptide chains are differentially associated through covalent disulfide bonds and a multiplicity of weak noncovalent forces that additively provide stability and maintenance of quarternary structure. Such forces are evident in experiments which revealed that upon mild reduction and alkylation, the four-chain structure remained intact and retained full antigen binding activity in neutral buffers.

In discussing subunit properties of Abs it should be stressed that biological and chemical symmetry exists within a single Ig molecule since both H and L chains are of the same class or subclass and primary structure, respectively (described below). Covalent disulfide bonds comprising Ig molecules can be categorized depending on their structural role and order of lability to reducing agents. First, intrachain disulfide bonds are located within each chain (H or L) and stabilize the domain structure. A basic structural rule in immunoglobulins is that domains are repetitive infrastructures that occur at a frequency of one per approximately every 110–115 amino acid residues beginning with the amino terminus of both H and L chains. Second, interchain disulfide bonds serve to link heavy and light chains covalently. Only one interchain disulfide bond links heavy and light chains, while a spectrum of one to several bonds crosslink the heavy chains and are dispersed throughout the Fc region (Figure 3-1).

Finally, disulfide bonds also form covalent bridges between the four-chain subunits of polymeric immunoglobulins as in secretory IgA or circulatory IgM (Figure 3-2). Chemically, the three types of disulfide bonds are titratable with increasing concentrations of thiol-reducing agents (mercaptoethanol, dithiothreitol, etc.). Intersubunit disulfide bonds involved in polymeric Ig structures are selectively reduced at low concentrations of reducing agent followed in order by interchain and finally intrachain bonds. The order of disulfide bond lability to reduction correlates with their structural interrelationship with the domain structures and solvent accessibility. Adjacent immunoglobulin subunits involved in polymeric structures, such as pentameric IgM, lack domain–domain interactions (Figure 3-2). Disulfide bonds involved in polymerization are therefore easily reduced and rapid diffusion of dissociated subunits inhibits bond reformation. In addition, the lack of intersubunit domain–domain interactions prohibits proper steric positioning of reduced sulfhydryls for reoxidation. Thus, alkylation is generally unnecessary with selective reduction of intersubunit disulfide bonds.

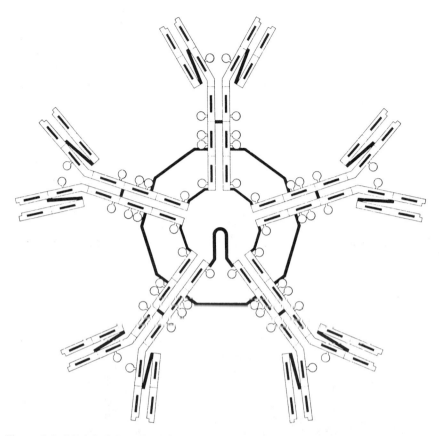

Figure 3-2. Model of the polymeric IgM antibody molecule. Disulfide bonds are noted as black bars (▬) and carbohydrate moieties as Ϙ . The J chain is visualized as a darkened loop (∩). (Figure reproduced from Ref 148 by permission.)

Reduction of interchain disulfide bonds is more easily achieved than with intra-chain bonds. Due to domain–domain interactions between H and L chains and partial sequestration from solvent (Figure 3-1), reduction requires higher concentra-tions of thiol reducing agents. Since unperturbed domain–domain interactions also prevent dissociation of H and L chains, higher concentrations of reducing agents are needed to insure that the equilibrium between reduced and nonreduced sulfhydryl groups is shifted toward the reduced state. Thus, alkylating agents are generally required to assure against reoxidation of reduced sulfhydryl groups involved in interchain linkages.

Finally, intrachain disulfide bonds require high concentrations of reducing agents to insure efficient reduction. Intrachain bonds are structurally buried within the relatively hydrophobic domain structure being inaccessible to solvent exchange. Efficient reduction of intrachain disulfide bonds is best achieved when isolated H and L chains are subjected to reducing agents. The fact that isolated chains are probably partially denatured[22] facilitates thiol reduction.

As depicted in Figure 3-1, domain–domain interactions occur between the amino-terminal half of the H chain (termed F_D) and the L chain. Such interactions also occur between domains constituting Fc fragments. However, no domain–domain interactions are operational between the two Fab fragments that comprise each immunoglobulin (Figure 3-1). Lack of such secondary forces explains in part the phenomenon of segmental flexibility inherent to different degrees in Ig molecules. Segmental flexibility is defined as the rotation of Fab fragments around the Fc axis between polar orientation to a more closely aligned "Y" configuration.

Although the carbohydrate content of immunoglobulins is complex it is relatively low (ranging from 2 to 12% by weight and dependent on Ig class). Polysaccharide moieties are most often covalently associated with constant region amino acid residues of heavy chains (Figures 3-1 and 3-2). The number, size, and chemical composition of carbohydrate moieties differs with each immunoglobulin class or subclass. Although the nature of the carbohydrates associated with Igs is not described in this chapter, chemical variations in carbohydrate content is the structural basis for what is termed Ig microheterogeneity. The latter explains the multiple protein bands obtained when homogeneous antibodies are subjected to isoelectric focusing analysis. The biological implications of microheterogeneity are not fully understood.

Immunoglobulin Isotypy

It is not possible in this chapter to discuss immunoglobulin classes and subclasses (referred to as isotypes) on a comprehensive phylogenetic basis, although the latter is important in assessing evolutionary significance and comparative properties of Igs.[23] Thus, only human and mouse Ig classes are described because of their obvious importance in immunology and cognate biotechnology. In human and mouse, five major isotypes or classes of H chains have been identified: γ, μ, α, δ, and ϵ. Immunoglobulin isotypic classifications are dictated by unique primary structures comprising each constant region of the heavy chains: IgG, IgM, IgA, IgD, and IgE. Within certain classes, variations in the prototypical amino acid sequence define important subclasses. Human IgG consists of four subclasses: IgG1, IgG2, IgG3, and IgG4; similarly mouse IgG has four: IgG1, IgG2a, IgG2b, and IgG3. Human IgA has two subclasses: IgA1 and IgA2.

Each Ig class and subclass exhibits specific effector functions that are direct consequences of the primary and three-dimensional structures associated with heavy-chain isotypes. Effector functions represent biological activities or properties such as antigenic distinctiveness, average serum concentration, serum half-life, complement binding and fixation, cell binding with specific membrane receptors, immunoglobulin hemeostasis (feedback inhibition), and transport of secretory Igs. Effector activities are part of an integrated dual function and permit antibodies to fulfill important biological roles. The extensive diversity, characteristic of the immune system, allows primary binding of a large spectrum of antigens. However, the initial binding must lead to antigen elimination physiologically which is based on a series of mechanisms activated subsequent to antigen binding.

Antibody light chains are constituted by two major isotypes: kappa (κ) and lambda (λ). In the mouse, λ has three defined subclasses: λ_1, λ_2, and λ_3. In the human, four nonallelic λ subclasses have been defined: λ_1, λ_2, λ_3, and λ_6.

Although isotypic determination can be established based on procurement of constant-region primary structures, it has been possible to elicit antibody reagents (both polyclonal and monoclonal) that are specific for Ig classes and subclasses of each species. Specific immunological reagents allow for a relatively rapid identification of isotypes in a variety of immunological assays.

The recent discovery of immunoglobulin-binding bacterial-derived proteins A and G has proved important since they preferentially distinguish species, class, and subclass of Igs. The Fc-binding proteins have proved important in differential purification of immunoglobulins.

Polymeric immunoglobulins represent multiples of the basic four-chain subunit structure through disulfide bridges as previously described. Immunoglobulin M forms covalent pentamers through formation of disulfide bonds linking each of five subunits (Figure 3-2). In addition, a polypeptide with a molecular weight of 16 kd, termed the J chain, is found covalently associated with the pentameric structure. A stoichiometric ratio of one J chain per IgM pentamer has been established. It is generally considered that the J chain is involved either in biosynthetic polymerization of the subunits or as a stabilizer of the pentameric structure. A portion of IgM molecules are hexamers when the J chain is absent

Another immunoglobulin serum IgA exists as a monomer, while IgA in biological fluid secretions (sIgA) is dimeric (polymeric). One J chain is found covalently associated with each sIgA dimer. Finally, an ancillary protein, termed secretory component (SC), which is synthesized and secreted by epithelial cells, is an integral part of the IgA dimeric structure.

Immunoglobulin Domain Structure

Delineation of immunoglobulin structure–function progressed proportionately with the historical transition from polyclonal to monoclonal Ig reagents. Homogeneous myeloma proteins proved indispensable stepping stones from polyclonal immunoglobulins to the current availability of hybridomas.[24] Extensive heterogeneity that characterized polyclonal immunoglobulins defied all but limited primary structural determinations. Human myeloma proteins, initially procured as clinical byproducts, proved amenable to amino acid sequencing. This was followed by Potter's important findings[25] that made routine the procurement of murine myeloma proteins. From a structure–function viewpoint, the most notable deficiency in studying myeloma proteins was the general lack of identifiable antigen binding specificity with an affinity considered biologically significant. This deficiency was rectified with the advent of hybridoma methodology.[24]

Comparative amino acid sequences of various homogeneous immunoglobulins among different species, classes, and subclasses of both H and L chains led to recognition of repetitive homology regions of 110–115 residues that contained intrachain disulfide bonds and a domain between conserved cysteines (Figure 3-1). The number of amino acids included within the domain varies but in general conserved cysteines span 60–65 amino acids.[26]

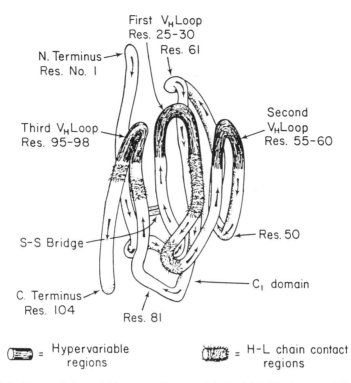

Figure 3-3. Heavy-chain variable-region immunoglobulin fold. The hypervariable regions are represented as shaded loops.

Antibody domains possess similar globular structures, referred to as the "immunoglobulin fold" (Figure 3-3), which is composed of differing layers of antiparallel β-pleated sheets stabilized by intrachain disulfide bonds (Figure 3-4). The repetitive domain theme in all immunoglobulins correlates with the chain size. The γ chain of IgG contains four domains (V_H, C_H1, C_H2, and C_H3), while L chains (both κ and λ) contain two domains. IgM and IgE possess five domains per heavy chain because of higher molecular weights of 72–75 kd.

The predominant structural feature of the repetitive domain is the antiparallel β-pleated sheet structure (Figure 3-4). Each constant domain is composed of two layers, each layer containing three and four antiparallel segments connected by loops or bends of various lengths. The variable domain differs in containing one five-stranded layer in place of the three-stranded layer. Thus, in Figure 3-4 the V and C domains resemble rotational allomers in that the interaction of each with the homologous domain of the other chain is via the five-stranded layer in the V domain, whereas in the C domain it is via the four-strand layer. Structurally C_H3 domains in Fc are similar to that of C_H1 domains, whereas C_H2 domains have somewhat different structures with minimal interactions between the C_H2 domains of the two H chains. The latter may be partly due to the presence of carbohydrates at the interacting interface.

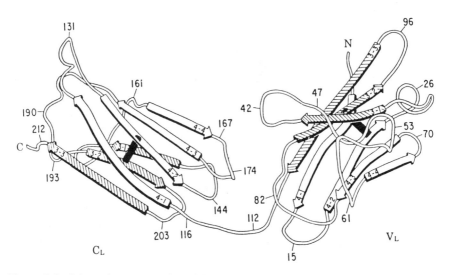

Figure 3-4. Schematic representation of the V_L and C_L domains. Arrows represent segments of primary structure forming the antiparallel β-pleated sheets. Numbers represent amino acid position and the black rectangles the intrachain disulfide bonds. The V domain describes the βββц ββц β-ββ ц β βββц βц βц βц β ц βββц βββц βρββц βββц βββц βββц βββц βββц β βββц βββц βββц β ββ ц ββц β pleated sheet rather than the five-stranded sheet described in the text. (Figure reproduced from Ref 149 by permission.)

The γ heavy chain features a hinge region between the second (C_H1) and third (C_H2) domains (Figure 3-1) that is proline rich, resulting in a rigid but linear double-stranded configuration. The hinge region is important biologically and biochemically since it serves as a pseudo-tether linking Fab and Fc fragments. This structural feature facilitates segmental flexibility in which the two Fab and Fc fragments tend to function independently. Segmental flexibility is probably important in the modulation of antigen binding (eg, avidity) and the biological expression of certain effector functions.[27,28]

Because of its exposed location, amino acid sequence, and length, the hinge region is relatively susceptible to proteolysis by enzymes, such as plasmin, papain, pepsin, and trypsin (Figure 3-1). Chemically, differential susceptibility has been advantageous in generating Fab, F(ab)$_2$, or Fc fragments.

Based on the concept that the domain is a basic structural immunoglobulin entity which can be traced phylogenetically, it has been proposed that antibodies and immunoglobulin-related molecules have evolved by duplication of a primordial gene encoding approximately 110 amino acids.[26] The domain-based immunoglobulin homology is characteristic of members of the immunoglobulin gene superfamily, such as T-cell receptors, MHC class-I and class-II molecules, Thy-1, and various cell-surface molecules.[29]

The domain theory[26] does not include quaternary relationships between H and L chains, which represent linear polymeric products through evolutionary duplication of the primitive domain unit. A particular interpretation of the domain theory can include a unique feature of the antibody system, the extensive affinity range (10^4 to

10^{12} M^{-1}). The expanded affinity and specificity expressed by antibodies significantly exceeds the average range of energy involved in enzyme–substrate interactions (mM to μM). However, it is not unreasonable to speculate that the evolutionarily derived primitive domain unit that became H and L chains originally exhibited catalytic activities with enzyme-like affinities or K_M values. However, in the eventual association of these two chains, which interestingly are translation products of two different chromosomes, the domains containing the active sites sterically interacted forming a site–site interface. In the process the low-affinity site characteristic of each chain became augmented when acting in concert and significantly higher affinities resulted. Subsequent to this evolutionary event genetic variability and diversity unfolded when binding and ligand clearance was selected for genetically. This concept is unproven but intriguing since in recent years the reverse conversion of antibodies to enzymes has gained popularity.[30]

Since primary structure dictates peptide folding and the three-dimensional structure of antibodies, it was necessary to generate significant data bases as a prelude to structure–function studies. Comparison of primary structures of many homogeneous proteins revealed that H and L chains were composed of variable (V) *N*-terminal and constant (C) *C*-terminal segments.[31] Variability is defined as the number of amino acids occurring at one position divided by the frequency of the most common amino acids at that position. With a sufficiently large data base it became evident that hypervariable segments within the V region of the light chain span residues 24–34, 50–56, and 89–97. In the heavy chain, hypervariable residues included 31–35, 50–65, 81–84, and 95–102. These hypervariable areas were designated complementarity-determining regions (CDRs) as they sterically form the antigen binding site of the V regions (Figures 3-3 and 3-4). Relatively conserved areas within the V regions were termed the framework (FR) regions.

In both light and heavy chains, the first and third CDRs begin after the first and second cysteine residues within the variable segment. Thus, the intrachain disulfide bonds of the V domains ensures spatial juxtaposition of the various CDR segments.

Crystallographic Studies of Immunoglobulins

The potential to systematically crystallize and compare immunoglobulins structurally was enhanced by the advent of hybridoma technology,[24] which permitted production of large amounts of homogeneous antibodies with defined specificities. Generation of monoclonal antibodies (Mab) to virtually any antigen was a major advancement for researchers seeking to decipher mechanisms involved in antigen–antibody interactions.

Crystallization of immunoglobulins appears to follow certain trends. First, despite adequate homogeneity, purity, and quantities, crystallization of undigested immunoglobulins has not been achieved with routine success. Second, crystallization of Fab fragments has proved relatively more successful than intact (undigested) Ig molecules. Third, addition of antigen (or ligand) facilitates crystallization of Fab fragments. The latter has led to a theory regarding stabilization of a specific conformational state by bound ligand facilitating crystallization.[32]

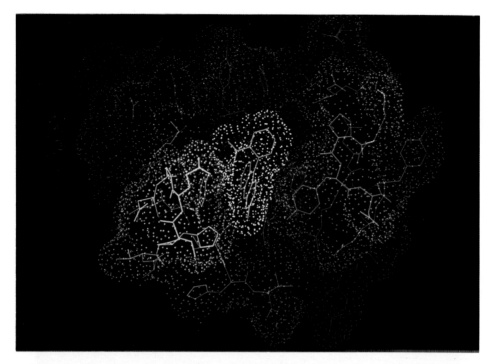

Plate 3-2. Three-dimensional depiction of fluorescein ligand (green) bound to the Fab fragment of anti-fluorescein Mab 4-4-20. Heavy-chain amino acid side chains are represented in pink, with blue dots depicting the van der Waals outline. Light-chain residues are shown in yellow, with red dots representing the van der Waals outline. (Provided by AB Edmundson.)

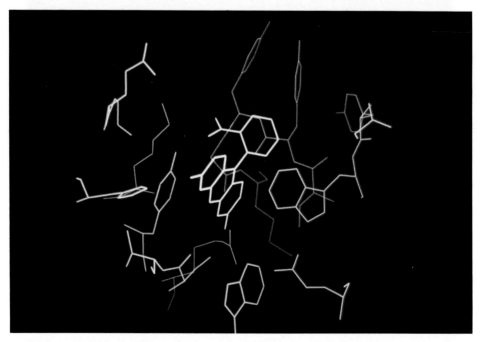

Plate 3-3. The hapten binding site of anti-fluorescein Mab 4-4-20. The fluorescein ligand is featured in white. Light-chain constituents are blue and heavy-chain constituents are blue and heavy-chain components are red. The xanthonyl (three planar rings) group of fluorescein is flanked by tyrosine L37 on the left and tryptophan H33 on the right. Tryptophan L101 forms the bottom of the site. Enolic oxygen atoms on opposite corners of the xanthonyl group point toward histidine L31 (left) and arginine L39 (right). The phenyl carboxyl group of fluorescein is located between tyrosines H103 (left) and H102 (right). (Provided by AB Edmundson.)

model protein antigens of known three-dimensional structure, such as lysozyme, myoglobin, influenza virus neuraminidase, and cytochrome C.[47]

The three-dimensional structure of a protein antigen–antibody complex involving lysozyme and an Fab fragment derived from a monoclonal anti-lysozyme antibody (D1.3) has been solved.[15] The interacting (lysozyme) epitope was discontinuous and conformational. The anti-lysozyme antibody site was relatively flat (cleftlike) with protrusions and depressions formed by amino acid side chains lining the cavity. Sixteen lysozyme and 17 antibody CDR residues made close contact through van der Waals forces and hydrogen bonds, forming a relatively tight antigen–antibody interface. The dimensions of the interface were about 30×20 Å, leading to exclusion of water molecules. Recently, analyses of another monoclonal anti-lysozyme Fab (HyHEL-5) bound to a different lysozyme epitope[48] were related to findings with D1.3. Differences existed in specific electrostatic interactions between charged residues on the antigen and on the antibody. Electrostatic interactions might contribute to the higher affinity of the HyHEL–lysozyme complex (2.5×10^9 M^{-1}) relative to the affinity of the D1.3–lysozyme complex (4.5×10^7 M^{-1}).

A myeloma protein of considerable interest is the human Bence-Jones dimer, (λ) Mcg, which has been crystallized as a dimer and the structure determined to 2.7 Å resolution.[49] The Mcg dimer binds a variety of aromatic and hydrophobic aliphatic compounds and binding studies have been compared both in crystals and in solution. Of special interest, the light chains comprising the Mcg IgG1 parent protein and the Bence-Jones dimer have identical primary structures, yet their three-dimensional structures exhibit conformational isomerism. One isomer in the Bence-Jones dimer is similar to the light-chain component of antigen binding (Fab) fragments, while the second isomer resembles the heavy-chain component. Thus, Mcg serves as a structural model for the Fab fragment in that it simulates the interactions of four domains. The Mcg active site can be visualized as a truncated cone in which the walls of the cavity are primarily aromatic in nature. Of the 21 side chains lining the Mcg cavity, 12 are aromatic: eight tyrosines and four phenylalanines.[50] Three negatively charged side chains line the rim, with no charged groups within the interior of the cavity. In a systematic search[49] for site-filling ligands compounds were diffused into the crystals (trigonal crystals grown in 1.9 mol/L ammonium sulfate, pH 6.2), and two binding sites were delineated. The main binding cavity exposed to solvent initially accommodated ligands such as 1-anilinonaphthalene-8-sulfonate. However, with time, the hydrophobic ligand diffused to a deep binding pocket beyond the floor of the main cavity. Ligands increasing in size from fluorescein to bis(N-methyl)acridine (lucigenin) to dimers of carboxytetramethylrhodamine were found to bind only to the main cavity of the Mcg site.

Recently a high-affinity anti-fluorescein monoclonal antibody (4-4-20) derived from a BALB/c mouse hyperimmunized with fluorescein–keyhole limpet hemocyanin was studied on a structure–function basis. Hybridoma 4-4-20 (IgG2a, κ) possessed an affinity of $2–3 \times 10^{10}$ M^{-1} for the fluorescyl ligand.[51,52] Other distinguishing features of the 4-4-20 Mab are listed in Table 3-1.

Table 3-1. Characterization of Monoclonal Antibody 4-4-20

Measurement	Value
Q_{max} (%)	96.4[a]
Absorption max (nm)	505[b]
Isoelectric point (pI)	7.4
Second-order assoc. rate $(M^{-1}s^{-1})$	5.0×10^6
Dissociation rate lifetime (s)	1683[c]
D_2O enhancement (%)	130.7 ± 1.8
Iodide quenching (%)	2.5[d]

[a]The 4-4-20 protein was titrated into 10^{-8} mol/L fluorescein, and fluorescence quenching measured after each addition. Reported Q_{max} values were extrapolated from a double reciprocal plot of fluorescence quenching vs. antibody concentraton.

The papain-derived Fab fragment of 4-4-20 was co-crystallized with ligand in polyethylene glycol (PEG) and 2-methyl-2,4-pentanediol (MPD) in forms suitable for x-ray analyses (2.5-Å resolution). Plate 3-1 presents the structure of the liganded Fab fragment derived from Mab 4-4-20. The Fab structure illustrates the lateral (trans) associations between H and L domains. The plate also shows the potential for weak longitudinal (cis) interactions between V and C domains of each chain. Since Plate 3-1 represents the structure of a liganded Fab fragment it is important to note significant differences between the V and C domains comprising the fragment. Both V domains appear relatively more densely structured than the C domains. Since the corresponding structure of the nonliganded form of 4-4-20 is not available, it remains unclear whether the differences noted are due solely to bound ligand.

In contrast, the C_H–C_L domain portion of the Fab is more loosely organized than

Table 3-2. Comparative Primary Structures of Heavy-Chain Variable Regions of Anti-Fluorescein Mabs 4-4-20 and 9-40

```
              1                    10                   20                  30
4-4-20        E V K L D E T G G G L V Q P G R P M K L S C V A S G F T F S
9-40          - - - - - - - - - - - - - - - - - - - - - - - - - - - - - -


              [-CDR 1-]                                 [- - - - - - - - - - - - - CDR 2 - - -
                                40                   50   52 a  b  c 53
4-4-20        D Y W M N W V R Q S P E K G L E W V A Q I R N K P Y N Y E T
9-40          - - - - - - - - - - - - - - - - - - - - - - - - - - - - - -


              - - - - - - - - - - - - - - - -]
                          60                   70                   80    82a  b  c 83
4-4-20        Y Y S D S V K G R F T I S R D D S K S S V Y L Q M N N L R V
9-40          - - - - - - - - - - - - - - - - - - - - - - - - - - - - - A


                                 [- - - CDR 3 - - - -]
                          90           100a b  c  d                       110
4-4-20        E D M G I Y Y C T G S Y Y G M D Y W G Q G T S V T V S S
9-40          - - - - - - - - - S Y G - H G A - - - - - - L - - - - A
```

Table 3-3. Comparative Primary Structures of Light-Chain Variable Regions
of Anti-Fluorescein Mabs 4-4-20 and 9-40

	1	10	20
4-4-20	D V V M T Q T P L S L P V S L G D Q A S		
9-40	– – – – – – – – – – – – – – – – – – – –		

——— CDR1 ———

	27a b c d e	30
4-4-20	I S C R S S Q S L V H S N G N T Y L R	
9-40	– – – – – – – – – – – – – – – – – – H	

	40	50
4-4-20	W Y L Q K P G Q S P K V L I Y K V	
9-40	– – – – – – – – – – – L – – – – –	

— CDR2 —

	60	70
4-4-20	S N R F S G V P D R F S G S G S G T D	
9-40	– – – – – – – – – – – – – – – – – – –	

	80
4-4-20	F T L K I S R V E A E D L G V Y F
9-40	– – – – – – – – – – – – – – – – –

——— CDR3 ———

	90	100
4-4-20	C S Q S T H V P W T F G G G T K L E	
9-40	– – – – – – – – – – – – – – – – – –	

4-4-20	I K
9-40	– –

the V_H–V_L domains with bound ligand. The primary structures of the H- and L-chain variable regions of 4-4-20 are presented in Tables 3-2 and 3-3, respectively. The amino acid sequences are compared to the primary structure describing the H- and L-chain variable regions of murine monoclonal anti-fluorescein antibody 9-40 (IgG, κ). The latter is idiotypically related (80–90%) to Mab 4-4-20 but possesses an affinity 1000-fold less (3-4 × 10^7 M^{-1}) and exhibits only 45.5% fluorescence quenching of the bound fluorescyl ligand. Table 3-4 emphasizes only the differences in the variable-region sequences between Mabs 4-4-20 and 9-40.

Plate 3-2 illustrates the active site of the crystallized Fab fragment of Mab 4-4-20. The site consists primarily of aromatic amino acids, such as tyrosine and tryptophan residues, enriched with basic arginine residues. Critical site-forming residues involved in the interactions with bound fluorescein are featured in Plate 3-3. The presence of aromatic and basic amino acid residues in the active site are consistent with binding of the aromatic and dianionic fluorescein ligand. As indicated previously, development of hapten systems that allow for direct comparisons of anti-

Table 3.4 Amino Acid Differences in the Heavy- and Light-Chain Variables Regions Comparing Anti-Fluorescein Mabs 4-4-20 and 9-40

		Residue Number									
		34	46								
Light chain	4-4-20	ARG	VAL								
	9-40	HIS	LEU								

		Residue Number									
		84	99	100	a	b	c	d	101	108	113
Heavy chain	4-4-20	VAL	GLY	SER	TYR	TYR	GLY	MET	ASP	SER	SER
	9-40	ALA	SER	TYR	GLY	TYR	HIS	GLY	ALA	LEU	ALA

body molecules that differ only in affinity (or any other parameter) will provide the basis for establishment of immunoglobulin structure–function principles.

Correlation of Hapten with Structure–Function of Specific Antibodies

The results of crystallization studies (Plates 3-1, 3-2, and 3-3) show that the important features and interactions evident within the antibody-active site need to be interpreted on the basis of various functional measurements that have been made in solution. The material presented is an attempt to supply background information concerning functional characterizations and to correlate such properties with the resolved structure (Plates 3-1, 3-2, and 3-3).

The fluorescein determinant has become one of the important haptens immunologically as an aid in beginning to understand rules of structure–function because of measurements that permit correlation of the two parameters. The system is emphasized here because of information presented in Plates 3-1, 3-2, and 3-3. The polyaromatic and dianionic nature of fluorescein conforms to properties generally considered necessary for immunogenicity. The size of fluorescein, as noted by a molecular weight of ~350 d, is important since solution studies have shown that fluorescein approximates a site-filling ligand.[53] The latter maximizes the number of intrasite interactions and directly effects affinity, as shown in Plates 3-2 and 3-3. The ligand's high fluorescence quantum yield (Φ) of 0.92 is beneficial in the development of sensitive fluorescent ligand binding assays, although the fluorescence lifetime of 4 ns is not sufficiently long to measure certain molecular events. Extensive studies[9] have shown that fluorescein is a potent hapten immunologically when covalently conjugated to T-cell (lymphocyte) dependent carriers, such as keyhole limpet hemocyanin (KLH). The immune response to fluorescein is significantly diverse. This phenomenon in all species studied to date (murine, lapine, avian, guinea pig, and bovine) necessitated employment of hybridoma methodology to dissect the response and generate homogeneous monoclonal antibody populations of defined specificity.[54]

Homogeneity of Monoclonal Antibody Active Sites

Monoclonality is a critical prerequisite in defining structure–function relationships. Monoclonal anti-fluorescein antibodies purified from either murine ascites fluid (in vivo) or from serum-free in vitro tissue culture were judged homogeneous by isoelectric focusing and linear kinetics describing the first-order dissociation rate.[55] In determining affinities of each monoclonal anti-fluorescein antibody the second-order association rate was assumed to be constant ($5.6 \times 10^6 \, M^{-1} \, s^{-1}$). The latter is slower than the rate assigned to diffusion-controlled reactions[56] and is probably attributable to the fact that the fluorescein ligand is a rigid ellipsoid (Plate 3-3) and therefore precise geometric orientation is required before binding can occur within the antibody active site. Based on a relatively constant association rate, antibody affinity is dictated by significant differences (logarithmic) in the dissociation rate.

A frequency plot of affinities for the characterized monoclonal antibodies elicited to the fluorescyl–KLH immunogen conform to a gaussian distribution with an average affinity of 4–$5 \times 10^8 \, M^{-1}$ (SD ± 4.5). Thus, when viewed as a population of antibodies, the hybridomas collectively simulate the classical heterogeneous hyperimmune response observed in serum analyses.[57]

Thermodynamics of the Anti-Fluorescein–Fluorescein Interaction

The thermodynamic properties exhibited by selected monoclonal anti-fluorescein antibodies have been described in detail.[14] In general, curvilinear van't Hoff plots were observed for all monoclonal anti-fluorescein antibodies studied, indicating that their standard enthalpy changes ($\Delta H°$) were temperature dependent. The anti-fluorescein–ligand interaction was also investigated in terms of unitary free energy (ΔG_u), standard enthalpy ($\Delta H°$), unitary entropy (ΔS_u), heat capacity changes ($\Delta C_p°$), and standard volume changes ($\Delta V°$). Analyses of thermodynamic properties revealed two competing forces in fluorescein binding. First, a hydrophobic effect was judged to be the thermodynamic driving force for fluorescein binding. Second, ligand binding restricts the mobility of active site residues, which makes an unfavorable contribution to $\Delta G°$. The latter forms the basis for hapten-induced conformational changes. The thermodynamic properties can be correlated with the active site structures presented in Plates 3-1, 3-2, and 3-3.

Properties of the Anti-Fluorescyl Site

Molecular mechanisms by which antibody-bound fluorescein undergoes a red spectral shift in its absorption spectrum and its fluorescence is quenched have been studied.[58] Displacement of λ_{max} ($\Delta 10$–20 nm) to the red correlates with polarity of the environment. The relative reduction in the quantum yield of fluorescein has been consistently $>80\%$ with polyclonal anti-fluorescein antibodies but has shown a significant range with monoclonal antibodies (35–99%). The degree of fluorescence quenching is therefore not constant and appears dependent on several factors. Screening of individual amino acids for the ability to quench fluorescein fluorescence in aqueous solution resulted in the finding that L-triptophan, and to a lesser extent L-tyrosine, were effective quenchers.[58] Stern-Volmer analyses and fluorescence lifetime (τ) measurements of tryptophan quenching revealed complex fluorescein–tryptophan dynamics (involving both static and dynamic components). In addition, titration of anti-fluorescein antibodies with fluorescyl ligand showed that fluorescence emission of excited tryptophanyl residues within the antibody active site were quenched. Collectively, these results suggested that tryptophan was involved either directly in fluorescence quenching or indirectly through energy transfer mechanisms within the antibody active site. Plates 3-2 and 3-3 show that tryptophan and tyrosine residues are important constituents of the anti-fluorescein active site, confirming the solution results.

Solvent perturbation studies have also been used to characterize both polyclonal and monoclonal anti-fluorescyl active sites further. Deuterium oxide, iodide, and oxygen have been employed in perturbation studies.[59–61] The relative fluorescence quantum yield of fluorescein bound to specifically purified high-affinity liganded polyclonal rabbit and chicken IgG antibody was significantly enhanced in deuterium oxide (D_2O) relative to the complex in aqueous (H_2O) solution. The degree of fluorescence enhancement correlated with the intrinsic affinity of polyclonal antibody for the ligand but the same correlation was not evident in examinations of individual monoclonal antibodies. Quantitatively, fluorescence enhancement in D_2O (95%) was identical for ligand bound to IgG and F(ab)$_2$ fragments derived from the same hybridoma. The isotope enhancement effect was not due to ligand dissociation as shown by a comparison of difference spectroscopy and equilibrium dialysis results in D_2O and H_2O buffers, and by similar enhancement of fluorescence with affinity-labeled antibody.[59] Identical extrinsic circular dichroism of antibody-bound fluorophore in D_2O and H_2O, coupled with the absence of a measureable isotope effect on the quenching of fluorescein by L-tryptophan, supported the contention that the D_2O effect was an excited state phenomenon.[59]

Comparative kinetic studies of ligand dissociation and D_2O enhancement were performed with both heterogeneous and homogeneous anti-fluorescyl antibodies.[61] Relatively high affinities of all liganded antibody preparations were determined by dissociation rate studies, demonstrating comparatively long lifetimes describing dissociation of bound fluorescein. In addition, rabbit polyclonal anti-fluorescyl preparations were found to display marked heterogeneity of dissociation rates, while mouse monoclonal anti-fluorescyl preparations exhibited a single linear off-rate, indicating homogeneity. Deuterium oxide fluorescence enhancement studies showed nonlinear kinetics with both heterogeneous and homogeneous antibody active sites. Temperature studies of ligand D_2O enhancement and dissociation rates using monoclonal anti-fluorescyl antibodies revealed similar, yet different activation energies (22.7 ± 0.8 and 20.2 ± 0.3 cal, respectively) for both phenomena. The studies demonstrated that the anti-fluorescein antibody active site consists of both solvent-accessible and relatively -inaccessible components, and that ligand binding involved both exchangeable hydrogen atoms and other unresolved interactions (Plates 3-2 and 3-3).

Differential accessibility of liganded high-affinity rabbit polyclonal anti-fluorescyl IgG antibody combining sites to the aqueous milieu has been investigated by solvent perturbation of the fluorescence of bound fluorophore.[60] Iodide, a dynamic quencher of fluorescein, was selected for use in such studies after examination of a number of water-soluble fluorescence quenchers. Quenching of antibody-bound fluorophore by iodide was measured with a number of liganded polyclonal anti-fluorescyl preparations, demonstrating partial solvent exposure of the fluorophore as well as heterogeneity of the high-affinity antibody populations. Fluorescence quenching, lifetime, and absorption spectroscopy provided evidence that the antibody-bound fluorophore quenched by iodide interacted with it directly and that anomalous binding of the anion to the surface of the protein, resulting in ground-state perturbations of the immunoglobulin, could not explain the results. Iodide quenching has proved useful in comparing the architecture of the anti-fluorescein sites between families of monoclonal antibodies.[52] Oxygen quenching studies with various monoclonal anti-fluorescyl antibodies (IgG) have revealed that the accessibility of bound ligand is a constant and independent of affinity.

In further studies, fluorescein isothiocyanate was reacted with purified rabbit polyclonal anti-fluorescyl antibodies under defined conditions[114] as a nonreversible affinity labeling reagent.[62] Relative to nonspecific antibody, significantly more ligand was conjugated to affinity-purified antibody and so was inhibited from further binding with radioactively labeled ligand. Fluorescyl ligand specifically conjugated to purified and absorbed antibody preparations exhibited a red spectral shift characteristic of specifically bound fluorophore. Fluorescence of ligand covalently conjugated to specific antibody was quenched about 95% relative to 90% for reversibly bound ligand. The quantum yield of the former is indicative of a thiocarbamyl linkage within the antibody active site. Fluorescence lifetime measurements by phase and modulation showed a close correlation between liganded and affinity-labeled antibody relative to free ligand and fluorescyl-conjugated nonantibody proteins. The fluorescein affinity label was not dissociated from the antibody active site upon denaturation of the protein in 6 mol/L guanidine–HCl. Thiol reduction, alkylation and resolution of immunoglobulin-derived H (γ) and L chains in two different dispersing agents showed that the ligand remained linked to either polypeptide. Fluorescyl ligand reversibly bound to high-affinity IgG (ie, nonaffinity labeled) was quantitatively released under conditions required for H- and L-chain production. The fluorescence of affinity-labeled ligand was enhanced in high concentrations of D_2O.[59] Similar studies showed that the cyanuric chloride derivative of fluorescein amine was also a stable affinity-labeling reagent.[63]

Normalization for Idiotypic Relatedness

Although monoclonal antibodies obtained from the same murine inbred strain or even the same individual animal are attractive reagents for comparative structure–function studies, interpretable results are not assured. The problem is that a random comparison of the primary structures of antibodies may yield differences too numerous and complex for conclusive analysis. In order to overcome this problem an additional normalization of available Mab must be made to facilitate comparative structural studies. To this end the generation of idiotype families has proved useful when coupled to hybridoma methodology.

Although idiotypic normalization is not a guarantee of structural homology suitable for structure–function interpretation, previous studies[64,65] suggested that selection of Ig molecules for the same specificity and the same idiotype implied common V regions (Tables 3-3, 3-4, and 3-5). Data further suggest that idiotypic normalization has resulted in the selection of Ig molecules with very similar properties. Assimilating information from selection of anti-fluorescein Mabs of the same specificity and a high degree of idiotypic cross relatedness (80% or greater), certain trends have been evident.[52] Although the intrafamily affinity range was approximately 1000-fold the molecules also differed significantly in percentage fluorescence quenching (Q_{max}) of the bound fluorescein ligand. The extent of spectral shift was similar and each antibody showed similar active site inaccessibility to iodine, similar percentage fluorescence enhancement in D_2O, as well as closely related fine-specificity binding patterns for fluorescyl analogs (erythrosin, eosin, and tetramethylrhodamine).[52]

Fragmentation of Monoclonal Antibodies for Structural Analyses

As indicated previously, the Fab fragment is an important reagent in structure–function analyses since comparative primary sequence studies emphasize the variable regions that convey antibody specificity. In addition, Fab fragments preferentially crystallize relative to the intact immunoglobulin, making it easy to obtain three-dimensional structural information. Such patterns in crystallization can be attributed to the relatively free and rapid motion of the Fc fragment around the hinge region.

Comparative studies conducted with purified liganded and nonliganded Fab preparations of each member of the idiotype family based on the 4-4-20 Mab prototype (Plate 3-1) revealed interesting results.[52,66] First, it was observed that the relative rate of digestion of the liganded Mab was greater than the nonliganded form. Second, the quantitative yield of Fab fragments was significantly higher with liganded antibody relative to digestion of the nonliganded molecule. Thus, ligand bound to the antibody active site within the Fab fragment apparently rendered the hinge region more accessible to the proteolytic action of papain. Bound ligand seemed to result in constriction of the Fab domains conveying resistance to prolonged digestion and theoretical yields of Fab fragments.

The rate of crystal growth by liganded Fab fragments can be characterized as relatively fast (weeks) compared to the nonliganded fragments, which has been slow (months) or inconsequential. Thus, as noted in papain digestion studies, the presence of ligand in the antibody active site facilitated crystal development and growth.

Antibody Allosterism

Recent structural resolutions of antigen–antibody complexes (as in Plate 3-1) have rekindled interest regarding conformational changes in the Fc region based on ligand binding. To date, successful crystallization, structural resolution, and comparative analyses of the same monoclonal Fab fragment with and without bound ligand has not been achieved. The experiment is vital in addressing questions regarding ligand-induced conformational changes. Conformational changes can be subdivided into various types. First, ligand may induce conformational changes within the variable domains forming the active site. Second, ligand-induced changes may be effected in the constant domains that constitute Fab fragments through binding in the variable domains. Third, conformational changes transmitted through the Fab fragment into the constant domains that comprise Fc fragments may also result. The latter would impact effector functions. Currently, no direct experimentation alludes to induced conformational changes because of the lack of comparative crystalline data. Claims of conformational changes are based primarily on successful crystallization of liganded Fab[15,45,48] and a comparison of the results with available nonliganded crystalline structures. No induced conformational changes in a liganded crystallized Fab were detected based on this approach.[15] However, conformational changes were noted in the lysozyme epitope upon antibody binding but not in the antibody molecule.[48]

Recently, it was concluded on the basis of an antibody complexed with influenza neuraminidase that changes in conformation were evident in both reactants (ie, Fab and bound antigen).[45] In neuraminidase C2 atoms of residues 368–371 were displaced approximately 1 Å when the bound structure was compared to the nonliganded conformer. A comparison of three different Fabs with the neuraminidase–Fab complex showed significant differences in the V_H–V_L domain pairing. Small sliding movements of one domain relative to the other (about 1 Å) were noted and the distances between the H- and L-chain CDRs were altered by ~4 Å. Thus, a "handshake" model was proposed in which antigen binding induces low-energy structural transitions within the Fab in the form of a sliding movement of the V_H and V_L domains. The sliding of domains and possible creation of various conformers potentially expands the range of specificities of an individual antibody molecule.[67] The differences in conclusions regarding conformational changes may depend on the energy of binding and other variables that await further delineation.

Quaternary interactions between adjacent domains have been found to be responsible for allosteric transitions within the Fab region. For example, it has been demonstrated that trans-interactions (ie, lateral) between C_L and C_H domains induce conformational changes in the V_H domain.[68] It has also been shown that association of V_L with V_H modulates reactivity of C_H1 with C_L through conformational changes probably transmitted through V_H–C_H1 contacts.[69] Energy transfer between adjacent variable and constant domains is presumably facilitated by segmental flexibility within the switch region.[70]

It has been proposed that a closing of the elbow bend and the resulting stiffening of the flexible antibody molecule by formation of longitudinal (cis) interactions may alter the Fc region.[71] The hypothesis was based on observations of an opened elbow angle in the intact IgG Kol molecule in contrast to a closed elbow angle within the liganded Fab fragment. This suggested that a closed elbow angle was characteristic of antigen-bound antibodies. Experiments designed to demonstrate such long-range effects have yielded negative results.[33,72] Observations of an open elbow angle in the D1.3 lysozyme and NC41–neuraminidase complex[15,45] weaken the theory. However, the plausibility of signal propagation from the variable to constant domains persists[73,74] and awaits significantly more data from the crystallization and analysis of appropriate Ig reagents.

Idiotypy: Definition and Structural Correlates

Antibody molecules can be defined antigenically in different ways. Previously, isotypic determinants within the constant regions of either H or L chains were described as determining Ig class or subclass. Importantly it has been found that immunogenic epitopes found in the area of the active site represent what is termed idiotypy (Id). "Idiotype" is a collective term broadly defined as a series of variable region antigens (idiotopes) associated with a single immunoglobulin or a group of structurally related immunoglobulins. Idiotypy was originally demonstrated by Oudin and Michel[75] and by Kunkel et al.[76] Quantitation of idiotypes was experimentally explored by Nisonoff and co-workers.[77]

Comparative studies of structurally related antibodies elicited to the same hapten have led to the identification of two classifications of idiotopes: (1) cross-reactive (IdX), recurrent or public idiotopes, and (2) individual idiotopes (IdI), nonrecurrent or private idiotopes.[78] The IdX epitopes are encoded by germline V genes and serve as serological markers for a single or a small group of related germline V_H or V_L gene products. The IdI determinants are considered somatic mutants of these germline genes. Direct proof of idiotype etiologies awaits definitive experimentation.

Idiotopes have been postulated to be involved in immunoregulation by serving as markers for communication between antigen-reactive cells in what is known as Jerne's network hypothesis.[79] In Jerne's theory, idiotopes are defined as antigenic autodeterminants that are recognized in the immune system and constitute an idiotypic cascade. Idiotypic and anti-idiotypic interactions have been classified according to topographical location of idiotopes on the V domains relative to their physical relationship to the antigen combining site (paratope).[80,81] Figure 3-5 outlines standard nomenclature associated with idiotypy. Anti-idiotypic antibodies of the α type (Ab2α) are directed against idiotopes distal to the paratope of Ab1. Anti-idiotypic antibodies that can interfere with antigen binding by steric hindrance are of the Ab2γ type. The Ab2β type are anti-idiotypic antibodies that bear idiotopes fitting in the antibody combining site of Ab1 and purportedly express an internal image of the antigen. The concept of anti-idiotypic antibodies bearing an internal image of the antigen has been an important research subject since it can be applied to the production of idiotype-based vaccines.[82] However, internal imaging has been a difficult concept to comprehend on a structural basis. An idiotype vaccine would have the distinct advantage of being devoid of harmful pathogens or undesirable contaminants. An anti-idiotypic antibody vaccine developed for type B viral hepatitis has been found to protect chimpanzees upon challenge with infectious hepatitis B virus.[83]

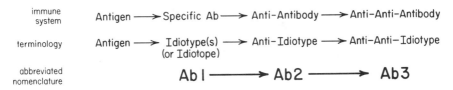

Figure 3-5. Idiotype nomenclature associated with the network hypothesis and described in the text.

There is widespread controversy as to whether the idiotype network is truly a regulatory physiological system (ie, immune response regulation by an intricate network based on idiotype–anti-idiotype interactions). A recent experiment with mice transgenic for a μ heavy-chain gene demonstrated increased production of endogenous immunoglobulins bearing the same idiotypic determinants as those specific for the transgene.[84] The authors concluded that the in vivo approach provided support for Jerne's network theory. Although direct experimental proof of the existence of a regulatory immune network is not available, idiotypes represent an important aspect of immunological theory and have proved important tools in determining immunoglobulin structural relatedness.

Because of the importance of idiotypes from both structural and genetic viewpoints (eg, markers for somatic mutational events) the identification of structural correlates of idiotopes have been vigorously pursued. Recombinations of H and L chains from functionally related murine myeloma proteins and monoclonal antibodies indicated that generally idiotypic determinants were conformational and required contributions of recombined autologous H and L chains for expression. Dependence of idiotypic expression on the specific pairing of autologous V-regions is not absolute since heterologous anti-galactan,[85] anti-Dnp,[86] anti-inulin,[87] and anti-arsonate[88] recombinant molecules were shown to express native anti-idiotypic structures, if reassociated H and L chains were derived from molecules sharing the same antibody specificity. Restoration of public idiotypes has been described for heterologous hybrid molecules constructed from MOPC 173 H chains and polyclonal L chains[89] and for T15$^+$ H chains assembled with irrelevant V_L domains.[90]

One approach used to define structural correlates of idiotopes has been to compare amino acid sequences of idiotypically related myeloma and hybridoma proteins.[91] This method was applied to anti-dextran antibodies, which are composed of a relatively invariable (λ) light chain. Both private, IdI(J558) and IdI(M104), and public idiotopes have been localized within the V_H segment and the D segment, respectively, of the V_H region.[92,93] Assignment of private idiotopes to the D segment has been confirmed using synthetic peptides as immunogens. Unadsorbed rabbit antisera to D-region peptides distinguished between M104 and J558 proteins possessing variable regions that differed by two amino acids.[94] A similar approach to mapping idiotypic determinants has been to select idiotypic variants using fluorescence-activated cell sorting and a subsequent comparison of their sequence to the prototype sequence. This method allowed localization of idiotopes to both the CDR2[95] and the D segment.[96] Neither approach described adequately distinguishes between the formation of the idiotypic determinant and amino acids for which a substitution yields conformational adjustments that allosterically influence expression and immunological reactivity of idiotypes.

An alternative method for predicting localization of idiotopes is based on studies of protein antigenicity that describe the surface of proteins as a continuum of potential antigenic sites.[97] When surface variability of V domains was plotted and compared with the variability plot by Wu and Kabat,[31] it appeared that the idiotope-determining region (IDR) only partially overlapped with the CDRs, and that framework regions might be an important factor in idiotypic determinant formation.[81]

x-Ray crystallographic coordinates of immunoglobulins have been used to compute surface regions accessible to a large spherical probe, comparable in size to an antibody domain.[98] The analysis was consistent with experimentally determined idiotopes that both hypervariable and framework residues were involved. Idiotype–anti-idiotope interactions may be analogous to the complementary, irregular, and flat large-surface association found in protein epitope–antibody complexes.[15] Experimentally defined idiotypic determinants may therefore overlap the H and L chains or V and C domains. Direct correlation of idiotypic determinants with the three-dimensional structure of Fab fragments has been achieved by immunoelectron microscopy studies.[99] A low-resolution three-dimensional model was constructed which suggested that idiotypic determinants were dispersed over the variable domains, extending from the CDRs to near the variable–constant switch region. Preliminary x-ray diffraction analysis of an idiotype–anti-idiotype immune complex has been reported.[100]

Idiotypy and Metatypy

In a recent study a syngenic polyclonal antibody population was elicited that preferentially bound the affinity-labeled liganded state of a high-affinity murine monoclonal anti-hapten antibody.[101] The antibody reagent reacted inefficiently with the nonliganded (idiotype) state of the homologous antibody and was unreactive with free hapten. The reagent was termed "anti-metatype" to distinguish it from reagents displaying anti-idiotype specificity. Furthermore, anti-metatype (Met) antibody did not react with the liganded form of an idiotypically unrelated murine monoclonal antibody of similar specificity and affinity. The idiotype–metatype interrelationship is portrayed in Figure 3-6.

As suggested previously, idiotypy may be conceptualized as an indicator of a conformational state or a series of states (to be described later in this chapter) existing in dynamic equilibrium within a non-liganded antibody site. In this context, metatype is viewed as a ligand-selected conformational state from a spectrum of dynamic states that characterize Ig molecules of a specific idiotype. The selected conformer may differ depending upon binding with homologous ligand or cross-reacting structural analogs.[32] Thus, metatypic states express energetically favorable three-dimensional structures resulting from the energy of interaction between the ligand and protein, thereby reflecting primary structures of H- and L-chain variable

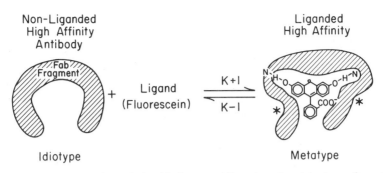

Figure 3-6. Hypothetical interrelationship between idiotypic and metatypic conformational states. The metatypic state is depicted with fluorescein bound to the antibody active site. (Figure reproduced from Ref 101 by permission.)

regions. The finding of a metatypic state directly attests to a conformational change in the variable regions upon ligand binding.

Role of Constant Domains

Using monoclonal anti-idiotope antibodies specific for MOPC 315 it was found that the Fv fragment was idiotypically deficient relative to the parent IgA molecule. These results contrasted with studies that showed that MOPC 315 idiotypic determinants were located on the Fv fragment of the Ab.[102] Restoration of public idiotypes has also been described for heterologous hybrid molecules constructed from MOPC 173 H chains and polyclonal L chains[89] and for T15+ H chains assembled with unrelated V_L domains.[90] The role of C_H1 and C_L domains in idiotypic expression has been examined.[103] Loss of idiotypic reactivity in rabbit antibody specific for micrococcal carbohydrates following incubation with low concentrations of reducing agents has been reported.[104] It was recently found that expression of certain T15-associated idiotypes was isotype dependent and required the specific interaction of α heavy chain.[105] Furthermore, a Cμ-restricted idiotypic determinant was also required for an anti-galactan antibody.[106] Additional data, implicating the C_H1 domain in maintaining proper folding of the V region, include a study of binding affinities of recombined V_H–L and V_H–V_L subunits. When these were compared to the affinity of the native riboflavin binding human IgG molecule, it was found that removal of the C_H1 domain decreased the ligand-binding affinity from 10^7 M^{-1} to 4×10^4 M^{-1}.[107] A previous report had shown that, for the Dnp-binding myeloma protein MOPC 315, the variable domains bound hapten with the same affinity as the native molecule. The differences in the two studies may be due to the relatively small size of Dnp compared to the riboflavin ligand. It is logical that the number of interactions between ligand and amino acids in the binding site varies with the size of the hapten. The riboflavin moiety may require both hydrogen bonding as well as hydrophobic interactions as previously documented for the structurally similar fluorescein molecule.[9] Cleavage of the C_H1 domain might destabilize the V region, decreasing interactions between contact residues in the binding site and the ligand.

Influence of various H-chain isotypes in the expression of idiotypic determinants was also indirectly investigated in serological analyses of class switch variants of hybridomas and myeloma cell lines. In one case, class switch variants were idiotypically identical to the parent Ig as judged by inhibition of binding of a polyclonal anti-idiotypic antiserum to the wildtype protein.[108] Another group reported a class switch variant of the MPC 11 myeloma protein that appeared to be idiotypically deficient relative to MPC 11 wildtype protein.[109] A partial amino acid sequence of the variant V_H domain (positions 21–50 and 99–129) indicated no changes in these regions compared to the parent V_H domain. However, somatic mutations in the V_H region could not be excluded.[110] In other reports, it was concluded that class switch variants isolated were idiotypically identical to the parent molecule.[111–113]

Longitudinal interactions involving C domains can be placed in the broader context of the Ig gene superfamily in view of the evolutionary conservation of the basic Ig domain structure. Additional evidence for the existence of conformational influences between adjacent domains emerges from the study of cytotoxic T lymphocyte recognition of allospecific determinants of the class-I major histocompatibility complex (MHC). x-Ray crystallographic analysis of a human MHC class-I molecule has revealed that the membrane-proximal region of the molecule contains two domains (α_3 and β_{2m}) with immunoglobulin folds, while the polymorphic membrane-distal region (α_1 and α_2 domains) forms a platform of eight antiparallel β strands topped by α helices.[114] Recently it has been suggested that the α_3 domain may conformationally influence expression of CTL antigenic determinants associated with the α_1 and α_2 domains.[115] Quarternary interactions between variable and constant regions of both the $\alpha\beta$ and $\gamma\delta$ T-cell receptors have been postulated based on conservation of the residues involved in the "ball and socket joint" of the V_H–C_H1 domains of the immunoglobulins, in the V_β, J_β, C_β and Y_γ, J_γ, C_γ gene segments.[44] It should be noted that C domains are not present in certain members of the immunoglobulin gene superfamily (eg, THY-1, CD8, CTLA4, etc).

Functional and Structural Implications of Variable Region Immunoglobulin Dynamic States

Since structure–function is usually viewed as a static phenomenon it is important to consider the implications of a more realistic dynamic perspective.

Structural dynamics within the antibody macromolecule can be inferred from studies that cite conformers in a variety of nonimmunoglobulin proteins as well as from direct experimentation with antibodies.[116,117] Before exploring the proposed importance of immunoglobulin (Ig) conformational dynamics, it is imperative to define structurally the dynamics in question, since in the relatively large antibody macromolecule, the capacity for multiple states is significantly high.[118] Three primary areas have been emphasized structurally within the intact Ig molecule for conformational changes. First, as previously stated immunochemists have debated conformational changes in the Fc region induced by antigen binding through covalently attached Fab fragments to explain effector functions.[28,119] Attempts to demonstrate such long-distance transmolecular conformational changes in the Ig molecule have met with only marginal success.[120–122] Second, conformational changes demonstrating fragment independence and segmental flexibility inherent in the Ig molecule have been experimentally established.[28,123–129] Finally, conformational transitions (isomerizations) within the variable Ig domains have been explored.[129]

Lancet and Pecht[130] initially suggested conformational transitions based upon a minimum mechanism in terms of conformational states, involving the antibody active site; each state purportedly binding ligands with different affinities. Based on kinetic evidence, they proposed that ligand binding shifted the isomeric equilibrium toward the energetically more favorable binding state. Thus, the concept of induced conformational transitions by ligand binding to the antigen binding site was established and has been reinforced in other studies.[14,130]

General Nature of Active Site Conformational States

The minimal mechanism scheme for hapten-specific homogeneous murine antibodies was based on the best fit of kinetic data to the g matrix (Figure 3-7A).[130,131] Although it is conceivable that a minimum number of conformational states that bind hapten may describe immunoglobulin MOPC 460, it should not be generalized that the minimum mechanism is characteristic of all antibodies. In fact the sum and nature of conformational states may vary with the geometry of the site (eg, cleft vs pocket). Kaivarainen et al[132] proposed several but limited numbers of fluctuating cavities.

In estimating the number and nature of conformational states associated with antibody active sites it is important first to consider local fluctuations in structure. Beginning with the dipeptide as a basic molecular entity capable of fluctuations in structure (bond vibrations and rotations, etc) and progressing with increased structural complexity to a macromolecular protein (such as antibody) two trends are evident. First, with increased complexity there is a concomitant increase in local fluctuations within the polypeptide chain(s).[133] Second, increased complexity leads to an augmentation of restrictions on the dynamics of the system. The biochemical nature of the immunoglobulin fold (Figure 3-3) would seem structurally consistent with such invoked restrictions. Thus, the genesis of energetically metastable conformational states within the Fab fragments can be traced to the nature and magnitude of time and local motions and fluctuations.

Based on these concepts conformational states can be viewed as relatively defined states stabilized by specific energy barriers. It has been proposed that energy barriers are not prohibitively large allowing the unliganded antibody active site to continuously exist in different conformational states. Antibody reactivity seemingly depends on such entropy so that the macromolecule can adapt to many situations and microenvironments. It would not seem advantageous for the antibody to exist in one frozen conformer as one can visualize at 0 K where there is no flexibility of the chains and entropy of the system equals zero (law of minimum energy).

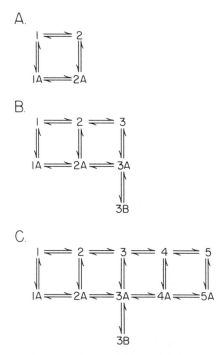

Figure 3-7. Various models illustrating variable-region immunoglobulin conformational states. (A) Two-state system.[130] (B) Hypothetical three-state model system, including isomerization to a unique liganded state (3B). (C) Five-state model system with state 3 being the preferred conformation for homologous ligand binding. In all models (A, B and C) states 1, 2, 3, etc, represent the nonliganded conformational state; 1A, 2A, 3A, etc, indicate liganded states that kinetically involve $k_1 + k_2$. State 3B is the proposed unique and crystallizable liganded conformers. (Reproduced from Ref 32 by permission.)

Activation enthalpies for the conformational transitions are in the range of 10 kcal mol^{-1}, yielding $T\Delta S$ of about 5 kcal mol^{-1} ($\Delta S = -17$ eu).[130]

Experimental Basis for Conformational States in Solution

The existence of variable-region conformational states can be established based on studies by Lancet and Pecht[130] and Herron.[134] Both studies relied on spectral rate measurements during the antigen–antibody interaction. Lancet and Pecht analyzed a low-affinity (3×10^5 M^{-1}) myeloma antibody while Herron studied a high-affinity (3×10^{10} M^{-1}) Mab. A two-step mechanism describing antigen–antibody interactions is essentially applicable to association processes in solution:

$$
A + B \underset{k_{-1}}{\overset{k_1}{\rightleftharpoons}} \overline{AB} \underset{k_{-2}}{\overset{k_2}{\rightleftharpoons}} C \tag{1}
$$

where A represents the Fab antibody binding site; B is ligand; $\overline{A}\overline{B}$ is an encounter complex, in which A and B form part of the solvation sphere of each other with no elementary interactions yet formed; and C is the final noncovalent complex. Using murine monoclonal as well as rabbit polyclonal anti-fluorescein antibodies, two-step association kinetics have been shown based on fluorescence quenching.[134] For high-affinity ($K_A = 10^{10}$ M^{-1}) hybridoma 4-4-20 (Plate 3-1), a technical lifetime of 71.5 s was measured for a linear slow component at 2°C, accounting for about 16% of the total observed fluorescence quenching.[134] This was preceeded by a resolvable linear fast component with a technical lifetime of 14.2 s, which accounted for 73% of the total fluorescence quenching. When the technical lifetimes were corrected for active site concentration and amount of bound fluorescein, a second-order association constant ($k_1 + k_2$ of Eq. 1) of 5.6 × 10^6 M^{-1}s^{-1} was derived. This value is consistent with previous conclusions of near-diffusion-controlled association rates. Since fluorescein can be viewed as rigid ellipsoidal ligand, proper rotational orientation may be required for binding, resulting in a binding rate slower than the diffusion-controlled rate.[135]

Based on temperature-jump experiments, the kinetics of binding of Dnp-lys with the low-affinity murine myeloma MOPC 460 has been measured.[130] Results showed two resolvable relaxation times, indicating a fast bimolecular hapten–protein association followed by a relatively slow monomolecular protein isomerization. The latter was indicative of conformational transitions. The fast association was kinetically and thermodynamically uncoupled from the slow isomerization and described kinetic reactions $k_1 + k_2$ (Eq. 1). Based on the fitting of relaxation time and amplitude data a minimum model was derived consistent with the schematic equilibria in Figure 3-7A. The scheme was consistent with an antigen-binding driven shift (and selection) in equilibrium for states 1A or 2A (Figure 3-7A). It was proposed that ligand bound (but not equivalently) to either states 1 or 2 caused a conformational shift consistent with the 1A ↔ 2A isomerization. The slow component observed in the temperature-jump experiments was considered evidence for such isomerization.

Based on careful documentation the physical interaction of antigen (ligand) with the specific antibody active site was viewed as a random pairing process of two complementary structures.[136] The antigen–antibody integration was characterized as the net result of a continuous and combined action of bonds forming and breaking due to various forces.

Interpretation of Kinetic Analysis of Various Conformer Models

Since the number or range of conformational states (viewed as discrete states or a continuum) has not yet been measured, one can hypothetically expand the number of states (eg, 2, 3, or 5 in Figure 3-10) to devise models to assess the effect of conformers on antibody function.

Kinetically, it is evident that conformational changes (continuum between hypothetical states 1, 2, and 3 in Figure 3-7B) take place in the 10^{-2} to 10^{-7} s range.[117] It is likely that ligand is bound preferentially to one of the conformers with high affinity (eg, state 3) or to all three conformers in decreasing affinity 3 > 2 > 1. The rate of isomerization between nonliganded conformers had not been measured.[129,134] Upon ligand interaction, kinetic studies suggest that two events occur. The first event is relatively fast (k_1 and k_2 in Eq. 1) and results in the formation of 1A, 2A, etc (Figure 3-7). Although the interaction of homologous ligand with each conformer may differ in affinity, the association rate (K_{on}) can be assumed to be relatively constant (ie, nearly diffusion controlled, $1-5 \times 10^6$ $M^{-1}s^{-1}$). The subsequent slow step previously recorded[129,134] would imply either isomerization between (1) 1A and 2A (Figure 3-7A); (2) 1A, 2A, and 3A (Figure 3-7B); (3) all five isomers in Figure 3-7C; or (4) the formation of 3B. To assess these options, it is important to consider isomerization kinetics. As mentioned previously, the rate of isomerization of the nonliganded conformers is 10^{-2} to 10^{-7} s, whereas the liganded conformers show a rate of isomerization of 10^{-2} to 10^{-4} s. Both rates may differ with the affinity of the interaction. It is interesting to hypothesize that the rate of isomerization is relatively faster in low-affinity sites, making it more difficult to stabilize with ligand. High-affinity sites might display a slower isomerization rate and would be stabilized more easily.

Analysis of the slow step showed linear kinetics in terms of fluorescence quenching, suggesting homogeneous kinetics indicative of a single event.[134] However, the single event must be interpreted on the basis of the number of conformers interacting with the ligand. If a minimum number of conformers is invoked, then the single step is likely to be the 1A ↔ 2A isomerization equilibrium. However, if the issue of multiple-ligand reacting conformers is addressed then the interpretation of the slow single step is more consistent with formation of a unique conformer 3B (Figure 3-7B and C). If 1A, 2A, and 3A exist in an isomerization equilibrium but with different rates between each step because of different affinities, the linear kinetics are not likely to be observed for the slow step. Thus, it would appear that the formation of a unique stable liganded complex 3B was observed.[134] The significance of the final state 3B in a multiple-conformer model is that it may act as an "equilibrium sink" which could remove or reduce the concentration of the intermediate complex 3A from the multiple-equilibria scheme in Figure 3-7 (B and C). The "equilibrium sink" is important in hypothetical considerations of an expanded model including five conformers (Figure 3-7C). As conformer 3A is converted to 3B in the five-conformer model the equilibrium shifts from 1A and 2A as well as from 4A and 5A in response to depletion of 3A. In a high-affinity interaction, 3B may be viewed as exhibiting a very slow dissociation rate consistent with values reported.[137] The relatively slow kinetics would indicate that the final conformational change is a major transition and not easily achieved, reflecting significant intrasite amino acid side chain modulations.[138]

If the rate of transition between 1A, 2A, and 3A is slow, similar to the 3A to 3B interconversion, the dissociation rates of the low-affinity interactions 1A and 2A would result in a partial regeneration of nonliganded conformers 1 and 2. The complexity of the various equilibria based on these transitions would result in nonlinear kinetics for the slow step. The observation of linear kinetics suggests quite the opposite. Thus, it is likely that the ligand bound to a preferred state (eg, state 3) triggers two events. State 3 can be viewed as the most favorable "energetically poised" conformer for ligand interaction. First the ligand would serve to capture the liganded state and, consequently, states 1 and 2 (Figure 3-7) would quickly convert to state 3 and bind ligand. The second step in the binding kinetics observed by both Herron[134] and Lancet and Pecht[130] would be consistent with a conformational transition into a unique liganded state (eg, state 3B in Figure 3-7 B and C). It is contended that it is liganded state 3B (Figure 3-7) that crystallizes readily as a homogeneous Fab population, with nearly all fragments fixed in the same conformational state.

Frequency of Active Site Conformational States Based on Equilibria Schemes

Initial considerations, as discussed in previous sections of this chapter, of the various conformational states were based on the assumption of equal frequency. Figure 3-7 suggests optimum binding to a hypothetical terminal conformer in a series of three different states. If the same linear series is expanded to multiple distinct states with the optimum binding state representative of an intermediate or average state, further implications are apparent. The multiple-state model suggests two extreme ways to analyze the distribution of the five conformers in the linear model. If one assumes equal rates of transition between each state, and adjacent states represent closely related conformers, then one might assume a normal distribution and unequal frequency. These assumptions would further indicate that extreme conformers are significantly different. A circular conformational equilibrium model would infer equal frequency of all states but the model is presumed flawed since extremely different conformers are not likely to be in isomeric equilibrium because of relatively extreme conformational (structural) and energetic differences.

If the linear model is correct (Figure 3-7) and a particular conformer preferentially binds the homologous ligand (ie, with highest relative affinity compared with the different conformers available), then that conformer may also be represented most frequently in the normal distribution scheme. Employing these assumptions, one can make the case for the unique liganded conformational state (3B in Figure 3-7B and C).

Role of Conformational States in Fab Crystal Formation

Recently, the crystallization process of Fab fragments derived from Mabs has been indicated to be facilitated by the presence of bound ligand.[66] Using fragments enzymatically derived from affinity-purified anti-fluorescein antibodies, it has become possible to crystallize univalent fragments in the liganded state (Plate 3-1). However, parallel studies conducted with nonliganded fragments showed insufficient crystal development. The presence of bound ligand appears to influence the rate, magnitude, and quality of crystal growth.[66] The latter refers specifically to development of crystals suitable for x-ray diffraction studies.

Such crystallographic information is consistent with the aforementioned concept that the purified nonliganded Fab molecule may exist in several conformational states. Stabilization of different conformations by different haptens has been suggested.[139] Pursuing this concept in terms of the three major nonliganded hypothetical conformational states (energetically metastable) illustrated in Figure 3-7B, the three proposed conformers may differ sufficiently in geometric properties that crystal lattice formation is inhibited. Thus, in effect, different conformers existing in such a mixture behave as noncrystallizable pseudocontaminants. Since bound ligand was the experimental variable in recent Fab crystallization studies,[66] it was suggested that the conformational states reside in the $V_L + V_H$ domains comprising the antigen binding site. It is difficult at this time to rule out ligand binding to only one conformer or all nonliganded states shown in Figure 3-7, but the number of ligand reactive conformers does significantly impact the model presented.

An interesting alternative that may explain in part the enhanced ability to crystallize liganded Fab fragments has been offered.[136] It has been suggested that the release of water molecules from polar sites upon ligand binding may decrease the dielectric constant, a concept consistent with promoting protein crystallization.

Biological and Chemical Implications of Variable Region Conformational States

The dynamics of multiconformational states in the variable region of the antibody molecule impacts many important areas related to the structure–function of the antibody macromolecule. This section summarizes certain areas in which consideration of multiconformational states may be pertinent.

First, as mentioned above, it is becoming evident that conformational states may be important in the crystallization of homogeneous antibody molecules. Perhaps successful crystallization of homogeneous antibodies means crystal lattice formation of only one conformer, bound ligand serving to produce such an enrichment. This would be analogous to stabilization of crystallizable myoglobin with the heme group. Knowledge of the various conformers may prove important in interpreting the secondary, tertiary, and quaterary structure of antibodies through x-ray diffraction analysis and may aid in a better understanding of the dynamics of antibodies in solution.[15] It is interesting to contemplate that crystallization of liganded low-affinity antibodies may prove more difficult than that of liganded high-affinity Fab fragments.

Second, it is conceivable that in the generation of anti-idiotype reagents, specificity may be directed toward a particular conformer (eg, most frequent state). Conformers may differ in their immunogenicity and expression of private and public idiotopes. Anti-idiotype interactions with idiotopes may serve to capture or "freeze" a particular conformer. If particular antibodies exhibit an extremely wide range of conformational states, it may explain why it is difficult in some cases to elicit polyclonal anti-idiotype or monoclonal anti-idiotope reagents.

It is important to note that the often observed ligand inhibition of idiotype–anti-idiotype interactions is perhaps further evidence for ligand-induced conformational changes.[140] Kabat[64] noted in idiotype studies with anti-oligosaccharide antibodies that idiotypic determinants in a cavity-type site are probably located on the outside

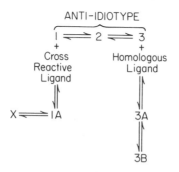

Figure 3-8. Model to explain cross-reaction of structurally related ligands with different conformers. The model conceptualizes that anti-Id reagents may be specific for various conformers. (Reproduced from Ref 32 by permission.)

of the antibody combining cavity. It was further suggested that filling the site with an oligosaccharide ligand caused conformational changes by which the idiotope configuration was altered. The latter is similar to the metatype experiments previously described.[101]

Third, Figure 3-8 addresses the possibility of cross-reactive ligand (structural analogs) binding to a different conformer than does the homologous ligand.[139] Since nearly all small ligand reactions display similar association rates (approaching diffusion controlled) this argues in favor of the model presented in Figure 3-8.[119,139] Different rates of association would argue for all ligands interacting with the same conformer, with the cross-reacting ligand (eg, rhodamine B) exhibiting a slower $k_1 + k_2$ than is the case with the homologous ligand fluorescein. However, the frequency of the cross-reactive conformer (State 1 in Figure 3-8) would of course influence the degree of binding observed. The model presented in Figure 3-8 differs from Figure 3-7 in that it suggests preferential ligand binding to only one "energetically poised" conformer. This is not to be considered in the absolute sense but as a matter of degree as previously suggested.

The concept of different conformational states and the ability of these conformers to react with homologous ligand in different ways (eg, affinity) or of specific conformers to react with structurally related (cross-reactive) ligands in essence increases the biological diversity of the immune response (Figure 3-8). It also provides insight into the different shapes assumed by the same site occupied with structurally different ligands.[49] Employing the multiple-conformer hypothesis, one must then view cross-reactivity and/or competitive inhibition measurements as involving two steps. First, dissociation of the homologous ligand from the liganded conformer (eg, state 3B) creating isomerization between the nonliganded states. Second, the isomerization equilibrium results in sufficient quantities of the proper conformer for heterologous ligand binding. In extreme (cross-reactive) excess, the conformer is selected through ligand binding. The balance between the two liganded conformers is recorded as percentage inhibition.

Fourth, if one considers ligand binding conformers as native conformational states, one must consider the relationship between the various conformers and denatured states (unreactive). Since antibody active sites are comprised of two polypeptide chains the denaturation → renaturation process may involve conformational drift.[141] However, it is not clear how conformational drift affects isomerization between the native conformation states.

Fifth, certain ligand-sensitive cryoglobulin properties may be explicable on the basis of the ligand "locking" the molecule into a conformational state that is not cryoprecipitable[142,143] or, conversely, a hapten-induced conformational change accompanying cryoprecipitation of an immunoglobulin.[144] Cryoprecipitation may reflect solubility of a particular conformer based on the presence or absence of ligand in the active site. Thus, cryoprecipitation is an expression of the enrichment of a given conformer much as in the crystallization phenomenon.

Single-Chain Antibody as a Structure–Function Model

This chapter has described certain aspects of the structure–function relationships within the antibody molecule. Segmental flexibility has been an important concept in delineating the roles of the Fab and Fc fragments. Importantly, Fab fragments possess the intrinsic binding properties of the intact Ab molecule. Thus, the four-domain structure that comprises the Fab fragment stabilizes the variable domains. This is expressed in the fact that the affinity for antigen in the Fab fragment simulates the parent molecule. As previously described, the Fab fragment is relatively resistant to further proteolytic digestion. However, it was shown that each domain within the four-domain structure exerts interdomain effects. The latter is best described in terms of idiotypic determinants and ligand binding. Recently, a new concept in synthetic antibody construction has emerged that should prove invaluable in assessing structure–function relationships involving H- and L-chain variable domains relative to the well-characterized Fab fragment. The concept termed "single-chain" antibody involves genetic engineering of Ab variable regions of known primary structure and specificity.[145,146] Through genetic engineering the Ig protein has been synthesized as a single-chain peptide involving only the antigen-binding variable regions of the prototype antibody. Thus, the variable regions of the single chain were synthesized with serine–glycine-rich synthetic linkers (14–15 amino acids) between the two regions. The linkers were designed to allow the synthetic peptide to fold after synthesis with the binding sites in proper orientation. The engineered single-chain antibody was expressed in bacteria (*Escherichia coli*) and then purified in the folded state. Although antigen-binding properties of the folded single-chain molecules did not perfectly simulate the activity of the parent molecule, significant binding was obtained.[145,146] The single-chain concept thus provides a reagent to study variable-domain interactions independent of constant domains as in the Fab fragment. From a structure–function viewpoint, certain questions raised in this chapter should be answered through proper exploitation of the single-chain antibody. It is also evident that the single-chain gene construct becomes an interesting genetic tool to be used in site-specific mutagenesis. Finally, one of the antibody molecules used in the single-chain studies was Mab 4-4-20, for which the crystal structure has been obtained as shown in Plates 3-1, 3-2, and 3-3 of this chapter. The single-chain antibody represents an exciting new development and expresses the promise of biotechnology in the future delineation of immunoglobulin structure and function.

Summary

The intent of this chapter was to provide both historical perspective and insight into the current status of structure–function relationships regarding the antibody macromolecule.

Despite a slow rate of progression, development of the rules and principles that dictate structure–function relationships operational in the antibody protein is a complex process, but one whose time has arrived. Elucidation of the principles

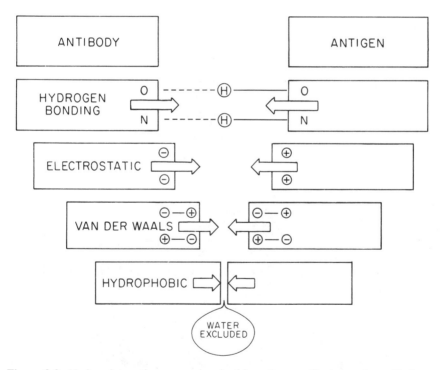

Figure 3-9. Various interacting groups involved in antigen–antibody reactions. Hydrogen bonds are based on formation of hydrogen bridges between atoms. Electrostatic forces result from attraction of oppositely charged groups. Van der Waals forces depend on the interaction between electron clouds (pictured as oscillating dipoles). Hydrophobic bonds are based on the association of nonpolar or hydrophobic groups. Distances between interacting groups vary with the type of bond and are illustrated on a relative basis. (Reproduced from Ref 148 by permission.)

involved is imperative since the unique properties of antibodies provides a potential unequaled in other protein systems. The inherent capacity to elicit specific antibody proteins to a wide variety of chemical structures and the concomitant provision of molecules of varying affinities to each structure represents a foundation for infinite inquiry.

As emphasized in the chapter, appropriate systems are being developed that will allow full exploration consistent with the unlimited potential of the immune system. Figure 3-9 summarizes the various intermolecule forces that nature employs to convey biological specificity. As documented in this chapter all these forces are operational in antigen–antibody binding. The immediate future will answer many questions regarding the integration of these forces in the expression of specificity. Undoubtedly, investigators will conclude that the same antibody specificity and affinity can be synthesized in many different ways. Such flexibility in the rules and principles of structure–function will permit integration of other important biological and biochemical properties into the structure of the antibody macromolecule.

References

1. Porter RR. *Biochem J*. 1959;73:119.

2. Amzel LM, Poljak, RJ, Saul F, Varga JM, Richards FF. *Proc Natl Acad Sci (USA)*. 1974;71:1427.

3. Amzel LM, Poljak RJ. *Annu Rev Biochem*. 1979;48:961.

4. Rajewski K, Takemori, T. *Annu Rev Immunol*. 1983;1:569.

5. Ruf J, Jonelle C, Rocca-Serra J, Monier D, Pierres M, Ju SLT, Dorf ME, Fougereau M. *Proc Natl Acad Sci (USA)*. 1983;80:3040.

6. Kraig E, Kronenberg M, Kapp JA, Pierce CW, Abruzzini AF, Sorenson CM, Samuelson LE, Schwartz RH, Hood LE. *J Exp Med*. 1983;158:192.

7. Tonegawa S. *Nature (London)*. 1983;302:573.

8. Eisen HN, Siskind GW. *Biochemistry*. 1964;3:996.

9. Voss EW, Jr. In *Fluorescein Hapten: An Immunological Probe*. Voss EW, ed. Boca Raton, FL: CRC Press Inc; 1984:3–14.

10. Jarvis MR, Voss EW. In *Fluorescein Hapten: An Immunological Probe*. Voss EW, ed. Boca Raton, FL: CRC Press Inc; 1984:131–154.

11. Kaartinen M, Griffiths GM, Hamlyn PH, Markham AF, Karjalainen J, Pelkonen LT, Makela O, Milstein C. *J Immunol*. 1983;30:937.

12. Kaartinen M, Griffiths GM, Markham AF, Milstein C. *Nature (London)*. 1983;304:320.

13. Griffiths GM, Berek C, Kaartinen M, Milstein C. *Nature (London)*. 1984;312:271.

14. Herron JN, Kranz DM, Jameson DM, Voss EW. *Biochemistry*. 1986;25:4602.

15. Amit AG, Mariuzza RA, Phillips SEV, Poljak RJ. *Science*. 1986;233:747.

16. Weigert M, Riblet R. *Immunopathology*. 1978;1:133.

17. Porter RR. *Science*. 1973;180:713.

18. Fleischman JB, Pain RH, Porter RR. *Arch Biochem Biophys* 1962;1:174.

19. Edelman GM. *J Am Chem Soc*. 1959;81:3155.

20. Fleischman JB, Porter RR, Press EM. *Biochem J*. 1963;88:220.

21. Nisonoff A, Wissler FC, Lipman LN, Woernley DL. *Arch Biochem Biophys*. 1960;89:230.

22. Cathou RE, Dorrington KJ. In Fasman GD, Timansheff SN, eds. *Biological Macromolecules, Subunits in Biological Systems, Part C,* Vol. I. New York: Marcel Dekker Inc; 1975:91.

23. Nisonoff A, Hopper JE, Spring SB. In *The Antibody Molecule.* New York: Academic Press Inc; 1975:264–345.

24. Kohler G, Milstein C. *Nature (London).* 1975;256:495.

25. Potter M. *Adv Immunol.* 1977;25:141.

26. Edelman GM, Gall WE. *Annu Rev Biochem.* 1969;38:415.

27. Klein M, Haeffner-Cavaillon N, Isenman DE, Rivat C, Navia M, Davies DR, Dorrington KJ. *Proc Natl Acad Sci (USA).* 1981;78:524.

28. Oi VT, Vuong R, Hardy J, Reidler J, Dangl J, Herzenberg LA, Stryer L. *Nature (London).* 1984;307:136.

29. Williams AF, Barclay AN. *Annu Rev Immunol.* 1988;6:381.

30. Pollack SJ, Nakayama GR, Schultz PG. *Science.* 1988;242:1038.

31. Wu TT, Kabat EA. *J Exp Med.* 1970; 132:211.

32. Voss EW, Dombrink-Kurtzman MA, Miklasz SD. *Immunol Invest.* 1988;17:25.

33. Davies DR, Metzger H. *Annu Rev Immunol.* 1983;1:87.

34. Jones PT, Dear PH, Foote J, Neuberger MS, Winter G. *Nature (London).* 1986;321:522.

35. Riechman L, Clark M, Waldmann H, Winter G. *Nature (London).* 1988;332:323.

36. Verhoyen M, Milstein C, Winter G. *Science.* 1988;239:1534.

37. Novotny J, Bruccoleri R, Newell J, Murphy D, Haber E, Karplus M. *J Biol Chem.* 1983;258:14433.

38. Matsushima M, Marquart M, Jones TA, Colman PM, Bartels K, Huber R. *J Mol Biol.* 1978;121:441.

39. Abola EE, Ely KR, Edmundson AB. *Biochemistry.* 1980;19:432.

40. Marquart M, Deisenhofer J, Huber R. *J Mol Biol* 1980;141:369.

41. Bennett WS, Huber R. *CRC Crit Rev Biochem.* 1984;15:291.

42. Navia MA, Segal DM, Padlan EA, Davies DR, Nao R, Rudikoff S, Potter M. *Proc Natl Acad Sci (USA).* 1979;76:4071.

43. Saul FA, Amzel AM, Poljak M. *J Biol Chem.* 1978;253:585.

44. Segal DM, Padlan EA, Gerson GH, Rudikoff S, Potter M, Davies DM. *Proc Natl Acad Sci (USA).* 1974;71:4298.

45. Colman PM, Laver WG, Varghese JN, Baker AT, Tulloch PA, Air GM, Webster RG. *Nature (London).* 1987;326:358.

46. Lesk AM, Chothia C. *Nature (London).* 1988;335:188.

47. Alzari PM, Lascombe M-B, Poljak RJ. *Annu Rev Immunol* 1988;6:555.

48. Sheriff S, Silverton EW, Padlan EA, Cohen GH, Smith-Gill SJ, Finzel BC, Davies DR. *Proc Natl Acad Sci (USA).* 1987;84:8075.

49. Edmundson AB, Ely KR, Herron JN. *Mol Immunol.* 1984;21:561.

50. Edmundson AB, Ely KR, Girling RL, Abola EE, Schiffer M, Westholm FA, Fausch MD, Deutsch HF. *Biochemistry.* 1974;13:3816.

51. Kranz DM, Herron JN, Voss EW. *J Biol Chem.* 1982;257:6987.

52. Bates RM, Ballard DW, Voss EW. *Mol Immunol.* 1985;22:871.

53. Voss EW, Eschenfeldt W, Root RT. *Immunochemistry.* 1976;13:447.

54. Kranz DM, Voss EW. *Mol Immunol.* 1981;18:889.

55. Herron JN, Voss EW. *J Biochem Biophys Meth.* 1983;8:189.

56. Pecht I. In Sela M, ed. *The Antigens,* Vol 6. New York: Academic Press Inc; 1982:1–68.

57. Herron JN, Voss EW. *Mol Immunol.* 1983;20:1323.

58. Watt RM, Voss EW. *Immunochemistry.* 1977;14:533.

59. Voss EW, Watt RM, Weber G. *Mol Immunol.* 1979;17:505.

60. Watt RM, Voss EW. *J Biol Chem.* 1979;254:1684.

61. Kranz DM, Herron JN, Giannis DE, Voss EW. *J Biol Chem.* 1981;256:4433.

62. Watt RM, Voss EW. *Immunochemistry.* 1978;15:875.

63. Watt RM, Voss EW. In Voss EW, ed. *Fluorescein Hapten: An Immunological Probe.* Boca Raton, FL: CRC Press Inc; 1984:177–181.

64. Kabat EA. In Green MI, Nisonoff A, eds. *The Biology of Idiotypes.* New York: Plenum Press; 1984:3–17.

65. Rudikoff S. In Green MI, Nisonoff A, eds. *The Biology of Idiotypes.* New York: Plenum Press; 1984:115.

66. Gibson AL, Herron JN, He X-M, Patrick VA, Mason ML, Lin J-N, Kranz DM, Voss EW, Edmundson AB. *Proteins.* 1988;3:155.

67. Stevens FJ, Chang C-H, Schiffer M. *Proc Natl Acad Sci (USA).* 1988;85:6895.

68. Klein M, Kells DIC, Tinker DO, Dorrington KJ. *Biochemistry.* 1977;16:552.

69. Alexandru I, Kells DIC, Dorrington KJ, Klein M. *Mol Immunol.* 1980;17:1351.

70. Edmundson AB, Ely KR, Abola EE. *Contemp Top Mol Immunol.* 1978;7:95.

71. Huber R, Deisenhofer D, Colman PM, Matsushima M, Palm W. *Nature (London).* 1976;264:415.

72. Metzger H. *Contemp Top Mol Immunol.* 1978;7:119.

73. Huber R. *Science.* 1986;233:702.

74. Huber R, Bennett WS. *Nature (London).* 1987;326:334.

75. Oudin J, Michel M. *Compt Rend Acad Sci (Paris).* 1963;257:805.

76. Kunkel HG, Mannick M, Williams RC. *Science.* 1963;140:1218.

77. Nisonoff A, Hopper JE, Spring SB. In *The Antibody Molecule.* New York: Academic Press Inc; 1975;444–496.

78. Bona CA. In *Idiotypes and Lymphocytes.* New York: Academic Press Inc; 1981:5.

79. Jerne NK. *Ann Immunol (Inst Pasteur).* 1974;125c:373.

80. Jerne NK. *Harvey Lect.* 1975;70:93.

81. Kieber-Emmons T, Kohler H. *Immunol Rev.* 1986;90:29.

82. Uytdehaag FGCM, Bunschoten H, Weijer K, Osterhaus ADME. *Immunol Rev.* 1986;90:93.

83. Kennedy RC, Eichberg JW, Lanford RE, Dreesman GR. *Science.* 1986;232:220.

84. Slaoui M, Urbain-Vansanter G, Demeur C, Leo O, Marvel J, Moser M, Tassignor J, Greene MI, Urbain J. *Immunol Rev.* 1986;90:73.

85. Manjula BN, Mushinki EB, Glaudemans CPJ. *J Immunol.* 1977;119;867.

86. Nusair T, Baumal R, Rosenstein R, Jorgenson T, Marks A. *Mol Immunol.* 1983;20:537.

87. Lieberman R, Vrana M, Humphrey W, Chien CC, Potter M. *J Exp Med.* 1977;146:1294.

88. Milner ECB, Capra D. *Mol Immunol.* 1983;20:39.

89. Schiff C, Boyer M, Milili M, Fougereau M. *Ann Immunol (Paris).* 1981;132c:113.

90. Desaymard CAM, Giusti AM, Scharff MD. *Mol Immunol.* 1984;21:961.

91. Davie JM, Seiden MV, Greenspan NS, Lutz CT, Bartholow TL, Clevinger BJ. *Annu Rev Immunol.* 1986;4:147.

92. Clevinger BJ, Schilling J, Hood L, Davie JM. *J Exp Med.* 1980;151:1950.

93. Schilling J, Clevinger BJ, Davie JM, Hood L. *Nature (London).* 1980;283:35.

94. McMillan S, Seiden MV, Houghten RA, Clevinger BJ, Davie JM, Lerner RA. *Cell.* 1983;35:859.

95. Bruggemann M, Muller HJ, Burger C, Rajewski K. *EMBO J.* 1986;5:1561.

96. Radbruch A, Zaiss S, Kappen C, Bruggemann M, Beyreuther K, Rajewsky K. *Nature (London).* 1985;315:508.

97. Benjamin DC, Berzofsky JA, East IJ, Gurd FRN, Hannum C, Leach SJ, Margoliash E, Michael JG, Miller A, Prager EM, Reichlin M, Sercarz EE, Smith-Gill SJ, Todd PE, Wilson AC. *Annu Rev Immunol.* 1984;2:67.

98. Novotny J, Handschumacher M, Haber E. *J Mol Biol.* 1986;189:715.

99. Roux, KH, Monafo WJ, Davie JM, Greenspan NS. *Proc Natl Acad Sci (USA).* 1987;84:4984.

100. Boulot G, Rojas C, Bentley GA, Poljak RJ, Barbier E, LeGuern C, Cazenave P-A. *J Mol Biol.* 1987;194:577.

101. Voss EW, Miklasz, SD, Petrossian A, Dombrink-Kurtzman MA. *Mol Immunol.* 1988;25:751.

102. Wells JV, Fudenberg HH, Givol D. *Proc Natl Acad Sci (USA).* 1973;70:1585.

103. Rinfret A, Horne C, Dorrington KJ, Klein M. *J Immunol.* 1985;135:2574.

104. Binion SB, Rodkey LS. *Mol Immunol.* 1983;20:475.

105. Morahan G, Berek C, Miller JFAP. *Nature (London).* 1983; 301:720.

106. Rudikoff S, Pawlita M, Pumphrey J, Mushinski E, Potter M. *J Exp Med.* 1983;158:1385.

107. Sen J, Beychok S. *Proteins.* 1986;1:256.

108. Radbruch A, Liesegang B, Rajewsky K. *Proc Natl Acad Sci (USA).* 1980;77:1980.

109. Inbar D, Hochman J, Givol D. *Proc Natl Acad Sci (USA).* 1972;69:2659.

110. Beyreuther K, Bovens J, Brüggenmann M, Dildrop R, Kelsoe G, Krawinkel U, Müller C, Nishikawa S, Radbruch A, Reth M, Siekevitz M, Takemori T, Tesch H, Wildner G, Zaiss S, Rajensky K. In Bona CA, Kohler H, eds. *Immune Networks.* Ann. N.Y. Acad. Sci. 1983;418:121.

111. Baumhackel H, Liesegang B, Radbruch A, Rajewsky K, Sablitsky F. *J Immunol.* 1982;128:1217.

112. Neuberger M, Rajewsky K. *Proc Natl Acad Sci (USA).* 1981;78:1138.

113. Thammana P, Scharff MD. *Eur J Immunol.* 1983;13:614.

114. Bjorkman PJ, Saper MA, Samraoui B, Bennett WS, Strominger J, Wiley DC. *Nature (London).* 1987;329:506.

115. Maziarz CT, Burakoff SJ, Bluestone J. *J Immunol.* 1988;140:4372.

116. Nemethy G. In *Subunits in Biological Systems,* Vol. 7. Timasheff SN, Fasman GD, eds. New York: Marcel Dekker Inc; 1975:1–90.

117. Careri G, Fasella D, Gratton E. *Annu Rev Biophys Bioeng.* 1979;8:69–97.

118. Edmundson AB, Ely KR, Abola EE. In Reisfield RA, Inman FP, eds. *Contemp Top Mol Immunol,* Vol. 7. 1988:95–118.

119. Winkelhake J. *Immunochemistry.* 1978;15:695.

120. Warner C, Schumaker V. *Biochemistry.* 1970;9:451.

121. Pilz I, Kratky O, Karush F. *Eur J Biochem.* 1974;41:91.

122. Metger H. In Reisfield R, Inman FP, eds. *Contemp Top Mol Immunol,* Vol. 7. 1978:119–152.

123. Noelken ME, Nelson CA, Bulkley CE, Tanford C. *J Biol Chem.* 1965;240:218.

124. Valentine RC, Green NW. *J Mol Biol.* 1967;27:615.

125. Zagyansky YA, Nezlin RS, Tumerman LA. *Immunochemistry.* 1969;6:787.

126. Kaivarainen AI, Nezlin RS. *Biochem Biophys Res Comm*. 1976;68:270.

127. Seegan GW, Smith CA, Schumaker VN. *Proc Natl Acad Sci (USA)*. 1979;76:907.

128. Luedtke R, Owen CS, Karush F. *Biochemistry*. 1980;19:1182.

129. Pecht I. In Sela M, ed. *The Antigens*, Vol. 6. New York: Academic Press Inc; 1982:1–68.

130. Lancet D, Pecht I. *Proc Natl Acad Sci (USA)*. 1976;73:3549.

131. Zidovatski R, Blatt Y, Glaudemans CPJ, Mantula BN, Pecht I. *Biochemistry*. 1980;19:2790.

132. Kaivarainen A, Kaivarainen E, Franek F, Olsovska Z. *Immunol Lett*. 1981;3:323.

133. Ikegami A. *Biophys Comm*. 1977;6:117.

134. Herron JN. In Voss EW, ed. *The Fluorescein Hapten: An Immunological Probe*. Boca Raton, FL: CRC Press Inc; 1984:49–76.

135. Hill TL. *Proc Natl Acad Sci (USA)*. 1975;72:4918.

136. Absolom DR, van Oss CJ. *Crit Rev Immunol*. 1986;6:1.

137. Watt RM, Herron JN, Voss EW. *Mol Immunol*. 1980;17:1237.

138. Romans DG, Dorrington KJ. *Fed Proc Soc Am Exp Biol*. 1985;45:738.

139. Hsia JC, Little JR. *FEBS Lett*. 1973;31:80.

140. Karplus M. In Venkataraghavan B, Feldman RJ, eds. *Macromolecular Structure and Specificity: Computer Assisted Modeling and Applications*. *Ann NY Acad Sci*. 1985;439:107–123.

141. Weber G. *Biochemistry*. 1986;25:3626.

142. Ballard DW, Kranz DM, Voss EW. *Proc Natl Acad Sci (USA)*. 1983;80:5071.

143. Dombrink-Kurtzman MA, Voss EW. *Mol Immunol*. 1988;25:1309.

144. Okada A, Nakanishi M, Tsurui H, Wada A, Terashima M, Osawa T. *Mol Immunol*. 1985;22:715.

145. Bird RE, Hardman KD, Jacobson JW, Johnson S, Kaufman BM, Lee S-M, Lee T, Pope SH, Riordan GS, Whitlow M. *Science*. 1988;242:423.

146. Huston JS, Levinson D, Mudgett-Hunter M, Tai M-S, Novotny J, Margolies MN, Ridge RJ, Bruccoleri RE, Haber E, Crea R, Oppermann H. *Proc Natl Acad Sci (USA)*. 1988;85:5879.

147. Cantor CR, Schimmel PR. In *Biophysical Chemistry*, Part 1: *The Conformation of Biological Macromolecules*. New York: W. H. Freeman & Co Inc; 1980:69.

148. Roitt I, Brostoff J, Male D. In *Immunology*. St. Louis, MO: The C. V. Mosby Co; 1985:5.4.

149. Nisonoff, A. *Introduction to Molecular Immunology*, 2nd ed, Sunderland, MA: Sinauer Assoc. Inc; 1984:85.

CHAPTER 4

Immunoglobulin Genes

Edward W. Voss, Jr.

Department of Microbiology, University of Illinois, 131 Burrill Hall, 407 S. Goodwin Avenue, Urbana, IL 61801 USA

Immunoglobulin Genes and Antibody Structure

Primary structural determinations of antibody molecules was virtually impossible until homogeneous immunoglobulins (initially myeloma proteins) became routinely available in purified form to replace polyclonal populations. The original determinations of immunoglobulin primary structures primarily characterized human and murine myelomas of various classes and subclasses. As the number of determined sequences increased, when primary structures within the same polypeptide chain were compared distinct variable and constant regions became apparent. However, the problem remained of accounting for antibody diversity requiring a theoretical 10^7 to 10^8 different specificities for immunological competency. Immunological information conflicted with important factual and theoretical considerations, creating a paradox regarding the nature of the genome involved in antibody synthesis and diversity. Extensive allotype studies showed that allotypic serological determinants were present on immunoglobulin chains of a given class but were independent of antibody specificity. Allotypes appeared to segregate as single Mendelian traits, suggesting the existence of a single gene for each chain and class of antibody molecule. Molecular biological concepts at the time aspired to the abstraction that "one gene encoded one polypeptide" and created a dilemma in immunogenetics.

In 1965 Dreyer and Bennett proposed a model designed to solve the paradox.[1] The model proposed that genes encoding the variable portion (ie, specificity) of immunoglobulin molecules were present in the germline repertoire and combined with the gene encoding the constant portion during B-cell (lymphocyte) differentiation. Experimental confirmation of the Dreyer and Bennett theory was based on the application of bacteria-derived restriction enzymes to immunoglobulin genome analyses. In an important series of experiments, Hozumi and Tonegawa[2] demonstrated somatic rearrangement of immunoglobulin genes based on different hybridization patterns in restriction digested germline embryonic DNA and MOPC 321 myeloma DNA (plasmacytoma) using radiolabeled purified MOPC 321 κ mRNA as the probe. In embryonic DNA the probe hybridized with different fragments which represented the variable and constant region exons separated by various sized introns. However, in the differentiated plasmacytoma genome the variable and constant regions were located in only a single relatively small hybridizable DNA fragment. This led to the significant conclusion that in the comparison of embryonic DNA with the differentiated cell genome the variable and constant regions had rearranged. These hallmark studies and important conclusions had an immediate and significant impact and an information explosion ensued concerning the generation of antibody diversity and the control of immunoglobulin gene expression.[3]

Variable-Region Genes

It is important to establish in this section that H-chain and both types of L-chain genes all reside on different chromosomes within the various animal species. Germline variable (V) regions of both H and L chains were found as assembled exons 5' to the C region coding sequences. Germline variable regions include two complementarity determining regions (CDRs) bracketed by framework regions.[4] Variable regions are completed by the joining of discrete DNA segments: the variable (V_H), diversity (D), and joining (J_H) for the heavy chain and the variable (V_L) and joining (J_L) for the light chain (illustrated in Figure 4-1). The V_H segment encodes a 5' hydrophobic leader peptide separated by a short intron from the exon encoding the V region, which includes CDR1 and CDR2 (see Figure 4-2). The third CDR is encoded by the combining of D and J_H segments. The L chain lacks a D segment, suggesting that less diversity is generated through exon rearrangement to form the light-chain variable region.

Assembly of randomly selected segments encoding the V region is linked to B-cell differentiation.[5-7] During B-cell maturation in the bone marrow, H-chain genes are assembled first at the pre-B-cell stage. Assembly proceeds in two distinct sequential steps: (1) D to J_H and (2) V_H to DJ_H (Figure 4-3). Rearrangement of V_L and J_L gene segments occurs with further B-cell differentiation. Light-chain rearrangement is apparently dependent on a successful $V_H DJ_H$ assembly and subsequent expression of H chains. Rearrangement of both L-chain loci (κ and λ) proceeds in an ordered sequential fashion in that κ-chain rearrangement preceeds λ-chain recombination. Such events obviously imply sophisticated control mechanisms involving interchromosomal communication. Thus, if a productive V_κ to J_κ recombination occurs in the differentiating B-cell the λ and J_λ remain in the nonrearranged germline configuration. If the V_κ to J_κ rearrangement is unsuccessful the recombination events proceed. In B-cell lines that produce λ chains, the J_κ–C_κ locus is generally found deleted or rearranged.

Despite a potential participation of three different chromosomes and multiple alleles in the expression of H and L chains, the principle of allelic exclusion predominates. The latter ensures that a given B-cell only produces single H and L chains, resulting in a functional antibody molecule with defined specificity. Alt (1984) proposed a feedback mechanism which ensured that when one effective

Ig Gene Organization:

1. Heavy Chain Genes:

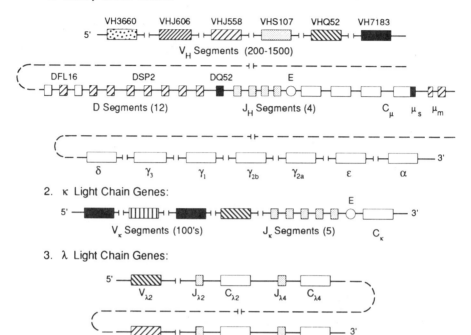

2. κ Light Chain Genes:

3. λ Light Chain Genes:

Figure 4-1. Organization of the murine immunoglobulin genes. Specific V_H gene segment families located on chromosome 12 are indicated by shaded boxes. The D, J, and C segments are located 3′ to variable exons. Kappa gene segments are indicated in a linear array (chromosome 6). The unique grouping of λ genes is indicated as they appear on chromosome 16. Heavy- and κ-chain enhancers are indicated by E. (Reproduced from Ref 4 by permission.)

rearrangement occurred further rearrangements (eg, the other allele) were prohibited.[8] Light-chain allelic exclusion appears regulated by the production of a functional L chain. "Functional" is defined as a light chain that can associate with a previously expressed H chain to form a stable complex and antibody active site.

Rearrangement of Ig V genes (referred to as the IgH locus) is apparently mediated by conserved recognition sequences that flank germline V, D, and J segments. Genomic recombination recognition elements are composed of a common palindromic heptamer or an A–T-rich nonamer separated by a nonconserved spacer of either 12 or 23 bp. The spacers define the plausibility of recombination in that joining of two segments is only allowed if the respective recognition element flanking one are separated by a 12-bp spacer and the other by a 23-bp spacer. Site-specific joining events at the molecular level are theoretically mediated by an enzyme system termed "recombinase."

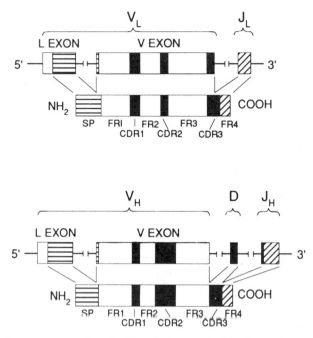

Figure 4-2. Rearrangement of murine V-region segments. The V_L and J_L gene segments are correlated with the light-chain polypeptide structure (top). The V_H, D, and J_H segments are aligned with the heavy-chain polypeptide structure (bottom). (Reproduced from Ref 9 by permission.)

Generation of Diversity

Antibody diversity is generated by a variety of somatic and germline mechanisms that operate either before or after immunogen stimulation. One source of diversity is attributable to the combinational rearrangement of V_H and V_L segments (Figure 4-1). The number of functional V genes per mouse haploid genome is not firmly established and varies with the increasing number of reported immunoglobulin primary structures. Current estimates indicate 2 V_λ genes approximately 300 V_κ and 200 V_H genes.[9] Such estimates vary with the experimental procedure. For example, Southern blot analyses, Ig sequence groupings, and V-gene-family analysis yield lower values than estimates based on nucleic acid hybridization studies. Thus, the question of expressed genes and silent genes remains unsolved. Combinatorial diversity is amplified by the presence of 12 D-gene segments and four J_H-gene segments in the IgH locus. The L-chain genome contains four J_λ and gene segments. A second source of diversity resides in the combinatorial association of expressed H and L chains. The latter represents an area of controversy. Some investigators have found no restriction in H- and L-chain pairings,[10] whereas in other cases restriction has been reported.[11] Heavy- and L-chain recombination experiments usually involve certain procedures that result in at least partial de-

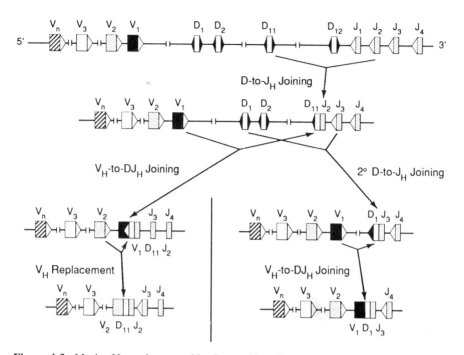

Figure 4-3. Murine V_H-region assembly. Recognition elements separated by a 23-bp spacer are indicated with open triangles. Filled triangles represent recognition elements separated by a 12-bp spacer. (Reproduced from Ref 4 by permission.)

naturation of the polypeptide chains. Such uncontrolled differences may account for the disparate results.

Diversity can be augmented at a third level, namely the joining mechanism of individual V region segments (ie, junctional diversity). Evidence has accumulated which suggests that joining mechanisms for V_L-J_L and V_H-D-J_H are imprecise generating V_H and V_L domains with differing amino acids and length within the junctional regions. A problem associated with junctional diversity is that it appears to be potentially biologically inefficient, since relatively large numbers of nonfunctional V genes could be generated that are "out-of-frame" with respect to the D, J_H, and V_H coding sequences. However such "out-of-frame" diversity may generate antibodies of various specificities and does not imply nonfunctionality. It has been shown that nucleotides are added at the V_H-D and D-J_H junctions. Nucleotides found at these junctions cannot be traced to germline sequences at the 3' end of the V_H segment, the 5' end of J_H or the 5' and 3' ends of the D segment.

Another source of V-region diversity is somatic mutation and is linked to the quality of the immune response.[12-15] Somatic mutation coupled with antigen selection is considered the principal mechanism in the phenomenon of affinity maturation.[16] The latter is defined as the observed increase in affinity with time after the initial immunogenic stimulation. Induction of somatic mutational processes is considered coupled to the IgM to IgG class switch. Thus, antibodies comprising hyperimmune responses are of the IgG class (or subclasses) and exhibit significantly higher affinity than antibodies associated with the early primary response.

Availability and maintenance of hybridoma cell lines of defined specificity in tissue culture for relatively long periods have provided an avenue to study time-dependent somatic mutational events. Obviously, in vitro studies are limited since the antigen selection phase is not operable. The studies are based on the premise that the primary structure of low-affinity IgM monoclonal antibodies leads to an approximation of the germline variable-region gene. The amino acid changes in the V genes of antibodies with time have been found consistent with somatic mutational events. Somatic mutation rates in V genes have been estimated as 10^{-3} to 10^{-4} bp^{-1} per cell per generation, which significantly differs from the background rate of 10^{-8} bp^{-1} per cell per generation associated with C-region genes. These values suggest a V-region-specific somatic hypermutation process.

One final mechanism of antibody diversity may reside at the protein level. It has been proposed that the associated variable domains of the expressed antibody molecule exhibit extensive conformational dynamics.[17,18] Selection of conformers may explain immunologic cross-reactivity, which in essence represents another form of diversity.

Thus, the immunologic repertoire generated by the cumulative effects of the different mechanisms involved in diversity is enormous. For example, with combinatorial joining, based on the assumption that V, D, and J segments assort randomly and independently during V-domain assembly, more than 10^7 combinations are possible ($200 \ V_HH \times 12 \ D \times 4 \ J_H \times 300 \ V_L \times 4 \ J_L$). Superimposed on this base value (10^7) junctional diversity and the other factors may increase estimatable diversity to $>10^9$. The significance of such a value can only be judged on what is necessary to constitute immune competence.

Constant-Region Genes and Class Switching

At the polypeptide level each final product consists of the V and C domains in one contiguous chain. Thus, after gene rearrangement the final processed mRNA for each chain consists of one exon containing all essential components.

The H-chain locus is of special importance since the same V region can be linked to various C_H genes during the stages of B-cell differentiation. In both murine and human gene systems H-chain isotype are encoded in linear clusters located 5' to the J_H segments. As shown in Figure 4-1 the $C\mu$ region is the most proximal C region relative to the V genes. The other C regions are located in a linear array 3' to the $C\mu$ region. The $C\mu$ and $C\delta$ regions are initially transcribed into a large mRNA transcript (containing the rearranged V region) which is subsequently and differentially processed to allow simultaneous expression of both μ and δ immunoglobulins on the surface of maturing B lymphocytes (Figure 4-4). Both μ and δ regions are associated with the same V domain. After immunogen stimulation of the competent B-cell a class switch generally occurs and is T-cell dependent (Figure 4-5). Subsequent expression of a H-chain isotype other than μ and δ involves a recombination event resulting in gene deletions at the DNA level. Although class switch induction

Heavy Chain Gene Expression:

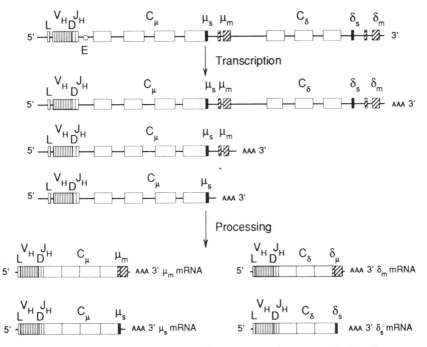

Figure 4-4. Expression of murine heavy-chain constant-region genes. The B-cells, express-ing both μ and δ C regions, produce transcripts containing Cμ and Cδ sequences. Primary transcripts are processed to generate mRNA species as indicated. (Reproduced from Ref 4 by permission.)

is ill defined, the recombination mechanism appears to be a set of repetitive se-quences located 5' to each set of C exons (except the δ exons). The repetitive sequences are referred to as switch (S) regions which are 2–10 kb in length and consist of short tandem redundant sequences. A looping out and deletion mecha-nism of class switching has been proposed based on analyses of spontaneously occurring switch mutants of a pre-B-cell line.[19]

Different polyadenylation sites at the 3' end of various exons have been consid-ered as the basis of control mechanisms to modulate processing of mRNA tran-scripts. Various polyadenylation sites are viewed as a means to control expression of alternate carboxy-terminal sequences that result in a secreted or membrane form of the Ig molecule.[20,21] During initial stages of B-cell differentiation the cell ex-clusively produces a membrane form of the heavy chain. After immunogen induc-tion and passage through division and differentiation states the secreted form is synthesized. Splicing may represent the level at which mRNA processing is regu-lated in the production of the alternate carboxy-terminal sequences of the H chains.

A nuclear factor present in surface IgM-bearing B-cells appears to induce splicing of the intron between the C_H4 exon and the membrane exon (Figure 4-4) and has

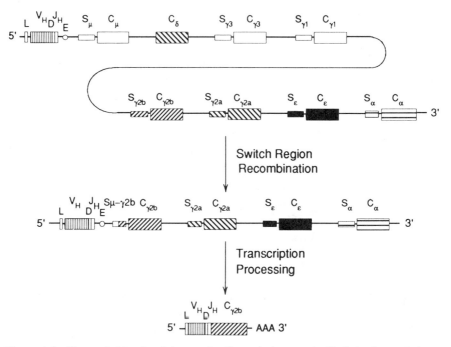

Figure 4-5. Class switching involving murine C_H region exons. An H-chain class switch to an IgG2b molecule is indicated. Heavy-chain C-region exons (boxes) are shaded to match the corresponding S region. (Reproduced from Ref 4 by permission.)

been inferred by microinjection of both a μ gene and B-cell nuclear extracts into *Xenopus* oocytes.[22]

Regulatory Genomes

Control of immunoglobulin gene transcription involves both the V-gene promoter and a transcriptional enhancer element. The V-gene promoter consists of a well-conserved TATA consensus sequence which determines the position of transcriptional initiation. Comparison of V-promoter-region sequences has revealed the presence of a consensus octanucleotide (ATGCAAAT) in the V_H promoters and its complement (ATTTGCAT) in the V_L promoters. The octanucleotide appears to be essential for transcriptional activity as deletion of the octanucleotide negates promoter function.

The V_H promoter confers lymphocyte lineage specificity to heterologous genes in transfection experiments. An additional heptameric sequence (CTCATGA) has been identified in the V_H promoter region.[23] The sequence is located 5′ to the conserved octamer.[24]

A second regulatory element in Ig genes is the enhancer (E) element located in the J–C intron of the H- and κ-chain loci. It is postulated that V–D–J or V–J recombination localizes a V-gene promoter near the enhancer, thus potentiating transcription. However, increased accumulation of heavy-chain mRNA in plasma cells is not related to enhancer activity but is regulated primarily by posttranscriptional processes. This suggests that the enhancer is only required to initiate transcriptional competence. Some sequences involved in cell-specific interactions have been identified in both IgH and k enhancers by DNA footprinting analysis. One such sequence is the ATTGCAT consensus sequence found in the V segment and other promoters. The gene encoding a κ-enhancer binding protein has been isolated.[25] It appears that induction of κ-chain expression by bacterial lipopolysaccharide or phorbol esters in B-cell lines harboring positively rearranged κ genes is correlated to appearance of a binding protein in nuclear extracts. The mechanism of action may involve posttranscriptional modification of a precursor form.

Summary

The unique germ-line array of immunoglobulin-related gene segments provides a basis upon which random associations generate a significant level of antibody diversity. Future studies employing molecular biological principles will lead to an elucidation of mechanisms involved in complex genetic processes, such as class switching, somatic mutation, and affinity maturation. Understanding of such processes will lead to modulation and control of the immune response as well as to molecular devices that can elucidate pathological states as in the various autoimmune syndromes.

References

1. Dreyer WJ, Bennett JC. *Proc Natl Acad Sci (USA)*. 1965;54:864.

2. Hozumi N, Tonegawa S. *Proc Natl Acad Sci (USA)*. 1976;73:3628.

3. Wu TJ, Kabat EA. *J Exp Med*. 1970;132:211.

4. Blackwell TK, Alt FW. In Hames BD, Glover DM, eds. *Molecular Immunology*. Oxford: IRL Press; 1988:1.

5. Alt FW, Blackwell TK, DePinho RA, Reth MG, Yancopoulos GD. *Immunol Rev*. 1986;89:5.

6. Yancopoulos GD, Alt FW. *Annu Rev Immunol*. 1988;4:339.

7. Reth M, Leclercq L. In Calabi F, Neuberger MS, eds. *Molecular Genetic of Immunoglobulins*. Amsterdam: Elsevier; 1987:111.

8. Alt FW. *Nature (London)*. 1984;312:502.

9. Brodeur P. In Calabi F, Neuberger MS, eds. *Molecular Genetics of Immunoglobulins*. Amsterdam: Elsevier; 1987:81.

10. Hamel PA, Klein MH, Smith-Gill, SJ, Dorrington KJ. *J Immunol*. 1987;139:3012.

11. Kranz DM, Voss EW. *Proc Natl Acad Sci (USA)*. 1981;78:5807.

12. Allen D, Cumano A, Dildrop R, Kocks C, Rajewsky K, Rajewsky N, Roes J, Sablitsky F, Siekevitz M. *Immunol Rev*. 1987;96:23.

13. Berek C, Milstein C. *Immunol Rev*. 1987;96:59.

14. Malipiero UV, Levy NS, Gearhart PJ. *Immunol Rev*. 1987;96:59.

15. Mansen T, Wysocki LJ, Margolies MN, Gefter ML. *Immunol Rev*. 1987;96:141.

16. Eisen HN, Siskind GW. *Biochemistry*. 1964;3:996.

17. Stevens FJ, Chang C-H, Schiffer M. *Proc Natl Acad Sci (USA)*. 1988;17:25.

18. Voss EW, Dombrink-Kurtzman MA, Miklasz SD. *Immunol Invest*. 1988;17:25.

19. Jäck, H-M, McDowell M, Steinberg C, Wabl M. *Proc Natl Acad Sci (USA)*. 1988;85:1581.

20. Galli G, Guise J, Tucker P, Nevins JR. *Proc Natl Acad Sci (USA)*. 1988;85:2439.

21. Guise JW, Lim PL, Yvan D, Tucker PW. *J Immunol*. 1988;140:3988.

22. Tsurvshita N, Ho L, Korn LJ. *Cell*. 1988;239:494.

23. Eaton S, Calame K. *Proc Natl Acad Sci (USA)*. 1987;84:7634.

24. Landolfi NF, Yin S-M, Capra JD, Tucker PW. *Nucl Acid Res*. 1988;16:5503.

25. Singh H, Lebowitz JA, Baldwin AS, Sharp P. *Cell*. 1988;52:415.

CHAPTER 5

Structure, Expression, and Function of Class-I Genes of the Human Major Histocompatibility Complex

Rakesh Srivastava and Michael E. Lambert

Department of Immunology, Scripps Clinic and Research Foundation, 10666 North Torrey Pines Road, La Jolla, CA 92037 USA

Introduction

The major histocompatibility complex (MHC), an important genetic component of the vertebrate immune system, has been identified in several species and consists of a linked cluster of structurally related as well as unrelated genes and gene families.[1] The human MHC (also referred to as human leukocyte antigens, HLA) extends over 3 million base pairs of DNA and resides on the short arm of chromosome 6 (6p21.3). The gene products of MHC are known to be intimately involved in various aspects of cellular and humoral immunity and a large number of diseases have been found to be in linkage disequilibrium with this region.[2,3] Three major families of genes have been identified in this complex: (1) the class-I genes, which encode the classical transplantation antigens (HLA-A, -B, and -C) and a family of several structurally related genes of unknown function; (2) the class-II genes, which are the structural homologs of the murine immune response genes; and (3) the class-III genes, which encode several components of the serum complement system (C2, Bf, C4A, and C4B) as well as the cytochrome P450 genes that encode steroid hydroxylases A and B. Recently, Levi-Strauss et al[4] have identified and mapped a novel gene of unknown function located between Bf and C4A. This gene, designated RD, is widely expressed among various tissues examined. The genes for tumor necrosis factor α and β have also been mapped centromeric to the B locus[5]. A series of genes designated BAT (B-locus associated transcripts) has been identified in close proximity to the HLA-B locus,[6] although, the function of these genes is not known. The hereditary hemochromatosis locus has also been mapped between the HLA-B and -A loci.[7]

This chapter presents a selective and critical overview of current and emerging thinking concerning the structure, expression, and function of class-I (MHC-I) genes. We have focused primarily on human MHC-I but refer, where appropriate, to studies of the murine MHC-I genes, which are currently better characterized overall than their human counterparts.

The HLA-A, -B, and -C Antigens

The study of the class-I MHC has been of considerable interest to both immunologists and molecular geneticists because of the complex mechanisms by which the polypeptide products derived from this region modulate cell–cell interactions in the elimination of foreign antigens.[8] The HLA-A and -B antigens are expressed on the surface of virtually all nucleated cells in noncovalent association with a non-MHC encoded protein, β2 microglobulin (β2m). A typical class-I heavy chain (the product of the HLA-A, -B, or -C loci) is a glycoprotein of an average molecular weight of approximately 42 kilodaltons (kd). The protein has a domain-like structure similar to that noted among various members of the immunoglobulin super gene family. The domain structure of class-I proteins is reflected in the molecular organization of the class-I genes, with a separate exon encoding each domain.[9] A transmembrane (TM) domain of approximately 25 amino acids is flanked by three extracellular domains ($\alpha 1$, $\alpha 2$, and $\alpha 3$, 90 amino acids each) on the amino terminus and a cytoplasmic tail of approximately 30 amino acids on the carboxy terminus.[10] The third external domain ($\alpha 3$, most proximal to the TM domain) displays amino acid sequence homology to the constant-region domains of the immunoglobulin molecules.

Recently, Bjorkmann et al[11,12] have solved the three-dimensional structure of one such protein, HLA-A2, at a resolution of 3.5 Å, and based on the available sequence data, the proteins derived from other class-I loci also are anticipated to conform to the same teritary structure. As revealed in these studies[11,12] the external domains of the globular class-I proteins are folded in such a way that the $\alpha 1$ and $\alpha 2$ domains not only interact with each other but also make interdomain contacts with both the $\alpha 3$ domain and β2m. While the folding of the $\alpha 1$ domain resembles that of $\alpha 2$ [an antiparallel beta (β)-pleated sheet with a long α helix], both the $\alpha 3$ and β2m domains form β-pleated sheets. As a net result of the interdomain contacts that provide the tertiary foldings, a large helical groove (25 Å long, 11 Å deep, and 10 Å wide) is created between the two α helices of the $\alpha 1$ and $\alpha 2$ domains. The base of this Bjorkman's groove is formed by eight strands of the β-pleated sheets that are also contributed by the $\alpha 1$ and $\alpha 2$ domains. This groove is postulated to be the "antigen binding pocket" and can accommodate short peptides up to 20 amino acids.

One of the striking features of the HLA-A, -B, and -C proteins is their high level of allelic polymorphism, which is unprecedented among other genes and gene families. Between 50 and 100 alleles have been estimated for the HLA-A and -B loci, respectively,[13] and 11 alleles have been identified at the HLA-C locus.[14] Many of the allelic class-I genes differ in their nucleotide sequences to such an extent that the encoded protein products of these genes are as different from each other as any given non-MHC protein differs between two species. Thus, as Klein[13] has pointed out, the HLA-A antigens of two individuals typed as A2 and A3, differ as much as the protein lactate dehydrogenase-A differs between mouse and pig. Several mechanisms have been proposed to account for the origin and maintenance of this high degree of polymorphism. These include (1) the trans-species hypothesis,[13] (2) the nonimmune selection process,[15] and (3) gene conversion.[16-18] Whatever the genetic mechanisms that control this diversity, the allele-specific changes present in the primary amino acid sequence of the class-I proteins are found to be mainly confined to the Bjorkman's groove, implying that this diversity may be of functional significance.

The involvement of HLA-A and HLA-B proteins in cellular immunity has been widely studied. These proteins serve as major determinants in skin and tissue graft rejection and also provide the context for antigen recognition by cytotoxic T lymphocytes (CTLs).[19] Although a physical association between a class-I protein and a foreign antigen has yet to be demonstrated, several lines of evidence indicate that invading foreign antigens are first degraded into small peptides before MHC molecules present them to CTLs. In fact, it has been shown that HLA-A2 molecules can provide the context for presentation of a synthetic polypeptide to CTLs.[20] Crystallographic studies by Bjorkman et al[11] have provided further evidence that there may be a physical association between the class-I molecules and these "foreign" peptides.

Unlike HLA-A and HLA-B molecules, however, little is known about HLA-C restricted CTLs.[21,22] In fact, it has been argued that HLA-C locus-derived proteins, because of certain structural features, may not serve as restriction elements. Instead, they may be vestigial or they may play a different role than those played by the HLA-A and HLA-B molecules.[23] A functional disparity between the HLA-A and -B and the HLA-C proteins is also apparent in that, unlike HLA-A and -B, HLA-C molecules have little or no influence on graft rejection.[24] Recently, Dill et al[25] have addressed the question of the functional significance of HLA-C molecules using transgenic mice as a model system. As with the HLA-A or HLA-B locus gene-containing transgenic mice,[26-28] however, the HLA-Cw3 transgenic mice were able to elicit HLA-Cw3-mediated graft rejection and induction of HLA-CW3-restricted CTLs against influenza and Sendai viruses. In light of these experiments, the precise role of the HLA-C locus must be reassessed.

Molecular Mapping of the Class-I Region

Until recently, the size of the human MHC was defined in terms of centimorgans, a unit of genetic distance between loci on the chromosome. The advent of pulsed field gradient electrophoresis techniques,[29] however, has greatly facilitated megabase-scale mapping of the human MHC at the molecular level. Thus, the minimum physical distance covered by this locus on the short arm of chromosome 6 has been estimated to be roughly three megabases,[30,31] which is in good agreement with the genetic distance (3 centimorgans). Almost half of this distance is occupied by the class-I region. In our preliminary studies[30] we reported that the entire human class-I region maps to a total of three Not I restriction enzyme-derived DNA fragments (1090 kb, 540 kb, and 190 kb). Subsequently, we demonstrated that the 190-kb fragment was linked to the 540-kb fragment,[32] although its orientation could not be defined from those experiments. The HLA-B locus was assigned to the 1090-kb fragment and the HLA-A locus to the 540-kb fragment using the locus-specific probes pRS30.4[33] and pHLA-2a.1,[34] respectively. A third class-I locus was identified on the small Not I fragment (190 kb) using a probe (pRS5.10) specific for a novel class-I gene designated RS5.[32] Based on genetic information that the majority of the human class-I genes map telomeric to the HLA-A locus[35] and those of the mouse map telomeric to the H-2D locus,[36,37] we tentatively proposed that the 190-kb fragment lay telomeric to the 540-kb fragment.[30] Although the linkage of these two fragments (540 kb and 190 kb) was experimentally proved, orientation was purely suggestive. Carroll et al[31] have further refined the Not I-generated map of the class-I region by using additional probes and have now conclusively placed the smallest of the three Not I fragments toward the centromeric side of the 540-kb fragment.

A series of HLA-A, -B, and -C locus-specific genomic probes has been used to further dissect the class-I region.[38,39] Pontarotti et al[39] have shown that each of the HLA-A, -B, and -C locus genes can be mapped with a high degree of precision on distinct SfiI or MluI restriction enzyme-generated DNA fragments derived from the MHC. They have calculated that the physical distance between the HLA-B and the HLA-C locus is 130 kb and have also mapped a class-I pseudogene (pHLA12.4) to within 200 kb of the HLA-A locus, although the orientation of this latter gene with respect to HLA-A is not clear. The region between HLA-C and HLA-A has not been mapped with greater accuracy, and it is estimated that the minimum distance between these two loci is approximately 1000 kb.[31] The majority of the nonclassical class-I genes are thought to map within 340 kb of the HLA-A locus[38] and at least one additional gene, HLA-328, has been mapped centromeric to HLA-A.[40] One important conclusion from the analysis by Chimini et al[38] is that, in contrast to the mouse class-I region, it appears that no extensive contraction or expansion in the human class-I region has occurred during evolution. Of the 16 HLA haplotypes tested, only one was found to have lost approximately 40 kb of DNA near the HLA-A locus. This deletion, which is further documented by cloning experiments, was always associated with the HLA-A24 haplotype.

The Number of Class-I Genes in Humans

The number of class-I related sequences in the human genome has been variously estimated, but there is no definitive count available for any given haplotype. Although this number may be as high as 30,[41] a minimum of 17 genes have been identified in a HLA heterozygous B-cell line, LCL 721 (typed A1–A2, B8–B5, C?–C?, DR3–DR1, DQw2–DQw1, DPw4–DPw2), based on the detection of 17 distinct bands by class-I cross-reactive probes in HindIII enzymatically digested genomic DNA from this cell line.[42] In the DNA of other cell lines, however, the number of HindIII fragments that harbor class-I-type sequences may range from as low as 12 to as high as 20.[43] Whether this difference in the number of HindIII fragments reflects differences in the number of class-I genes among various cell lines or simply reflects polymorphism at the HindIII sites is not known. It should be noted that a class-I polymorphism with respect to the enzyme EcoRI does exist. While the HLA-B27 gene, derived from cell line 3.1.0, resides on a 6.8-kb EcoRI fragment (see Table 5-1), it was identified on a 4.3-kb EcoRI fragment in another study.[44] Our cloning experiments using the HLA hemizygous cell line 3.1.0 (typed A2, B27, Cw1) and the HLA homozygous cell line JY (A2–A2, B7–B7, Cw?) clearly indicate that the number of class-I-related sequences is higher than 17 in these two lines. Our analysis is based primarily on EcoRI-generated fragments of genomic DNA that define individual human class-I genes or gene fragments. A summary of the class-I clones isolated in this study is presented in Table 5-1 and, as shown in column 4, genes from each of the reported class-I loci (HLA-A, -B, -C; HLA12.4; RS5; and HLA6.0) are represented in this collection. A few of the clones contained more than one class-I sequence. The sizes of the EcoRI fragments that represent individual class-I genes (or gene segments) range from ~2 to >20 kb, which matches well with the size of the EcoRI bands detected on the genomic southerns obtained from these cell lines (our unpublished data).

Although there is as yet no clear consensus concerning the total number of class-I genes in humans, the mapping data indicate that the differences, if any, in the number of class-I genes in various HLA haplotypes may not be as extensive as has been found in the case of different haplotypes in the murine MHC. The mouse strain with b haplotype has 26 genes,[36] as opposed to 33 genes in the d haplotype.[37] In the f haplotype, nine class-I genes in the Qa region are deleted.[45]

The Nonclassical Class-I Genes

In both the human and murine MHC, a large number of "nonclassical" class-I genes, ie, genes derived from loci other than those that encode transplantation antigens, have been identified and mapped. However, a very limited distribution of data exists on the serological detection of the products of these genes. In the mouse, the non-H2-K, -D-L class-I genes have been divided into Qa and TL subgroups.[46] Several strains of mice have been studied for the organization of the Qa–TL region and each has been found to contain varying numbers of genes in this portion of the MHC.[45] The Qa antigens are primarily expressed on a subset of lymphoid cells[46,47] and some of the Qa-region genes are expressed as secretory molecules.[48,49] The TL molecules are selectively expressed in actively dividing cortical thymoctyes and in certain thymic leukemias.[50,51] No function has been attributed, however, to either of these murine gene products,[52] although our understanding of mouse class-I gene expression is far from complete. Hunt et al[53] have reported that as many as 14 different class-I genes are expressed in the thymus, although only five could be defined by the available serological reagents. The same investigators have also found that the brain, earlier considered to be devoid of class-I molecules, expresses three different class-I genes. The most recent studies of the Qa–TL region have revealed that several of these nonclassical class-I genes are expressed as ubiq-

Table 5-1. Summary of the Class I Cosmid Clones

No.	Clone Designation[a]	Size of RS29-positive EcoRI Fragments[b] (kb)	Intensity of Hybridization	Overlaps and Identity to the Known Class-I Loci[c]
1	CosRS1*	26–29.0	Strong	=7=31
2	CosRS2*	~26.0	Strong	
3	CosRS3*	7.8	Strong	=8
4	CosRS4	ND	Strong	
5	CosRS5	18.0	Strong	RS5, HLA-6.2 (E)
6	CosRS6	6.4, 4.5	Strong/strong	=18=LN11=HLA12.4
7	CosRS7	~23.0	Strong	CD1-like
8	CosRS8*	~8.0	Strong	=3
9	CosRS9*	~7.8	Strong	
10	CosRS11*	~7.8	Strong	
11	CosRS12	2.5	Strong	Rearranged
12	CosRS13	1.5	Strong	Rearranged
13	CosRS14	8, 3.6	Strong/weak	
14	CosRS17	2.3	Strong	Rearranged
15	CosRS18*	6.4	Strong	=6=LN11
16	CosRS19	~15.0	Weak	
17	CosRS21	2.8	Weak	Rearranged
18	CosRS22	7.1, 3.5	Weak/weak	
19	CosRS23	~20.0	Strong	
20	CosRS24	6.4	Strong	
21	CosRS25	6.4	Strong	
22	CosRS26	6.4	Strong	HLA-CW1
23	CosRS27	~6.0	Strong	HLA-6.0
24	CosRS28	6.4, 11.0	Strong/strong	HLA-A2 (6.4kb)
25	CosRS29	6.4	Strong	
26	CosRS31	>15.0	Strong	=1=7
27	CosRS32	3.5	Strong	HLA-B27 (truncated)
28	CosRS34	6.8	Strong	=40
29	CosRS35	~6.0	Strong	
30	CosRS36	~7.0	Strong	
31	CosRS37	7, 11.0[d]	Strong/strong	
32	CosRS38	6.8	Strong	HLA-B27
33	CosRS39	6.8	Strong	HLA-B27
34	CosRS40	~7.0	Strong	=34
35	CosRS41	ND	Strong	
36	CosRS42	ND	Strong	
37	CosRS43	ND	Strong	=39
38	CosRS44	ND	Strong	=38
39	CosRS45	ND	Strong	
40	CosRS46	ND	Strong	
41	CosRS47	ND	Strong	
42	CosRS48	ND	Strong	

[a]Clones marked * were derived from the JY cell line.

[b]RS29 is a panHLA genomic probe alleleic to LN11. ND = not determined.

[c]= Marks overlapping cosmid clones containing identical genes as determined by EcoRI + PstI double-digestion blotting patterns.

[d]The 7-kb EcoRI fragment from CosRS37 hybridizes strongly to the B-locus-specific oligonucleotide probe.

uitously as their classical (H2K, D–L) counterparts.[54-57] A few of these genes have complex modes of expression by which the same gene encodes membrane-bound or secretory molecules in different tissues.[58] Studies of cDNA cloning have revealed that some of the genes derived from the TL region encode class-I proteins that are three amino acids shorter in the α2 domain as compared to the corresponding regions in the H2K, D–L polypeptides.[59] The functional significance, however, of these proteins still remains unknown. It also appears that the numerical count of the nonclassical class-I type sequences in mice is far from clear. Livant et al[60] have estimated that there are approximately 60 class-I-type sequences in mice by the "probe excess titration" method. Although this number is significantly higher than that defined by the cloning experiments,[36,37] it cannot be overlooked in light of these more recent findings. Despite the fact that saturation cloning of the mouse MHC has been carried out, two additional expressed class-I genes,[53] as well as an additional subfamily of several divergent class-I genes, have subsequently been discovered in several strains of mice.[61] A gene, designated Hmt, that encodes a maternally transmitted antigen is also thought to be a divergent member of the class-I gene family and it has been found in linkage disequilibrium with the TL region.[62]

The human class-I region is similarly composed of more genes than can be serologically defined. The total number of class-I genes in humans is estimated to be between 20 and 30.[41] Although no categorization of these additional genes has been made into Qa- or TL-equivalent regions, possible human analogs of the mouse Qa and TL antigens have been reported, primarily on the basis of tissue distribution and biochemical characteristics. For example, an antigen named T6[63] is a marker molecule for immature T lymphocytes[64] and certain T-cell leukemias.[65] Several features of the T6 antigen (eg, tissue distribution and biochemical properties) are akin to those of the murine TL molecule.[66] A detailed characterization of the peptide maps of the T6 antigen, however, did not reveal any significant homology to the murine TL antigens.[67] Subsequently, molecular cloning experiments have demonstrated that the genes encoding such antigens do not map to the HLA complex[68] but instead constitute a separate gene family residing on chromosome 1. The nucleotide sequence analyses of these genes revealed no striking homology to the mouse TL region genes or to the human class I genes. Thus, a true human analog of the TL antigen has yet to be identified. The thymic differentiation marker M241 is another example of a human-TL-like antigen,[69] and a set of novel class-I-like molecules has been identified in the T-cell line MOLT-4.[70]

Fauchet et al[71] have described an exhaustive serological study in which over 1000 different alloantisera obtained from multiparous women were used to detect novel class-I molecules. Of particular interest was the antiserum designated 101RE. This antiserum specifically precipitated a novel class-I molecule that escaped detection by the HLA framework antibody W6–32. The molecule recognized by 101RE had a lower molecular weight when compared to the known class-I antigens and was expressed in association with β2m. The expression of this molecule was restricted to phytohemagglutinin (PHA)-stimulated T-cell blasts. Although the gene encoding such an antigen has not been identified, its linkage to the HLA complex was apparent from the fact that it segregated with the HLA haplotypes. Similar results were also obtained in another study[72] in which PHA blast-cell-restricted expression of novel class-I molecules was shown to be in linkage disequilibrium with the HLA-A haplotypes.

Are the Non-HLA-A, -B, and -C Genes Human Counterparts of Mouse Qa–TL Genes?

At the genetic level, the mode of evolution of the human class-I gene family apparently resembles that seen in the mouse. It has been proposed that the murine Qa–TL region genes have been generated by a duplication event in which the sequences of the two functional loci, H2K and D–L have multiplied to generate an array of structurally homologous genes. Although this argument has been contested,[73] a similar multiplication event at the HLA-A, -B, and -C loci would explain the multiplicity of class-I-type sequences observed in the human MHC. There is, however, clearly no evidence that the non-HLA-A, -B, -C genes are human equivalents of the mouse Qa–TL genes. At least seven non-HLA-A, -B, and -C genes have been sequenced in recent years and none displays any striking homology to the Qa–TL region genes of mice.[32,74–78] In fact, as mentioned earlier,[68] it has been recently shown that the family of genes that encodes the putative human TL antigens does not map to the HLA locus. Also, the mouse Qa–TL region shows a high degree of contraction and expansion, ie, different strains of mice carry varying number of genes in this region,[45] while no such differences were noticed in the size of the human class-I region, as estimated by recent pulsed field electrophoresis mapping studies.[38] Similarly, on an evolutionary scale, a definitive pattern in the length of introns differentiates the H2K, D–L genes from the Qa–TL genes in mouse.[79] Such a correlation, however, cannot be made between the HLA-A, -B, and -C and the non-HLA-A, -B, -C genes. Finally, it has been demonstrated by DNA hybridization studies that the genetic homolog of the mouse Qa–TL region is not conserved even in different strains of mice[45] and other rodents.[80] With these facts in mind, therefore, and since there are no functional criteria by which to define the Qa–TL genes, caution should be taken whenever comparing the human non-HLA-A, -B, and -C genes with the mouse Qa–TL genes.

The Structure of Non-HLA-A, -B, and -C Genes

To date, the structures of three non-HLA-A, -B, and -C locus genes and their alleles have been determined and each of these genes has shown a pattern of exon–intron organization similar to that found in the HLA-A, -B, and -C locus genes. These three non-HLA-A, -B, and -C loci include HLA12.4,[74] RS5[32] (renamed HLA-E[77]), and HLA6.0.[78] Each of these genes has been shown to encode polypeptide products upon transfection into murine or human cells. The cDNA clones corresponding to an allele of HLA12.4 (M Chorney, personal communication), RS5 (Ref 76 and our unpublished data) and HLA6.0 (A Swaroop and H Shukla, unpublished results) have been isolated. Evidence, however, is lacking for the expression and tissue distribution of the corresponding protein products. As shown in Figure 5-1, the

FIRST EXTERNAL DOMAIN (α1)

```
        1         10        20        30        40        50        60        70        80        90
RS5     ---LK-H---------S-------N----V----M--S----RSARDTA-IF-VN----A-----
HLA6.0  -----SAA-------A--M----------V----EE-RNT-HA---MNLQ-------
HLA12.4 R-----TM--A---D--------D---E---M-R--K--N--C--A-E-NLRIA------G
CONSENSUS GSHSMRYFYTSVSRPGRGEPRFIAVGVDDTQFVRFDSDAASPRMEPRAPWIEQEGPEYWDRETQIVKAQSQTDRESLRTLRGYYNQSEA
```

SECOND EXTERNAL DOMAIN (α2)

```
        91        100       110       120       130       140       150       160       170       180
RS5     -----W-H-EL---F----E-F------LT------V--L-SEQ-SND-SE-DDQ-----D------HK--K---LHL
HLA6.0  S---W-I--L-S----E------L------------SK-C--N--R-----H-----M---
HLA12.4 ---M-S---------PF--E-H----------M--R---R-V--EF--R--------
CONSENSUS GSHTLQRMYGCDVGPDGRLLRGYHQYAYDGKDYIALNEDLRSWTAADTAAQITQRKWEAARVAEQLRAYLEGTCVEWLRRYLENGKETLQRA
```

THIRD EXTERNAL DOMAIN (α3)

```
        183       190       200       210       220       230       240       250       260       270
RS5     E---------------------Q--GH------G------G------E-V---
HLA6.0  ----VF-Y------I----V----V------G------E-M---
HLA12.4 ---M-----------------------G-------E----
CONSENSUS DPPKTHVTHHPISDHEATLRCWALGFYPAEITLTWQRDGEDQTQDTELVETRPAGDRTFQKWAAVVVPSGEEQRYTCHVQHEGLPKFLTLRW
```

TRANSMEMBRANE REGION

```
          280         290         300         310
RS5       KPASQPTIVGIIA:GLVLLGSVVS GAVVAAVIWRKKSS
HLA6.0    KQS-L----M--V-A---V-AA--T -A---L-K---
HLA12.4   E-S---------VA--T -------M-K---

HLA-A2    E-S-------F-A-IT ------M-R---
HLA-A3    ELS--------A-IT -----M-R---
HLA-B7    E-S---SV----V-:FAV-AV--I ----MC-R---
HLA-B27   E-S-S-V----V-:AV-AV--I ----MC-R---
HLA-CW3   E-S-------V----AV-AVLAVL---V-MC-R---
CONSENSUS EPSSQPTIFVGIXA:GLXXLXVVXX GAVVAAVMXRRKSS
```

CYTOPLASMIC DOMAIN ONE   **CYTOPLASMIC DOMAIN TWO**

```
                320                    330
RS5       GGKGGSYSKAE            WSDSAQGSESHSL:::
HLA6.0    D:::::::::             :::::::::::::
HLA12.4   DR-----Q-A            S-N----DVSLTA::

HLA-A2    DR-----Q-A            S-----DVSLTACK
HLA-A3    DR-----TQ-A           S-----DVSLTACK
HLA-B7    -------Q-A            C-----DVSLTA::
HLA-B27   -------Q-A            C-----DVSLTA::
HLA-CW3   -----C-Q-A            S-N---DESLIACK
CONSENSUS XXKGGSYSQAA           XSDSAQGSDVSLTAXX
```

Figure 5-1. Divergence in the amino acid sequences of nonclassical class-I proteins. Amino acid sequences derived from the nucleotide sequences of three nonallelic, nonclassical class-I genes are compared with the "consensus" class-I amino acid sequence as reported by Parham et al.[85] Amino acids are represented by a single-letter code. A dash (—) indicates similarity to the consensus and a colon (:) indicates a gap. Sequences are taken from Ref32 (RS5; note: a sequencing discrepancy in the α1 domain of RS5 is shown corrected), Ref78 (HLA6.0) and Ref74 (HLA12.4).

amino acid sequences of these putative proteins, as deduced from the genomic and cDNA sequences, show strong homology to the classical class-I proteins. Although similar in organization to the HLA-A, -B, and -C genes, each of these three loci has certain unique features. These include:

1. Unlike HLA-A, -B, or -C, which encode transmembrane proteins, HLA12.4 was shown in transfection studies to encode an intracellular protein.[81] This is apparently because of the lack of a cystein residue at position 164. A cystein residue at this position may therefore be a prerequisite for the secondary and tertiary foldings of those class-I proteins, which bind β2m and are subsequently transported to the cell surface. A genomic clone allelic to HLA12.4 has recently been isolated and sequenced.[82] This gene, designated JY8, has acquired a single base deletion in the exon that encodes the α-3 domain, so the protein encoded by JY8 differs in its primary amino acid sequence when compared with the amino acid sequence of the HLA12.4-encoded protein. This difference in amino acid sequences, however, does not abolish the allelic nature of the two genes (HLA12.4 and JY8). Nucleotide deletion–insertion events that alter the protein reading frames are not unprecedented among class-I alleles, especially in the case of nonclassical class-I genes. Another allele of HLA12.4, designated LN11A,[75] has acquired several deletions and insertions that alter the reading frame. A single nucleotide variation (deletion–insertion) in the exon that encodes the signal sequence in the murine Q4 alleles has also been reported.[49] Some of the murine TL genes have acquired a nine-base pair deletion at a stretch in the exon that encodes the α2 domain[59] and thus, although the reading frame remains unaltered, the encoded protein would have an α2 domain that is shorter by three amino acids.

2. The novel gene designated RS5[32] has several unique features that distinguish it from other class-I genes. In contrast to the promotor elements of all the reported human class-I genes, the sequence of the "TATA" box in RS5 has not undergone the A → C transition at the second nucleotide and so resembles the TATAAA sequence found in the mouse class-I genes. However, a second "TATA" box, resembling those in other human class-I genes (TCTAAA), is present upstream from this TATAAA sequence. Another feature of RS5 that resembles that found in the mouse class-I genes is the positioning of a protein synthesis initiation codon in the first exon, which results in a shorter signal sequence. The gene RS5 has also acquired a frameshift mutation in the seventh exon and so encodes a divergent protein with a shorter cytoplasmic tail. The gene is transcribed along with an Alu insertion element at the 3' end, which provides a novel site for poly (A) adenylation. The nucleotide sequence-derived amino acid sequence of the putative RS5 protein displays a high level of divergence in its primary structure as compared to those of the HLA-A, -B, and -C antigens (see Figure 5-1).

Recently, the sequence of a novel gene, designated HLA6.2 or HLA-E has been reported.[77] The level of nucleotide sequence homology between RS5 and this gene is of the same order as that seen between the allelic class-I sequences and which is unprecedented among the nonallelic genes.[83] Each of the unique features of RS5 as discussed above are also conserved in HLA6.2. The true allelic nature of these genes

```
                              280                                    290                              300
RS5      A-- --- G-- --- --- --- --- --- A--    -T- C-- --T -GA TCT GTG ::: ::: --- --- --T
JTW15    A-- --- G-- --- --- --- --- --- A--    -T- C-- --T -GA TCT GTG ::: ::: --- --- --T
HLA6.2   A-- --- G-- --- --- --- --- --- A--    -T- C-- --T -GA TCT GTG ::: ::: --- --- --T

HLA6.0   --- -A- --- -T- --- --- A-- --T        -T- T-- --T --CA ::: --- GTA --- --C --C

P12.4    --- --A --- --- G-- --- --- --- ---    T-- --T -A CT- --- GTG --- ACT --- --C
LN11     --- --A --- --- T-- T-- --- --- ---    A-- --T -A CT- --- GTG --- ACT --- --C
JY8      --- --A --- --- --- T-- --C --- ---    --- --T -A CT- --- GTG --- ACT --- --C

JY328    --- --A --- --- --- --- A-- --- ---           --T --- ::: --T --- CTA GGA GCT GTG --C

HLA-Cw1  GAG CCG TCT TCC CAG CCC ATC CCC ATC GTG GGC ATC GTT GCT GGC  CTG GCT GTC CTG GCT GTC CTA GCT ::: GTC CTA GGA GCT GTG GTG
HLA-Cw2  --- -A- --- --- --- --- --- --- --- --- ---    --- --- --- --- --- --- --- --- --- --- --- --- --- --- --- --- --- ---
HLA-Cw3  --- -A- --- --- --- --- --- --- --- --- ---    --- --- --- --- --- --- --- --- --- --- --- --- --- --- --- --- --- A--
HLA-CX52 --- --- --- --- --- --- --- --- --- --- ---    --- --- --- --- --- --- --- --- --- --- --- --- --- --- --- --- --- --C
HLA-A2   --- --- --- --- --- --- --- --- A-- --- ---    --- --T --C CT- -G: ::: --- --- GTG A-- ACT --- --- --- --- --- --- --C
HLA-A3   --- -T- --- --- --- --- --- --- A-- --- ---    --- --T --C CT- -G: ::: --- --- GTG A-- ACT --- --- --- --- --- --- --C
HLA-A11  --- -T- --- --- --- --- --- --- A-- --- ---    --- --T --C CT- -G: ::: --- --- GTG A-- ACT --- --- --- --- --- --- --C
HLA-Aw24 --- --A --- G-- --- --- --- --- A-- --- ---    --- --T --C CT- -G: ::: --- --- GTG A-- ACT --- --- --- --- --- --- --C
HLA-B7   --- --- --- G-- --- --- --- --T --- --- ---    --- --T G-C CTA --C: ::: --- --- --T -GTG A-C --- --- --- --- --- --- ---
HLA-B27  --- --- --- --- T-- --- --- --T --- --- ---    --- --T G-C CTA --C: ::: --- --- --T -GTG A-C --- --- --- --- --- --- --C

                       310
RS5      --- -C- --- --- --A -G- --- --A --- --- --- --- --- --- --- --- --- ---
JTW15    --- -C- --- --- --A -G- --- --A --- --- --- --- --- --- --- --- --- ---
HLA6.2   --- -C- --- -T- --A -G- --- --A --- --- --- --- --- --- --- --- --- ---

HLA6.0   --- -C- --- --- C-- --- --A A-- --- --- --- --- --- --- --- --- --- ---

P12.4    --- --C- --- -A- --G --- --A --- --- --- --- --- --- --- --- --- --- ---
LN11     A-- --A- --- -A- --G --- --A --- --- --- --- --- --- --- --- --- --- ---
JY8      --- --C- --- -A- --G --- --A --- --- --- --- --- --- --- --- --- --- ---

JY328    A-C -C- A-- --- --- --- --- --- --- --- --- --- --- --- --- --- --- ---

HLA-Cw1  GCT GTT GTG ATG TGT AGG AGG AAG AGC TCA
HLA-Cw2  --- --- --- --- --- --- --- --- --- ---
HLA-Cw3  --- -T- --- --- --- --- --- --- --- ---
HLA-CX52 --- --- --- --- --- --- --- --- --- ---
HLA-A2   --- --C- --- -G- --- --- --- --- --- ---
HLA-A3   --- --C- --- -G- --- --- --- --- --- ---
HLA-A11  --- --C- --- -G- --- --- --- --- --- ---
HLA-Aw24 --- --C- --- -G- --- --C --- --- --- ---
HLA-B7   --- --- --- --- --- --- --- --T --- ---
HLA-B27  --- --- --- --- --- --- --- --T --- ---
```

Figure 5-2. Locus-specific regions in the nucleotide sequences of various class-I genes. The nucleotide sequences of exon V, which encodes the transmembrane domain of class-I proteins, are shown compared. Brackets indicate allelic genes, dashes indicate identity to the sequence of HLA-Cwl, and colons indicate gaps. Oligonucleotide stretches that define locus specificity are boxed. The sequences were obtained from references as follows: RS5,[32] JTW15,[76] HLA-6.2,[77] HLA-6.0,[78] p12.4,[74] LN11,[75] JY8,[83] JY328,[82] HLA-Cwl and HLA-Cw2,[23] HLA-Cw3,[113] HLA-CX52,[114] HLA-A2,[83] HLA-A3,[115] HLA-A11,[116] HLA-Aw24,[117] HLA-B7,[83] HLA-B27.[118]

Table 5-2. Locus-Specific Amino Acids[a]

	Residue Number					
Antigen	52	138	183	189	239	268
RS5	Met	Thr	Glu	Val	Gly	Glu
JTW15	Met	Thr	Glu	Val	Gly	Glu
HLA6.2	Met	Thr	Glu	Val	Gly	Glu
HLA6.0	Val	Thr	Asp	Val	Gly	Glu
P12.4	Met	Met	Glu	Met	Gly	Glu
HLA-A	Ile	Met	Asp	Met	Gly	Lys
HLA-B	Ile	Thr	Asp	Val	Arg*	Lys
HLA-C	Val	Thr	Glu	Val	Gly	Glu

[a]Comparison of the amino acid residues in nonclassical class-I proteins at positions identified to be locus specific among classical class-I proteins. It should be noted that because of the inclusion of nonclassical class-I sequences here, no HLA-A and HLA-C specific residue can be found at these positions, contrary to the analyses of Parham et al.[85] Only the genes allelic to HLA-B have a specific residue, (position 239) as marked with an asterisk.

is reflected by the following additional facts: As seen in Figure 5-2, there is a 100% match in the two sequences in regions that have been identified as being locus specific in class-I genes.[84] Similarly, at each of the six amino acid positions identified to be locus specific in class-I proteins[85] both the genes RS5 and HLA6.2 encode identical amino acid residues (see Table 5-2). Also, the HLA6.2-specific probe E.a (derived from the coding sequence of HLA6.2) shares more than 97%

```
  1  CTGCCTTGTGTGCGACTGAGATGCAGGATTTCCTCACGCCTCCCCTATGT   50
     ||||||||||||||||||||||||||||||||||||||||||||||||||
  1  CTGCCTTGTGTGCGACTGAGATGCAGGATTTCCTCACGCCTCCCCTATGT   50

 51  GTCTTAGGGG.ACTCTGGCTTCTCTTTTTGCAAGGGCCTCTGAATCTGTC   99
     ||||||||||  |||||||||||||||  ||||||||||||||||||||||
 51  GTCTTAGGGGAACTCTGGCTTCTCTTTCTGCAAGGGCCTCTGAATCTGTC  100

100  TGTGTCCCTGTTAGCACAATGTGAGGAGGTAGAGAAACAGTCCACCTCTG  149
     ||||||||||||||||||||||||||||||||||||||||||||||||||
101  TGTGTCCCTGTTAGCACAATGTGAGGAGGTAGAGAAACAGTCCACCTCTG  150

150  TGTCTACCATGACCCCC.TTCCTCACACTGACCTGTGTTCCTTCCCTGTT  198
     ||||||||||||||||| |||||||||||||||||||||||||||||||||
151  TGTCTACCATGACCCCCGTTCCTCACACTGACCTGTGTTCCTTCCCTGTT  200

199  CTCTTTTCTATTAAAAATAAGAACCTGGGCAGAGTGCGGCA           239
     ||||||||| ||||||||||||||||||||||||||||||||
201  CTCTTTTCT.TTAAAAATAAGAACCTGGGCAGAGTGCGGCA           240
```

Figure 5-3. Nucleotide sequence comparision of the two allelic genes RS5 and HLA-6.2 in the region from which the HLA-6.2-specific probe E.a was derived.[77] The sequence on the top represents E.a and that at the bottom, RS5.[32] The two sequences show a difference of only five nucleotides.

1 2 3 4 5

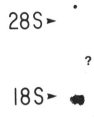

28S▸

?

18S▸

Figure 5-4. Northern blot analysis of RNAs from human cell lines using a 30-nucleotide oligomer probe specific for RS5. Five micrograms of poly(A)+ mRNA was electrophoresed in lanes 1–3 and 40 μg of total cytoplasmic RNA was used in lanes 4 and 5. Hybridization was carried out at 42°C in 6XSSC. The blot was washed with 2XSSC and 0.1% NaDodSO$_4$ at 55°C. Order of lanes: 1, JY; 2, MOLT-4; 3, SU; 4, HuT 78; 5, HuT 102. The minor species of transcript marked with "?" was consistantly and reproducibly observed in several different preparations of poly(A)+ mRNA from the JY cell line.

homology with the corresponding region of the gene RS5 (see Figure 5-3). This homology is well within the documented range of heterogeneity at the 3' ends of the class-I alleles.[82] The probe E.a, with only five nucleotic differences in its entire stretch when compared with the corresponding region of the RS5 sequence, could not distinguish between the RNA transcripts generated from the two genes. Since the probe E.a detects only a single gene among different haplotypes[77] and since both genes have been mapped identically,[31] it is certain that the two genes are derived from the same locus.

Expression studies carried out using either oligomeric or genomic probes derived from RS5 have revealed multiple-sized transcripts generated from this gene (Figure 5-4, Refs 32, 76, 77). The consistant observation of heterogeneously sized RS5 specific mRNA as well as the variable levels of RS5 expression observed among different tissues may reflect complex regulatory mechanisms governing the control of RS5 expression. A close examination of the genomic RS5 sequence in fact reveals the presence of several promotor-like elements in the 5' noncoding region.

As yet, however, no studies have been undertaken to determine whether transcription of RS5 can be initiated from multiple start sites.

3. A distinct feature of the gene HLA6.0[78] is the presence of a termination codon in the sixth exon. Thus, the putative HLA6.0 protein would lack a large part of its cytoplasmic tail.

Insertion of Alu Sequences in the Class-I Genes

A large part of the mammalian genome is occupied by noncoding sequences and various repeat elements whose function is not well understood. In humans, the most abundant of these repeat elements are the Alu sequences.[86] A typical member of the human Alu family is approximately 300 bp in length and is repeated up to 500,000 times per haploid genome. It has been recently demonstrated that Alu sequences are mobile within the mammalian genome[87] and thus, by transposition, may contribute to genetic variability.[88] Allelic variation generated by Alu insertions has in fact been found in several genes, including globin,[89] immunoglobulin,[90] and a cardiac hormone, pronatriodilatin.[91] Given the high copy number of Alu, it is therefore not surprising that, statistically, both the mouse and the human class-I regions have been found to contain a fair share of these repeat elements in their intergenic DNA sequences. In some cases, however, the insertion of Alu sequences has occurred intragenically, within the class-I genes themselves. These insertion events, which occur in both introns and exons, have been used as molecular markers to define the evolutionary history of the class-I region.[73] Thus, contrary to the commonly held view, Duran and Pease[73] have demonstrated that the origin of the murine Qa–TL region predates the origin of the H-2D–L region. These conclusions were primarily drawn by a careful analyses of Alu insertion events at the 3' noncoding ends of the class-I genes among several H-2 haplotypes of the mouse.

Perhaps of more significance is the observation that H-2D–L and certain TL-region genes in mice[92,93] and a non-HLA-A, -B, -C gene in humans[32,76,77] are transcribed colinearly with an Alu sequence. The sites for polyadenylation at the 3' end of the mature mRNAs in such cases are provided by these Alu sequences (multiple-Alu sequences have also been reported in the mature mRNAs derived from the human Low Density Lipoprotein receptor gene).[94] Although these insertions occur in the coding sequence, they occupy the untranslated region and therefore do not alter the reading frame of the mRNA. A possibility exists, however, that the insertion of Alu sequences, in both the coding and the noncoding regions, may have functional significance in controlling class-I gene expression. It has been shown that class-I genes that are cotranscribed with Alu sequences can be selectively activated in certain viral transformation processes.[95] Since Alu sequences can independently transcribe from their own RNA polymerase III promoters, the encoded antisense polynucleotide stretches may modulate the processing and translation of mRNAs by hybridizing with Alu-sequence-containing regions. When transcribed in "sense," these sequences could compete for transacting factors that are needed for the processing of pre-mRNAs. Korenberg and Rykowski[96] have also suggested that Alu sequences define HTF islands (see Hpa II Tiny Fragments) that are proposed to be associated with expressed genes.[97] On a more global basis, Alu sequences have been shown to serve as "attachment points" for the nuclear matrix[98] and thus may serve in controlling the topology of DNA.

Locus Specificity: The Nonclassical Class-I Genes Follow the Same Rules as Their Classical Counterparts

The nucleotide sequences of all the reported class-I genes are highly homologous.[83] Any one of the genes can be used as a DNA probe to isolate the other members of this family. Individual class-I genes can be distinguished in DNA blot analyses by a judicious choice of restriction enzymes. The analysis of the mRNA products derived from individual class-I genes cannot be accomplished, however, with pan-HLA class I DNA probes, because of the codominant expression of similarly sized homologous transcripts from different loci. Thus, a need to identify locus-specific nucleotide sequences in the coding domains of the class-I genes became apparent. Davidson et al[84] have compared the available nucleotide sequences of a limited number of class-I alleles from the HLA-A, -B, and -C loci and have found that a stretch of 27 nucleotides in the fifth exon that encodes the transmembrane domain shows a level of divergence that can define locus specificity among the HLA-A, -B, and -C loci. Oligonucleotide probes derived from this region have been used successfully to study the expression of HLA-A, -B, and -C genes.[84] As sequences of more class-I genes became available, we have further extended this comparison of the nucleotide sequences and, as shown in Figure 5-2, the original conclusions of Davidson et al,[84] as drawn for classical class-I genes, also hold true for each of the three nonclassical class-I loci reported to date. Thus, we were able to synthesize oligonucleotide probes specific for the alleles of RS5, HLA12.4, and HLA6.0.

Parham et al[85] have defined locus-specific amino acid residues present in the three extracellular domains of the HLA-A, -B, and -C molecules. In this analysis, protein sequences of 39 alleles from the HLA-A, -B, and -C loci were compared and positions 52 (α1 domain); 138, 183 (α2 domain); and 189, 239, and 268 (α3 domain) were identified as representing locus-specific residues. However, all the three loci were not different at each of these positions. The consensus pattern that emerges from such an analysis is that, of the three loci, two always have identical amino acids at a given position, whereas the third has a unique residue. However, when this analysis was carried out, the sequences of non-HLA-A, -B, and -C loci were not taken into consideration. As shown in Table 5-2, upon inclusion of such sequences, each of the three amino acid residues originally identified as being HLA-C specific (positions 52, 183, and 268) no longer defines such a specificity toward the C locus. Similarly, no HLA-A-specific residue can be identified at any of the six positions. It remains to be seen whether the only remaining amino acid residue specific for HLA-B (Arg-139) will retain this specificity once more sequences become available from the non-HLA, -B, and -C loci. As shown in Table 5-2, no residue specific for any of the three nonclassical class I loci emerged at any of the positions identified by Parham et al.[85]

Accessory Molecules Involved in the Expression of the Nonclassical Class-I Proteins

Our transfection experiments have indicated that, although the RS5 protein is expressed at a high level in the cytoplasm of transfected mouse L cells,[32] it is not transported to the cell surface. The presence of transfected human β2m in these mouse cells, however, led to transient cell-surface expression of the protein, although the level of expression was far lower than that observed with the transfected HLA-B7 or HLA-A2 genes. We have repeatedly observed, however, that cell-surface expression of the RS5 protein cannot be stably maintained in transfected cell lines after serial passage (as monitored by FACS analyses with the HLA framework antibody W6–32). One possibility is that, unlike transiently transfected cells, the stably transfected cell lines do not express this protein at the cell surface in a configuration that can be recognized by W6–32. A polyclonal class-I antiserum, K455,[151] was efficient, however, in recognizing the cell-surface expression of RS5 in the transfected human HLA-null cell line 72.221 (our unpublished studies). Similarly, a xenoantiserum[67] raised against a mixture of several T and B cells also detected cell-surface expression of RS5 in transfected murine cells. Another possibility remains, that an accessory molecule(s) in addition to β2m may be needed for efficient transport across the cell membrane. In many ways, however, transfection may be an artificial system, in which the background of the recipient cell and its microenvironment largely determine the mode of expression of transfected DNA, without reflecting upon the true nature of its expression and function in any given tissue.

Recently it has been shown that, in activated T lymphocytes, a small fraction of HLA-like molecules are expressed in physical association with an integral membrane protein designated CD8 (mol wt 32–34 kd).[99] A possibility exists that this small subpopulation of the class-I proteins consists of the less studied nonclassical class-I heavy chains, such as those encoded by the clone RS5 or HLA6.0. Although there are no data to establish the functional relevance of the association of CD8 with class-I proteins, several speculations have been made. These include its involvement in (1) increased interaction between effector cytotoxic T cells and target cells and (2) recycling of class-I molecules. Bushkin et al[99] have shown a physical association between HLA-like molecules and CD8 molecules of the same cells. The possibility exists, however, that this interaction is of general importance even between class-I molecules and CD8 molecules of different cells, and it may play a role in the processes of cell–cell communication.

Since class-I–CD8 interactions are observed only upon activation of T cells, it is possible that the activation process leads to dissociation of bound β2m from the intracellular pool of class-I molecules, followed by replacement with CD8 molecules, before transport of class-I molecules to the cell surface. The observation that a large proportion of the RS5-equivalent HLA6.2 protein is mostly expressed intracellularly (in stably transfected human cells[77]), despite the presence of a perfect transmembrane domain in its structure, may imply that a mechanism is operative in which a molecule other than β2m is needed for the efficient transport of the RS5 protein to the cell surface. Two points are noteworthy here. First, the CD8-associated HLA-like molecules that have been found on activated T cells represent only a minor fraction of the total class-I molecules, possibly hinting that they are the non-HLA-A, -B, -C-type class-I proteins, which are poorly expressed when compared to the constitutively expressed HLA-A, -B, -C proteins. This is further supported by our RNA blotting experiments with several human cell lines, which indicate that the expression of the RS5 gene is probably several hundredfold less than that of the HLA-A, -B, -C genes (our unpublished data). Second, activated T cells have been shown to induce cell-surface expression of the nonclassical class-I proteins.[71,72] This latter observation is further substantiated by our isolation of a cDNA clone for RS5 from activated T-cells (our unpublished data).

Functional Significance of Non-HLA-A, -B, and -C Genes

Data are insufficient to assign any functional role to the non-HLA-A, -B, and -C locus genes. If tissue distribution is any criterion for expected function, the CD1 genes (rather than the non-HLA-A, -B, -C genes) should be the functional equivalents of the mouse TL genes. Any prediction of the functional significance of these genes at present can only be speculative. In view of the fact that some of the silent class-I genes may be induced in tissue culture in response to the mitogens, to protein synthesis inhibitors such as cycloheximide, or by the DNA-damaging agents (see Cellular Stress and MHC-I Expression), it appears that the expression of these genes is under tight regulation through both cis- and trans-acting regulators. If expressed, the encoded proteins may be able to elicit a function similar to that of the HLA-A, -B, and -C locus proteins because of their immense structural similarities. The nonclassical class-I genes may serve as a reservoir of functional restriction elements (class-I proteins) that have the same capabilities as their classical counterparts, but the immune system may only make use of these additional proteins under certain physiological conditions, such as cellular stress (see Cellular Stress and MHC-I Expression). The consideration that these genes serve as a "reservoir of functional proteins," if true, would be physiologically more relevant and meaningful in terms of immune function than considering them as solely a consequence of nonadaptive gene amplification events. This latter function is significant only in terms of evolutionary change and has no immediate bearing within an individual's lifespan.

New experimental approaches are needed to discern the function of the non-HLA-A, -B, -C genes. Recently, some laboratories have undertaken "reverse genetics" approaches to studying the expression of the non-HLA-A, -B, and -C genes. In these experiments, cloned class-I genes were transfected in mouse cells and novel class-I products were identified using either HLA framework antibodies or xenoantisera. The first evidence for expression of a nonclassical class-I gene derived from the HLA complex was reported by Paul et al.[43] In this study, a cosmid clone (P2B2) containing a novel class-I gene was transfected in mouse cells (J27) that had been previously transfected with total human DNA and selected for the expression of human β2m.[100] Although the novel class-I gene contained in the clone P2B2 hybridized strongly to a pan-HLA DNA probe (pDP001),[101] indicating strong sequence conservation, the encoded protein product of this gene was not recognized by any of the monomorphic class-I heavy-chain monoclonal reagents used. Further serological studies have revealed that this gene is selectively expressed in PHA-activated HLA-A2-positive T cells.

As revealed in the studies by Paul et al,[43] the lack of appropriate serologic reagents has prevented the identification of some of the novel class-I protein products encoded by the nonclassical class-I genes. However, in contrast to the protein encoded by the clone P2B2, the product of another nonclassical class-I gene, RS5, is recognized by the HLA framework antibodies W6–32[32] and K455 (our unpublished data).[151] This observation was further confirmed in experiments in which an allele of RS5 was used in transfection studies.[77] Two additional novel class-I genes, designated HLA6.0 and HLA5.4, also encode proteins that are recognizable by the HLA framework antibody W6–32.[102] These serological observations, as well as the strong nucleotide sequence homology of the genes RS5 and HLA6.0 to the classical class-I gene sequences (the sequence of HLA5.4 is not known), support the conclusion that the nonclassical class-I proteins have conserved secondary and tertiary structures that resemble their classical counterparts. Therefore, it is reasonable to assume that if the non-HLA-A, -B, -C class-I molecules have any function, they may exert it by way of cell–cell interactions in a fashion similar to that of the classical class-I antigens. However, they may have remained undetected because of their relatively nonpolymorphic nature.

Two major components of cellular immunity are self-tolerance and T-cell restriction. Both of these functions are governed by the known class-I antigens. The ability of the non-HLA-A, -B, and -C class-I gene products to elicit these physiological functions, however, has not been tested. Evidence is only now beginning to emerge for the possible involvement of novel class-I proteins in T-cell restriction in the mouse.[57] Owing to their structural homology with classical transplantation antigens, it is likely that these molecules are recognized by alpha–beta (α–β) T-cell receptors (TCR) or by a receptor system of similar origin. Non-α–β TCR-like molecules have also been reported in both mouse and human.[103–105] Of particular interest is the T-cell receptor designated gamma–delta (γ–δ) TCR. The subunit structure of this receptor is highly similar to that of the α–β TCR[103,104] and, like the α–β TCR, this receptor is also associated with CD3 molecules, which are considered to be signal transduction vehicles. Although, under certain conditions, γ–δ TCRs can recognize classical class-I proteins as a ligand,[106] the true ligands for the γ–δ TCR are by and large unknown.

The distinctive tissue distribution of the γ–δ TCR has led to speculations concerning its function. Recent commentaries by Janeway and his colleagues[107,108] have invoked the possibility of the involvement of nonpolymorphic (nonclassical) class I proteins in γ–δ TCR-mediated immune surveillance. Earlier it was shown that the γ–δ TCR is selectively expressed on a very small subpopulation of T cells that do not express either CD4 or CD8 marker proteins. The function of this subset of T cells, termed "double negatives," is not known. Recently, it has been shown that a substantial proportion of this population of γ–δ TCR-bearing T cells is represented by dendritic epidermal cells (DEC) in mice.[109,110] Subsequently, Bonneville et al[111] have discovered that an additional population of murine lymphoid cells, termed intestinal intraepithelial lymphocytes (IELs), are also enriched in γ–δ but, unlike the epidermal cells, IELs are CD8[+]. This phenotype would then resemble that of the α–β TCR-bearing T cells that are restricted by classical class-I proteins. Upon comparing the γ–δ receptors of these two populations (DECs and IELs) it was found that the γ chains in the two cases migrated differently when subjected to one-dimensional polyacrylamide gel electrophoresis. Further analyses revealed that the genes encoding the γ-chains in DECs had different molecular rearrangements than those seen in IELs. Thus, the γ-chain in IEL is encoded by the Vγ7 gene segment and that in the DEC by Vγ5. Both of these genomic rearrangements are distinct from those seen in mature thymocytes that utilize Vγ4. The heterogenity in V-region usage of the γ-chain genes in different tissues may be a reflection of the functional diversity of the γ–δ receptor. Of particular interest is the γ–δ receptors on IELs. The cytolytic activity of IELs has already been demonstrated.[112] Because of their CD8[+] nature, a true analogy can now be made between the ligands of γ–δ TCRs of IEL and α–β TCRs of CD8[+] T cells. However, relatively restricted usage of V genes in IEL may be a reflection of the fact that the γ–δ TCRs bind a ligand that is not as polymorphic as the ligands for α–β TCRs. The observation that the nonclassical class-I proteins are nonpolymorphic raises a possibility that they serve as ligands for the γ–δ TCRs.

Recent studies by Lambert et al (see Cellular Stress and MHC-I Expression) have shown that ultraviolet light C (250 mms) (UVC) and several other DNA-damaging agents can augment the expression of a select group of class-I proteins, possibly including the nonclassical determinants. It is proposed that these novel antigens serve as marker molecules for the damaged cells that are recognized by a specific set of cytotoxic T cells. The T cells recognize the novel class-I proteins either alone or in association with a "self"-peptide generated in response to cellular DNA damage. A role for UVC-induced nonclassical class-I proteins in such a process of immune elimination is an attractive possibility in light of the fact that skin, which is the most exposed part of the body to the UVC component of sunlight, is enriched by the extra thymic population of γ–δ TCR-bearing T cells. It is conceivable that under conditions of chronic damage to epidermal cells, damaged cells are selectively removed following induced expression of novel class-I proteins and γ–δ TCR-mediated cell lysis.

Molecular Approaches to the Study of Expression of Novel Class-I Genes

Despite large-scale cloning of the human class-I region, it is not clear how many of the 20 or more genes identified as belonging to the class-I family are actually expressed. Transfection experiments, in one case, revealed that only three such

Table 5-3. Oligonucleotide Primers Specific for Various Exons

No.	Sequence	Specificity
1	5′CACTCCATGAGGTATTTC3′	5′ region of exon 2. Using this primer, exon 2 can be sequenced in 5′–3′ direction.
2	3′CGATGATGTTGGTCTCGCTCC5′	3′ region of exon 2. Using this primer, exon 2 can be sequenced in 3′–5′ direction.
3	3′TCTTGCCCTTCCTCTGCGACGACGTCGC5′	3′ region of exon 3. Using this primer, exon 3 can be sequenced in the 3′–5′ direction.
4	3′TCGGGGAGTGGGACTCTACCC5′	3′ region of exon 4. Using this primer, exon 4 can be sequenced in the 3′–5′ direction.
5	3′TTCCCCACTCCTCACCCCAGACTC5′	5′ region of V intron. Using this primer, exon V can be sequenced in 3′–5′ direction.

genes may be expressed.[102] This, however, does not exclude the possibility that many of the transfected genes may not have been expressed because of tissue- or cell-specific barriers. Because of the lack of information concerning tissue-specific class-I expression, a global approach to identify all potentially expressed class I genes would be to first determine the nucleotide sequence of each member of this family. Although this would be an arduous task, as each of the genes occupies approximately 4 kb of DNA, an alternative would be to determine only the sequence of the exons in each of the genes, which would involve the sequencing of approximately 1.6 kb of DNA from each clone. In order to facilitate the sequencing of these restricted areas, it would be advantageous to have available exon-specific sequencing primers that could be universally used for every member of this family. From the available sequences of several class-I genes, we have determined that stretches of 18 or more conserved nucleotides can be identified among class-I genes at the boundaries of the exons and introns. Based on these sequences, exon-specific sequencing primers have been designed, and a list of such primers is given in Table 5-3. On the assumption that these sequences are conserved among other class-I genes, these primers would be valuable in rapid sequencing of the class-I genes. It should be noted, however, that even if these primers hybridize to various class-I genes, they may not prove to be suitable for sequencing, as it has been noted that even a single base pair mismatch within the primer–template hybrid can render DNA polymerase inactive in extending DNA synthesis.[116]

A comprehensive compilation of sequence data would be useful in identifying intact, truncated, and pseudogenes. Sequence data can also be used to predict whether the product of a given gene is cell bound or secreted. Thus, the presence of an inframe stop codon in the fifth exon can always be considered a diagnostic feature of genes that encode secretory class-I molecules. Alternative RNA splicing of some class-I genes has also been reported, both in normal cells and in a variety of tumors,[119,120] and the protein products of such splicing events are expressed as novel secretory molecules. Nucleotide sequence data may be helpful in identifying other such unusually placed splicing signals.

Comparative sequence analyses would provide further insights into the exon-shuffling events that have occurred between class-I genes during the course of evolution.[18] The mechanisms for the generation of allelic polymorphism at the human class-I loci remain undefined, although parallels are often made with the murine system, where gene conversion seems to be an operative mechanism underlying the generation of genetic diversity. A variety of mutants have been isolated in the mouse to demonstrate the exchange of stretches of nucleotides between the class-I genes located several thousand base pairs apart.[17] The available nucleotide sequence data were informative in identifying the "donor" and "acceptor" genes involved in these gene conversion events. Although there is no direct evidence for gene conversion events among the human class-I genes, the presence of allelic subtypes strongly indicates that a mechanism similar to gene conversion may be operative. When the nucleotide sequences of the genes of the two subtypes of HLA-B27 antigens (HLAB27w and HLAB27k) were compared, a pattern of gene conversion-like events was noticed.[121] When the sequence comparison was extended to non-HLA-B27 genes, a putative donor gene was also identified. Sequence data from every member of this gene family would be helpful in studying the frequency of such gene conversion events.

The identification of "intact" novel class-I genes from sequence analyses would also shorten the list of class-I genes for which functional studies should be undertaken. Production of transgenic mice for each of these novel class-I genes may be an important step in the study of the role of these genes in immune function. Transgenic mice have been successfully used to express the antigens derived from each of the three well-characterized HLA loci, namely HLA-A,[26] -B,[27] and -C.[25] It remains to be seen, however, whether the non-HLA-A, -B, and -C locus-derived proteins can also be tolerably expressed as transgenes. One important question that remains is the influence of these transgenes on the TCR (both $\alpha-\beta$ and $\gamma-\delta$) repertoire of the recipient mice. A bias toward any of the known V-region gene usages in these mice could lead to design of experiments to dissect further the molecular mechanisms underlying the phenomenon of selective use of the TCR repertoire. Transgenic animals would also serve as an excellent system to determine whether these novel proteins have any influence on graft rejection and whether they can serve as restriction elements in the process of antigen recognition.

Regulation of Human MHC-I Expression

Expression of MHC-I has been well studied and shown to be regulated over development, as well as during viral infection, viral transformation, and cellular transformation, and in response to specific substances, including interferons.[122] Recently, however, it has become clear that MHC-I expression is also regulated by exposure to several forms of cellular stress, including DNA damage[123] and ethanol treatment.[124] These observations suggest the possibility that the induction of MHC-1 is regulated in response to changes in cellular physiology brought about by agents or regimens that perturb cellular metabolism. In the following sections we review current thinking concerning the regulation of MHC-I expression, and in particular the emerging understanding of the involvement of specific cis-acting DNA regulatory elements and trans-acting factors in MHC-I transcriptional control.

Developmental Regulation of MHC-I Expression

Previous studies have demonstrated that the MHC-I represents a family of developmentally regulated genes. For example, MHC-I antigens are not expressed on the cell surface of the nonfertilized egg or on early mouse embryos.[125] Neither are they expressed on undifferentiated embryonal carcinoma (EC) cells, although in vitro differentiation of these cells, induced by such chemicals as retinoic acid or dibutyrl cAMP,[126,127] results in cell-surface expression of MHC-I. Otherwise, MHC-I is expressed on most adult somatic cells, with the exception, for example, of neurons.

Regulation of MHC-I expression over development may involve multiple mechanisms. Although there is no evidence for major rearrangements of murine H-2 genes during development,[128] there is evidence that changes in H-2 expression during chemically induced differentiation of EC cells is correlated with partial demethylation.[129] Suprisingly, increased expression specifically of the H-2K gene in differentiated F9 cells is correlated with an *increase* in gene methylation.[130] Expression of MHC-I over development may also be mediated by the action of interferons. Expression of MHC-I in mouse embryos has been found, for example, to be responsive to interferons, although this effect appears to be stage specific.[131] This finding has led to the hypothesis that developmentally regulated expression of MHC-I is controlled, in part, by endogenous production of interferons and by the expression of interferon receptors.[132]

Effects of Viral Infection, Viral Transformation, and Cellular Transformation

A considerable body of evidence suggests that viral infection and viral transformation can alter class-I expression. A comprehensive review of this topic has recently been presented by Brown et al.[122] Studies of the effects of several transforming viruses, including DNA and RNA viruses, indicate that levels of MHC-I expression can be regulated both up and down, depending on the specific virus and the specific stage of viral infection or viral transformation.[122] The effects seen among viruses at any one stage are also not consistent: Several viruses, such as radiation-induced leukemia virus (RadLV), human adenovirus type 12 (Ad12), and Moloney murine leukemia virus (MuLV), down regulate MHC-I expression following viral transformation, whereas both polyoma virus (Py) and simian virus 40 (SV40) enhance expression. Likewise, Harvey sarcoma virus (HSV) infection down regulates MHC, whereas infection by most other viruses is seen to enhance expression.

Studies with experimental tumor models have previously led to the description of a functional role for MHC class-I molecules in tumor progression and metastasis.[133–135] Studies with the murine methylcholanthracene-induced T10 fibrosarcoma cell line as well as AKR thymomas indicate that re-presentation of the H-2K^k allele, following gene transfer into metastatic subclones that are not expressing this gene, leads to loss of metastatic potential in stably transformed recipient clones. This loss of metastatic potential is thought to reflect the essential role of this allele as a restriction element for cytotoxic T-cell-mediated tumor cell lysis.

The involvement of MHC class-I alleles in metastatic potential has also been shown, however, to be dependent on the relative expression of different class-I alleles. Although transfection of highly metastatic T10 fibrosarcoma subclones with the H-2K^k gene reduces tumorigenicity and metastasis in syngeneic mice, transfection of nonmetastatic clones with a different allele, H-2D^k, leads to acquisition of metastatic potential. Recently, Alon et al[136] have further demonstrated that transfection of the H-2D^k gene into nonmetastatic lines leads not only to acquisition of metastatic potential but to a pronounced reduction in the expression of both Kirstenras mRNA and p21 protein. By contrast, the introduction of the H2-K^k allele reduced tumorigenicity and abolished metastasis but had no effect on Ki-ras expression. These studies demonstrate that the acquisition and loss of metastatic potential involving altered expression of different MHC class-I alleles may reflect multiple functions of these gene products in tumor selection.

Independent evidence that suppression of MHC class-I antigen production can contribute to tumorigenicity has also been obtained from studies of adenovirus type 12 transformation of rodent cells.[133] Cells transformed by adenovirus type 12 were found to be oncogenic by virtue of having escaped from T-cell immunity, by reduced expression of class-I gene products.

Recent studies, however, have called into question the association between lowered MHC-I expression and increased tumorigenicity.[137] Haddada and co-workers[137] have concluded that the expression of either high or low levels of MHC-I antigens is, at most, a minor factor in the differences observed among over 30 adenovirus and SV40-transformed hamster cell lines tested in their tumor-inducing capacity in naive, immunocompetent, syngeneic or allogeneic adult hamsters.

An alternative model of the involvement of MHC-I in tumorigenicity suggests a correlation between decreased MHC-I expression and an increased susceptibility to natural killer (NK) cells.[138] It has been hypothesized that tumorigenic cells with reduced levels of MHC-I have reduced tumorigenicity because they are eliminated from the host by endogenous NK cells. A recent study indicates that this may not be a general mechanism, however.[138] In this study MHC-I loss variants of the murine hepatoma cell line BW7756 were transfected with the H-2k^b gene to generate H-2k^b expressing clones. Natural killer cell, CTL and tumor challenge studies of these transfected tumor cells indicate no correlation between MHC-I levels and NK susceptibility and/or tumorigenicity. This study, as well as recent studies using BL6 melanoma cells, indicate that the correlation between low MHC-I expression, tumorigenicity, and high NK sensitivity may only be applicable to a subset of all tumors.

To date there has been little systematic study of the role of MHC class-I antigens in progression of human malignancies, and particularly in neoplasms of epithelial origin. A limited number of studies of both human breast carcinoma[139] and human retinoblastoma[140] do confirm, however, that some human tumors show a reduced expression of certain MHC antigens. In these studies only polymorphic MHC molecules were examined.

In addition to studies which indicate that transfection of specific MHC class-I alleles into certain rodent tumor cell lines can decrease their tumorigenicity in vivo, there is further evidence that treatment of these rodent lines with specific biological response modifiers, including immune interferon, can also transiently reduce tumorigenicity by augmenting the expression of MHC class-I antigens.[141]

We are not aware, however, of any studies to evaluate the prognostic value of MHC class I in the progression of any single type of human malignancy. Although we would stress that both tumor progression and metastasis are multistep, multifactor processes,[142] of which altered MHC class-I expression is only one mechanism, there is sufficient genetic evidence, from experimental rodent systems, to suggest that comprehensive molecular studies of MHC involvement in human tumor progression may be of value.

Cellular Stress and MHC-I Expression

It is now clear that several forms of environmental cellular stress are themselves capable of inducing elevated and enhanced expression of MHC-I. This includes ethanol stress[124] and cellular DNA damage.[123]

Singer et al[124] have found that ethanol can enhance the cell-surface expression of MHC-I antigens in a number of different mouse and human cell lines. These investigators have found that in ethanol-treated mouse L cells the increased cell-surface expression of MHC-I is also accompanied by an increase in steady-state mRNA levels. These effects were detected at an effective ethanol concentration of 1%, suggesting that this modality of induction may be of physiological significance. In a recent follow up study these same investigators have, in fact, demonstrated evidence of increased MHC-I expression on human peripheral blood lymphocytes during acute ethanol intoxication.[143]

Recently, we have demonstrated an enhancement of MHC-I protein synthesis by DNA damage in cultured human fibroblasts and keratinocytes.[123,144] In these studies we have used the QUEST system of standardized high-resolution two-dimensional protein gel electrophoresis (HR2D), quantitative analysis, and computer-based protein database development.[145,146] Specifically, we compared the effects of UVC and benzo[a]pyrene–trans-7,8-dihydrodiol-9,10 epoxide (BPDE) in the normal fetal lung fibroblast strain LI58, as well as three DNA repair deficient strains, GM5509 (Xeroderma Pigmentosum Group A),[147] GM1389 (Xeroderma Pigmentosum Variant),[148] and GM1915 [A Familial Hypercholesterolemia Hyperlipoproteinemia strain deficient for initiation of UVC- and BPDE-induced unscheduled DNA repair synthesis (UDS)].[148,149] In addition, we studied the effects elicited in the SV40 DNA-transformed human keratinocyte line SVK14[150] by UVC, BPDE, N-Methyl-N''-nitro-N-nitrosoguanidine (MNNG), and 7,12-dimethylbenz-[a]anthracene (DMBA). To test whether DNA damage-inducible proteins are under negative regulation, we have also compared the inducible patterns of change elicited by DNA damage with the changes induced by single, low doses of the protein synthesis inhibitor, cycloheximide (CHX).

Initially, we examined the effects of UVC and CHX on MHC-I expression after exposure of quiescent, confluent cultures of LI58 cells. Shown in Plate 5-1 are computer images of the regions containing MHC-I from the HR2D patterns of total cell lysates prepared from control, UVC-treated, and CHX-treated cells. As seen, UVC and CHX both induced the synthesis of MHC-I within 4 h. Induction of MHC-I in resting cultures of nondividing LI58 cells suggests that the increase in synthetic rate is not a secondary consequence of DNA damage or CHX-induced arrest of DNA synthesis but is, instead, a direct consequence of treatment with either regimen. The identity of the MHC-I products was determined by direct immunoprecipitation of MHC-I products from CHX-induced LI58 cells, using the anti-framework MHC-I rabbit sera K-455.[151]

To further test whether MHC-I induction in human fibroblasts by DNA damage is dependent on specific DNA lesions or on DNA repair, we examined the effects of both UVC and BPDE in exponentially growing cultures of four human fibroblast strains, including LI58 and the DNA damage-sensitive strains GM5509, GM1915, and GM1389. Both UVC and BPDE induced MHC-I expression in LI58 cells within 4 h, indicating that the triggering signal for induction was not restricted to DNA lesions induced by UVC damage. The UDS-defective lines GM5509 and GM1915 and the UDS-competent, postreplication repair-defective line GM1389 exhibited highly altered patterns of MHC-I induction. In particular, higher average ratios of MHC-I induction in the repair-defective lines suggests a positive correlation between an increased sensitivity to DNA damage and the extent of MHC-I induction.

Finally, we examined patterns of MHC-I expression induced in the SV40 DNA-transformed human keratinocyte line, SVK14, after exposure to several different DNA-damaging regimens. Although the overall number of K-455-reactive MHC-I products detected in total cell lysates patterns of this transformed cell type was lower than for any of the primary fibroblast strains tested, all DNA damage regimens tested, as well as CHX, induced MHC-I. Induction of MHC-I was also observed after treatment with ultraviolet light A (UVA) (345–440 nm), although the dose used was greater than 1000 times that of UVC. The metabolic inhibitor hydroxyurea (5 m mol/L) alone did not induce MHC-I overall, again indicating that arrest of DNA synthesis is insufficient for MHC-I induction. Time course studies demonstrated a persistence of these effects to 24 h after exposure.

Our studies demonstrate that MHC-I induction is part of the cellular stress response elicited in human fibroblasts and keratinocytes by several classes of DNA-damaging agents. The ability of CHX to induce MHC-I suggests that this induction may serve as a probe for the action of a cellular stress response pathway in mammalian cells under negative regulatory control. Recent studies indicate that mouse H-2K and D mRNA are transcriptionally induced by protein synthesis inhibitors, including CHX (R Zeff and S Nathenson, personal communication), and that RNA synthesis inhibitors can synergize with γ-interferon in the transcriptional induction of MHC-I in human K562 leukemia cells.[152] These findings are consistent with the

AP1

```
                                                                                        GT G G-- -
                          ******                                     C          T-               G T  G G-- -
HLA B7    GGACTCAGGCAGACAGTGTGACAAAGAG-GCTTGGTGT-AGGAGAAGAGAGGGATCAGGACGAAGTCCCA-GGCCCG-GACGG-GGCTCTCAGGGT
JY328
HLA A2    A                 G     --T G C  C        CAC  A C      G       G        G   CA G  TT
```

NF-KB   IRE

```
                                          ***************  *******************                   TC C
                                                                                        C C         CC C
                              A       T      G C          T                              T T C  TCT   C A
HLA B7    CTCAGGCTCCGAGGGCCGCGTCGCAATGGGGAG-CGCAGCGTTGGGGATTCCCACTCCCTGAGTTTCACTTCTTCT-----CCCAACTTGTG
HLA Cw3                                                                                  T T C  TCT   C A
JY328
HLA A2        C   A - G T   A G T    T C  C          -A T GC                              T T  CCTGCT   C AC
HLA A3        C   A T T    AA G T    T C  C          -A T GC                              T T C CCTGCT
```

```
                                                                   G C   CCNN               GG        T
                                            C GAATG   A        A    A                            CT-- T
HLA B7    TCGGGTCCTTCTTC-TAGGATACTCGTG-ACGCGTCCCACTTCCCACTCCCATTGGGTATTGGA--TATCTA--GAAGCCAATCAGCGTCGCC
HLA Cw3                     C GAATG   A -    A -   - G C  G-TTC AG              C-
JY328     A                 C  -    AC       GA G T     - G C G  T C GA
HLA A2    A                 A C -   AC G     GA G T       G C G  T C GA                            T   T
HLA A3                                                                                            T   T
```

"CCAAT"

"TATAA"

```
HLA B7    GCGGTCCCA-GT-TCTAAAGTCCCCAGCACCCACCCGGACTCAGAGTCTCCTCAGACGCCGAG-
HLA Cw3   A       G     G        GT              T   C
JY328     A       G     G        GT
HLA A2            G GG  C           G           G   T  C
HLA A3            G T      C  G                 G   T  C           G
```

Figure 5-5. Regulatory motifs in the 5' upstream region of human MHC-I genes. The nucleotide sequences of five class-I genes have been aligned. Dashes indicate gaps. IRE, interferon response element; AP1, AP1 consensus binding sequence; NF-*k*B, NF-KB consensus binding sequence. The sequences were obtained from references as follows: HLA-B7 (note: a sequencing discrepancy in the IRE region of B7 is shown corrected),[83] HLA-Cw3,[113] JY328,[82] HLA-A2,[83] and HLA-A3.[115]

Interferon (IFN)-inducible transcription of MHC-I genes has been demonstrated to be mediated by a cis-acting regulatory element, the interferon response element (IRE).[153] Ozato and co-workers[154] have recently demonstrated that this IRE binds a constitutive nuclear factor that is present in lymphocytes and fibroblasts even in the absence of IFN treatment. Following induction, two new binding activities were detected, one of which requires de novo protein synthesis. The sequence requirements for protein binding identified in this study have shown a motif, 5'-AGTT-TCNNT(C)TC(T)CT-3', which is found present in both MHC-I genes (see Figure 5-5) and other IFN-inducible genes[155] and which represents the basic structural requirement for specific binding of nuclear factors and for transcriptional induction.

Baldwin and Sharp[156] have identified two transcription factors, NF-*k*B and H2TF1, which interact with a single regulatory sequence present in the mouse H2-2k[b] promoter. Significantly, they have shown that NF-*k*B, an inducible B-cell factor that binds the *K* immunoglobulin light-chain gene enhancer, also binds the H2TF1 regulatory sequence. The DNA binding activity of NF-*k*B has itself been shown to be inducible in pre-B cells by lipopolysaccharide (LPS), in non-B cells by phorbol 12-myristate B-acetate (TPA), and in T cells by mitogens. Recent studies[157] have further demonstrated that enhancer binding of NF-*k*B is CHX inducible and is mediated by a posttranslational mechanism involving the cytoplasmic inhibitor I kB. As shown in Figure 5-5 the NF-*k*B–H2TF1 enhancer sequence is also found present in the 5' flanking region of the human B7, Cw3, JY328, A2, and A3 alleles. The high degree of sequence conservation between these alleles in this enhancer and in its location is striking and suggests that NF-*k*B may play an important role in transcriptional control of human MHC-I gene expression.

The binding sites for a transcription factor designated as AP1 (Activator Protein-1) are also present with a high degree of homology in the 5' flanking region of human MHC-I genes. As shown in Figure 5-5 one conserved site is located upstream from the transcriptional start and is present as a 6/7 match with the AP1 consensus enhancer. Studies of the murine H-2 gene indicate that AP1 sequences present in the enhancer are in fact capable of binding specific murine nuclear factors.[158] Recent studies have also demonstrated that c-fos and c-jun (the fos-associated protein p39) are capable of interacting to stimulate transcription of AP1-responsive genes.[159-161] Whether the murine H-2 AP1 binding nuclear factors and c-fos–c-jun are one and the same has not been determined, however.

The relationship between c-fos–c-jun and the AP1 binding sequence may be of significance in understanding MHC-I regulation. It has previously been reported, for example, that c-fos gene expression is positively correlated with MHC-I expression in both murine tumor cells and human leukemic cells.[162] Feldman and co-workers have investigated the requirement of c-fos expression for gamma-interferon inducibility of H-2K in the metastatic mouse 3LL carcinoma-derived cell line D122 and find that increased MHC-I expression is preceded by activation of c-fos. These studies have been confirmed by transfection studies in which c-fos has been shown to activate the H-2K gene directly. Feldman et al have also demonstrated that during chemically induced maturation of human leukemic cells to macrophages fos gene expression was induced, followed in turn by cell-surface expression of MHC-I.[162]

Another feature of the 5' region of MHC-I genes sequenced to date is the presence of "HTF (Hpa II tiny fragments) islands," DNA sequences in which CpG is abundant and nonmethylated.[163] It has been previously been argued that these HTF islands function to distinguish regions of the genome that are constantly available for interaction with nuclear components.[164] In the case of human MHC-I it appears that HTF islands are detected only in the expressed genes A, B, and C, although they are also present in the pseudogene HLAp12.1.4.[163] Recent evidence suggests, however, that HLAp12.1.4 is in fact a transcribed gene (M Chorney, personal communications). The HTF islands present in an additional 20–30 other human MHC-I genes are methylated, which supports the view that these genes may not be expressed.

At least two negative regulatory elements (NREs) have been identified in MHC-I genes. In mouse, an NRE has been found in the H2-L gene, which functions only in undifferentiated embryonal teratocarcinoma (F9) cells.[165] After retinoic acid induction of F9 differentiation, however, this element acts instead as a positive enhancer. An NRE has also been identified in the 5' flanking region of a gene, PD1, which encodes a porcine classical transplantation antigen.[166] This NRE reduces PDI expression 5- to 10-fold and also functions on a heterologous simian virus 40 (SV40) promoter. These investigators have proposed[166] that the PDI NREs also interact with positive regulatory elements and that their functions are mediated by trans-acting cellular factors. The possible interaction of a labile transcriptional repressor with the PDI NRE is suggested by the further observation that PDI transcription is CHX inducible and that this induction is mediated by the NRE sequence itself (D Singer, personal communication).

In addition to the enhancer elements mentioned above, several investigators have pointed to the presence of further regulatory motifs present in the 5' region of certain human MHC-I genes. This includes a sequence present uniquely in JY328 (position −470 to −529) with strong homology to the previously identified viral enhancer element GGTGTGGAAAG (B Duceman, personal communication). In addition, multiple copies of a tandem duplicate repeat, Py CAGG, are highly conserved among these genes. The specific function of these elements in transcriptional regulation of MHC-I has not been determined, however.

Regulation of Human MHC-I Expression and MHC-I Function

It is clear that MHC-I gene expression is highly regulated, in response to both exogenous and endogenous stimuli, and that transcriptional control of MHC-I gene expression is dependent on the interplay of multiple trans-acting transcriptional factors with several distinct cis-acting DNA sequence motifs. Despite this emerging appreciation of the complexity of mechanisms underlying control of MHC-I expression, there is as yet no clear understanding of the role that these various mechanisms play in determining the overall cellular function(s) of the MHC-I products.

At least three major questions remain concerning the significance of induced changes in MHC-I expression. First, it is unclear how or whether *quantitative* changes in levels of expression of specific MHC-I products can effect MHC-I function, particularly in regard to antigen presentation and immune selection. Although quantitative differences in basal levels of MHC-I expression among different cell types have previously been observed, the significance, if any, of modulating these levels is unknown. Second, it is as yet unclear whether quantitative changes in levels of class-I expression are of significance in the absence of antigen presentation. As mentioned above, for example, the ability of cellular stress, such as DNA damage, to enhance MHC-I protein synthesis may provide a mechanism to target damaged cells for immune elimination, but it is not known whether this also requires presentation of self-antigens. As discussed below, if MHC-I functions are more broadly defined to encompass roles beyond antigen presentation, then quantitative modulation of MHC-I levels per se may be sufficient to invoke functional responses. Third, it is as yet not clear how or whether *qualitative* differences in MHC-I expression affect cellular functions. It is apparent from studies of the role of specific murine H-2 alleles in tumorigenicity that the ratios of expression of different class-I genes can have a profound effect on cell recognition by CTLs. Detailed studies of the differential effects of stimuli, including interferons, on the relative expression of specific sets of human MHC-I genes are required to permit a more detailed assessment to be made of the significance of inducible class-I expression.

Although the classic view of MHC-I function centers on its central role in mediating graft rejection and as restriction elements in antigen presentation to CTLs, there is growing evidence that MHC-I may also play a functional role in several other immunologic and nonimmunologic cellular processes. Indeed Flaherty[15] has suggested that involvement in such nonimmune cellular processes may define as important an overall function for MHC-I as that per se in immune processes. This includes direct association between MHC-I antigens and hormone receptors, including insulin receptor, EGF receptor, and leutenizing hormone receptor; direct participation in the activation of both T cells and B cells; mediation of cell adhesion; a role as receptors for certain viruses; chemosensory functions; and the ability to interact with endogenous substances, such as γ-endorphin, and exogenous substances, such as penicillin. Dasgupta and Yunis[167] have in fact recently suggested that these various roles depict the function of MHC-I in immune regulation as a special case of a more generalized cellular function.

There is evidence, for example, that MHC class-I glycoproteins are involved as regulatory molecules in membrane-associated receptor systems.[168–173] Studies of the interactions between mouse class-I MHC antigens and the insulin receptor[168] have shown that both H-2K and H-2D molecules can be found in association with subpopulations of the insulin receptor, although there is as yet no clear biological or physiological understanding of the significance of these associations.

There is also evidence that MHC-I plays a functional role in activation of both T and B cells. Dasgupta and co-workers[167] have demonstrated that anti-class-I antibodies can inhibit PHA-induced T-cell mitogenesis by blocking an early event in a Ca^+-dependent pathway of cell activation. In addition, it has previously been shown that monoclonal antibodies directed against MHC-I and β2m are capable of suppressing primary mixed lymphocyte reactions and anti-T3, lectin, and virus-induced T-cell activation.[174,175] In further studies Dasgupta and co-workers[167] have reported that this suppression is mediated by inhibitory factors produced by monocyte adherent cells as a direct consequence of antibody binding to MHC-I, which demonstrates a ligand-receptor-like function for MHC-I on adherent cell surfaces. In recent studies these same investigators have demonstrated that MHC-I molecules present on monocytes–macrophages in fact behave like receptor molecules in that they are internalized. Approximately 30% of MHC-I molecules present on the cell surface were found to be endocytosed within 1 h. Internalization was mediated by coated pits and coated vesicles and the endocytosed molecules were transferred from endosomes to trans-golgi reticulum and trans-golgi cisternae, suggesting recycling back to the cell surface.[176]

In studies of the role of MHC-I in the proliferation of human B lymphocytes, Taylor et al[177] have demonstrated that anti-HLA class-I can inhibit the T-cell-independent proliferation of B cells. Specifically they have tested the ability of three monoclonal antibodies, including W6–32, to inhibit proliferation of human B cells stimulated by the T-independent mitogen *Staphylococcus aureus,* although not proliferation induced by the phorbol ester phorbol-12-myristate 13-acetate (PMA). These investigators have suggested that MHC-I are involved in the regulation of human B-lymphocyte proliferation and may regulate a critical event preceding the up regulation of protein kinase C activity.

There is also evidence for a specific association between MHC-I and the CD8 molecules of human suppressor-cytotoxic cells.[178] This association is due, at least in part, to disulfide bonding. Although the significance of this association is not clear it has been suggested that intercellular recognition between the CD8 of T cells and the class-1 of accessory or target cells may be regulated by CD8–class 1 complex formation on suppressor-cytotoxic T cells, and specifically by the cleavage of CD8–class-1 disulfide bonds.

The overall significance, however, of HLA class-I involvement in cellular processes besides those of antigen presentation and CTL-mediated cell lysis remains to be determined.

Summary

The recent solution of the three-dimensional structure for HLA-A2[11,12] has provided important new insights into the structure–function relationships of a classical class-I protein. The extension of this analysis to other classical class-I antigens is likely to improve our understanding of the functional significance of high levels of allelic polymorphism, which are unprecedented in the class-I gene family.

Perhaps of equal significance are the recent findings that the human class-I family includes several nonclassical, nonpolymorphic genetic determinants, including the gene RS5.[32] This observation raises anew questions concerning the overall cellular functions of the class-I products. As we have discussed, nonclassical class-I products may serve in several novel capacities. These include; (1) a role as a "reservoir of functional proteins'' that have the same capabilities as their classical counterparts but are utilized only under special physiological conditions; (2) a role as ligands for γ–δ TCRs, a function that has been proposed by Janeway and his colleagues.[107,108] This would be consistent with our hypothesis that the nonclassical determinants may be an integral part of the cellular stress response induced in epidermal cells by regimens that perturb cellular metabolism, including DNA damage; (3) a role in interacting with the integral membrane protein CD8.[99] As mentioned above, the CD8 associated HLA-like molecules that are found on activated T cells represent only a minor proportion of the total class-I molecules, possibly hinting that they are the nonclassical class-I proteins, which are poorly expressed when compared to the constitutively expressed HLA-A, -B, -C proteins.

Our understanding of the function of the classical class-I molecules themselves has recently been expanded to encompass involvement in cellular processes beside those of graft rejection and as restriction elements in antigen presentation and CTL-mediated cell lysis. As reviewed above, this includes a role for class-I glycoproteins as regulatory molecules in membrane-associated receptor systems[168] and in the mitogenic activation of both B and T cells.[167,177] These various roles depict the function of MHC-I in immune regulation as a special case of a more generalized cellular function.[167]

Finally, it is clear that MHC-I genes are highly regulated, in response to specific classes of exogenous and endogenous stimuli, and that inducible class-I expression is mediated by the interaction of specific trans-acting factors with cis-acting DNA regulatory motifs located in the 5' end of the class-I genes themselves. Of particular interest are recent observations by ourselves and others that cellular stress, including ethanol treatment[124] and DNA damage,[123] can enhance the synthesis of class-I proteins, and that class-I expression may in part be under negative regulation, since expression has been found to be inducible by protein synthesis inhibitors, including cycloheximide (Ref 123; D Singer, personal communication). Examination of the regulatory elements present in the 5' nontranscribed region of several human class-I genes has revealed the presence of multiple sequence motifs, including those required for AP1 binding and NF-kB binding (see Figure 5-5). These observations raise the possibility that class-I expression may be mediated by the action of one or more known gene products, including c-fos and/or c-jun, either individually or in physical association with one another,[159] and NF-kB.[157] Studies are currently underway in our laboratories to investigate the involvement of these gene products in inducible human class-I expression.

Acknowledgments

Work cited from the authors' own laboratories was supported by NIH grants CA 47519 and AI26334-01A2. We are grateful to A. Palestini for typing the manuscript and for comments provided by J McDonald, Z Ronai, and V Lotteau.

References

1. Klein J. *Natural History of the Major Histocompatibility Complex.* New York: Wiley-Interscience; 1986.

2. Svejgaard A, Platz P, Tyder LP. *Immunol Rev.* 1983;70:193.

3. Thomson G, Nicholas FW, Bodmer WF, O'Neill ME, Hedrick PW. *Tissue Antigens.* 1985;26:293.

4. Levi-Strauss M, Carroll M, Steinmetz M, Meo T. *Science.* 1988;240:201.

5. Nedwin GE, Naylor SL, Sakaguchi AY, Smith D, Nedwin JJ, Pennica D, Doeddel DB, Gray PW. *Nucl Acids Res.* 1985;13:6361.

6. Spies T, Blanck G, Bresnahn M, Sands J, Strominger JL. *Science.* (in press).

7. Edwards CQ, Griffen LM, Dadone MM, Sholnick MH, Kushner JP. *Am J Hum Genet.* 1986;38:805.

8. Paul WE, ed. *Fundamental Immunology.* New York: Raven Press; 1984.

9. Lawrance SK, Smith CL, Srivastava R, Cantor CR, Weissman SM. *Science.* 1987;235:1387.

10. Rodey GE, Fuller TC. *CRC Crit Rev Immunol.* 1987;7:229.

11. Bjorkman PJ, Saper MA, Samraoui B, Bennel WS, Strominger JL, Wiley DC. *Nature (London).* 1987;329:506.

12. Bjorkman PJ, Saper MA, Samraoui B, Bennel WS, Strominger JL, Wiley DC. *Nature (London).* 1987;329:512.

13. Klein J. *Human Immunol.* 1987;19:155.

14. Bodmer WF, Albert E, Bodmer JG, Dupont B, Mach B, Mayr WR, Sazasuki T, Schreuder Gm, Th, Svejgaard A, Terasaki PI. In Dupont B, ed. *Histocompatability Testing 1987.* New York: Springer Verlag; 1988.

15. 15. Flaherty L. *Human Immunol.* 1988;21:2.

16. Kourilsky P. *Biochimie.* 1983;65:85.

17. Nathenson SG, Galibter J, Pfaffenbach GM, Zeff RA. *Annu Rev Immunol.* 1986;4:471.

18. Holmes N, Parham P. *EMBO J.* 1985;4:2849.

19. Lust JA, Kumar V, Burton RC, Bartlett SC, Bennett M. *J Exp Med.* 1981;154:306.

20. Gotch F, Rothbard J, Howland K, Townsend A, McMichael A. *Nature (London).* 1987;326:881.

21. Grunnet N, Kristensen T, Krismeyer-Nielson F. *Tissue Antigens.* 1976;7:301.

22. Malissen B, Kristensen T, Goridis C, Madsen M, Mawas C. *Scand J Immunol* 1981;14:213.

23. Gussow D, Rein RS, Meyer I, Hoog WD, Seemann GHA, Hochstenbach FM, Ploegh HL. *Immunogenetics.* 1987;25:313.

24. Albrechtsen D, Moen T, Flatmark A, Halvorsen S, Jakobsen A, Jervell A, Solheim BG, Thorsby E. *Transplant Proc.* 1981;13:924.

25. Dill O, Kievits F, Koch S, Ivanyi P, Hammerling GJ. *Proc Natl Acad Sci (USA).* 1988;85:5664.

26. Bernhard EJ, Le AT, Barbosa JA, Lacy E, Engelhard VH. *J Exp Med.* 1988;168:1157.

27. Kievits F, Ivanyi P, Krimpenfort P, Berns A, Ploegh HL. *Nature (London).* 1987;329:447.

28. Taurog JD, Lowen L, Forman J, Hammer RE. *J Immunol.* 1988;141:4020.

29. Smith CL, Cantor CR. *Nature (London).* 1984;319:701.

30. Lawrance SK, Smith CL, Srivastava R, Cantor CR, Weissman SM. *Science.* 1987;235:1387.

31. Carroll M, Katzman P, Alicot EM, Koller BH, Geraghty DE, Orr HT, Strominger JL, Spies T. *Proc Natl Acad Sci (USA).* 1987;84:8535–8539.

32. Srivastava R, Chorney MJ, Lawrance SK, Pan J, Smith Z, Smith CL, Weissman SM. *Proc Natl Acad Sci (USA).* 1987;84:4224.

33. Srivastava R, Lawrance SK, Smith CL, Cantor CR, Weissman SM. *Trans Assoc Am Physicians.* 1986;99:1.

34. Koller BH, Orr HT. *J Immunol.* 1985;134:2727.

35. Orr HT, DeMars R. *Nature (London).* 1983;28:534.

36. Steinmetz M, Winoto A, Minard K, Hood L. *Cell.* 1982;28:489.

37. Weiss EH, Golden L, Fahrner K, Mellos AL, Devlin JJ, Bullman H, Tidens H, Bud H, Flavell RA. *Nature (London).* 1984;310:650.

38. Chimini G, Pontarotti P, Nguyen C, Toubert A, Boretto J, Jordan BR. *EMBO J.* 1988;7:395.

39. Pontarotti P, Chimini G, Nguyen C, Boretto J, Jordan BR. *Nucl Acids Res.* 1988;16:6767.

40. Duceman BW, Ness D, Rendo R, Chorney MJ, Srivastava R, Greenspan DS, Pan J, Weissman SM, Grumet FC. *Immunogenetics.* 1986;23:90.

41. Driesel AJ, Romer K, Schunter F, Laryea MD, Schnieder EM, Sernet PW, Hende J, Basler M, Kompf J. *Immunogenetics.* 1985;21:529.

42. Koller BH, Geraghty D, Orr HT, Shimizu Y, DeMars R. *Immunol Res.* 1987;6:1.

43. Paul P, Fauchet R, Boscher MY, Sayagh B, Masset M, Medrignac G, Dausset J, Cohen D. *Proc Natl Acad Sci (USA).* 1987;84:2872.

44. Krimpenfort P, Rudenko G, Hochstenbach F, Gussow D, Berns A, Ploegh HL. *EMBO J.* 1987;6:1673.

45. O'Neill AE, Reid K, Garberi JC, Karl M, Flaherty L. *Immunogenetics.* 1986;24:368.

46. Flaherty L. In Dorf M, ed. *Role of the Major Histocompatibility Complex in Immunobiology.* New York: Garland Press; 1981:35.

47. Harris RA, Hogartly PM, Penington DG, McKenzie IFC. *J Immunogenet.* 1984;11:265.

48. Kress M, Cosman D, Dhoury G, Jay G. *Cell.* 1983;34:189.

49. Robinson PJ, Bevec D, Mellor AL, Weiss EH. *Immunogenetics.* 1988;27:79.

50. Boyse EA, Old LJ. *Annu Rev Genet.* 1969;3:269.

51. Old LJ, Stockert E. *Annu Rev Genet.* 1977;17:127.

52. Klein J, Figueroa F, Nagy ZA. *Annu Rev Immunol.* 1983;1:119.

53. Hunt SW, Bronson KA, Cheroutre H, Hood L. *Fifth HLA and H-2 Cloning Workshop,* Les Avants, Switzerland, 1986.

54. Palmer MJ, Frelinger JA. *J Exp Med.* 1987;166:95–108.

55. Transy C, Nash SR, Wantine BD, Cochet M, Hunt III SW, Hood L, Kourilsky P. *J Exp Med.* 1987;166:341–361.

56. Robinson PJ. *Proc Natl Acad Sci (USA).* 1987;84:527–531.

57. Aldrich CJ, Rogers JR, Rich RR. *Immunogenetics.* 1988;28:334.

58. Stroynowsky I, Soloski M, Low MG, Hood L. *Cell.* 1987;50:759–768.

59. Chen YT, Obata Y, Stockert E, Old LJ. *J Exp Med.* 1985;162:1134.

60. Livant D, Blatt C, Hood L. *Cell.* 1986;47:461.

61. Singer DS, Hare J, Golding H, Flaherty L, Rudikoff S. *Immunogenetics.* 1988;28:13.

62. Rogers JR, Smith R III, Huston MM, Rich RR. *Adv Immunol.* 1986;38:313.

63. Terhorst C, van Agthoven A, LeClair K, Snow P, Reinherz E, Schlossman S. *Cell.* 1981;23:771.

64. Reinherz EL, Schlossman SF. *Cell.* 1980;29:821.

65. Reinherz ER, Kung PC, Goldstein G, Levey RH, Schlossman SF. *Proc Natl Acad Sci (USA).* 1980;77:1588.

66. Vitetta ES, Uhr JW, Boyse EA. *J Immunol.* 1978;114:252.

67. Bushkin Y, Chorney MJ, Diamante E, Fu SM, Wang CY. *Mol Immunol.* 1984;21:821.

68. Martin LH, Calabi F, Milstein C. *Proc Natl Acad Sci (USA).* 1986;83:9154.

69. van de Rijn M, Lerch PG, Knowles RW, Terhorst C. *J Immunol.* 1983;131:851.

70. Kahn-Perles B, Wietzerbin J, Caillol DH, LeMonnier F. *J Immunol.* 1985;134:1759.

71. Fauchet R, Boscher M, Bouhallier O, Merdrignac G, Genetet B, Termel P, Charron DJ. *Human Immunol.* 1986;17:30.

72. Crepaldi T, Peruccio D, Leechi M, Resegotti L, Guerra M, Funaro A, Richiardi P. *J Immunogenet.* 1987;14:219.

73. Duran LW, Pease LR. *J Immunol.* 1988;141:295.

74. Malissen M, Malissen B, Jordan BR. *Proc Natl Acad Sci. (USA).* 1982;79:893.

75. Biro PA, Pan J, Sood AK, Kole R, Reddy VB, Weissman SM. *Cold Spring Harbor Symp Quant Biol.* 1983;42:1082.

76. Mizuno S, Trapani JA, Koller BH, Dupont B, Yang SY. *J Immunol.* 1988;140:40024.

77. Koller BH, Geraghty DE, Shimizu Y, DeMars R, Orr HT. *J Immunol.* 1988;141:897–904.

78. Geraghty DE, Koller BH, Orr HT. *Proc Natl Acad Sci (USA).* 1987;84:9145–9149.

79. Ronne H, Widemark E, Rask L, Peterson PA. *Proc Natl Acad Sci (USA).* 1985;82:5860–5864.

80. Rogers JH. *EMBO J.* 1985;4:794.

81. Jordan BR, Caillol D, Damotte M, Delovitch T, Ferrier P, Kahn Perles B, Kourilsky F, Layet C, Bouiteiller PL, Lemonnier FA, Malissen M, N'guyen C, Sire J, Sodoyer R, Strachan T, Trucy J. *Immunol Rev.* 1985;84:73.

82. Duceman BW, Wang AM. *Nucl Acids Res.* 1988;16:10391.

83. Srivastava R, Duceman BW, Biro PA, Sood AK, Weissman SM. *Immunol Rev.* 1985;85:93.

84. Davidson WF, Kress M, Khoury G, Jay G. *J Biol Chem.* 1985;260:13414.

85. Parham P, Lomen CE, Lawlor DA, Ways JP, Holmes N, Coppin L, Salter RD, Wan AM, Ennis PD. *Proc Natl Acad Sci (USA).* 1988;85:4005–4009.

86. Kariya Y, Kato K, Hayashizaki Y, Himeno S, Tarui S, Matsubara K. *Gene.* 1987;53:1.

87. Lin CS, Goldthwait DA, Samols D. *Cell.* 1988;54:153.

88. Lambert ME, McDonald JF, Weinstein IB, eds. *Eukaryotic Transposable elements as mutagenic agents.* Cold Spring Harbor, NY: Cold Spring Harbor Laboratory; 1988.

89. Baralle FE, Shoulders CC, Goodbourn S, Jeffreys A, Proudfoot NJ. *Nucl Acids Res.* 1980;8:4393.

90. Straubinger B, Osterholzer E, Zachau HG. *Nucl Acids Res.* 1987;15:9567.

91. Nemer M, Chamberland D, Sirois D, Argentin S, Drouin J, Dixon RAF, Zivin RA, Condra JH. *Nature (London).* 1984;312:654.

92. Kress M, Barra Y, Seidman JG, Khoury G, Jay G. *Science.* 1984;226:974.

93. Pontarotti PA, Mashimo H, Zeff RA, Fischer DA, Hood L, Mellos A, Flavell RA, Nathenson SG. *Proc Natl Acad Sci (USA).* 1986;83:1782.

94. Yamamoto T, Davis CG, Brown MS, Schneider WJ, Casey ML, Goldstein JL, Russel DW. *Cell.* 1984;39:27.

95. Majello B, La Mantia G, Simeone A, Boncinelli E, Lania L. *Nature (London).* 1985;314:457.

96. Korenberg JR, Rykowski MC. *Cell.* 1988;53:391.

97. Bird AP. *Nature (London).* 1986;321:209.

98. Neuer-Nitsche B, Lu X, Werner D. *Nucl Acids Res.* 1988;16:8351.

99. Bushkin Y, Demaria S, Le J, Schwab R. *Proc Natl Acad Sci (USA).* 1988;85:3985–3989.

100. Kavathas P, Herzenberg LE. *Proc Natl Acad Sci (USA).* 1983;80:524.

101. Sood AK, Periera D, Weissman SM. *Proc Natl Acad Sci (USA).* 1981;78:616.

102. Shimizu Y, Geraghty DE, Koller BH, Orr HT, DeMars R. *Proc Natl Acad Sci (USA).* 1988;85:227.

103. Brenner MB, McLean J, Scheft H, Riberdy J, Ang S-L, Seidman JG, Devlin P, Karangel MS. *Nature (London).* 1987;325:683.

104. Borst J, van de Griend RJ, van Oostveen JW, Ang S-L, Melief CJ, Seidman JG, Bolhuis RLH. *Nature (London)*. 1987;325:683.

105. Nagasawa R, Gross J, Kanagawa O, Townsend K, Lanier LL, Chilleer J, Allison JP. *Immunology*. 1987;138:815.

106. Matis LA, Corn R, Bluestone JA. *Nature (London)*. 1987;330:262.

107. Janeway CA Jr. *Nature*. 1988;333:804.

108. Janeway CA Jr, Jones B, Hayday AC. *Immunol Today* 1988;9:73.

109. Koning F, Stingl G, Kokoyama WM, Hidekazu Y, Maloy WL, Tschachler R, Shevach EM, Coligan JE. *Science*. 1987;236:834.

110. Stingl G, Koning F, Hidekazu Y, Yokloyama WM, Tschachler E, Bluestone JA, Steiner G, Samelson LE, Lew AM, Coligan JE, Shevach EM. *Proc Natl Acad Sci (USA)*. 1987;84:4586.

111. Bonneville M, Janeway CA, Ito K, Haser W, Ishida I, Nakanishi N, Tonegawa S. *Nature (London)*. 1988;336:479.

112. Klein JR. *J Exp Med*. 1986;164:309.

113. Sodoyer R, Damotte M, Delovitch TL, Trucy J, Jordan BR, Strachan T. *EMBO J*. 1984;3:879.

114. Takata M, Inoko H, Asako A, Haranaka M, Watanabe B, Tsuji K, Iri H. *Immunogenetics*. 1988;28:265.

115. Strachan T, Sodoyer R, Damotte M, Jordan BR. *EMBO J*. 1984;3:887.

116. Cowan EP, Jelachich ML, Biddison WE, Coligan JE. *Immunogenetics*. 1987;25:241.

117. N'guyen C, Sodoyer R, Trucy J, Strachan T, Jordan BR. *Immunogenetics*. 1985;21:479.

118. Szots H, Riethmuller G, Weiss E, Meo T. *Proc Natl Acad Sci (USA)*. 1986;83:1428.

119. Krangel MS. *EMBO J*. 1985;4:1205.

120. Krangel MS. *J Exp Med*. 1986;163:1173.

121. Seemann GHA, Rein RS, Brown CS, Ploegh HL. *EMBO J*. 1986;5:547.

122. Brown GD, Choi Y, Pampeno C, Meruelo D. *CRC Rev Immunol*. 1988;8:175.

123. Lambert ME, Ronai ZA, Weinstein IB, Garrels JI. *Mol Cell Biol*. 1989;(in press).

124. Parent LJ, Ehrlich R, Matis L, Singer DS. *FASEB J*. 1987;1:469.

125. Buc Caran MH, Condamine H, Jacob F. *J Embryol Exp Morphol*. 1978;47:149.

126. Morello D, Gachelin G, Dubois P, Tanigaki N, Pressman D, Jacob F. *Transplantation*. 1978;26:119.

127. Morello D, Gachelin G, Daniel F, Kourilsky P. *Cold Spring Harbor Symp Quant Biol*. 1983;10:421.

128. Lew AM, Lillehoj EP, Cowan EP, Maloy WL, Van Schravendijk MR, Coligan JE. *Immunology*. 1986;57:3.

129. Daniel-Vedele F, Morello D, Benicourt C, Transy C, Le Bail O, Plata F, Kourilsky P. *EMBO J*. 1984;3:597.

130. Tanaka K, Appella E, Jay G. *Cell*. 1983;35:457.

131. Ozato K, Wan Y-J, Orrison BM. *Proc Natl Acad Sci (USA)*. 1985;82:2427.

132. Yarden A, Shure-Gottlieb H, Chebath J, Revel M, Kimchi A. *EMBO J*. 1984;3:969.

133. Bernards R, Schrier PL, Houwling A, Bos JL *Nature (London)*. 1983;305:776.

134. Katzav S, De Baestselier P, Tartakovsky B, Feldman M, Segal S. *J Natl Cancer Inst*. 1983;71:317.

135. Wallich R, Bulbuc N, Hammerling GJ, Katzav S, Segal S, Feldman M. *Nature (London)*. 1985;315:301.

136. Alon Y, Hammerling GJ, Segal S, Bar-Eli M. *Cancer Res*. 1987;47:2553.

137. Haddada H, Sogn JA, Coligan JE, Carbone M, Dixon K, Levine AS, Lewis AM. *J Virol.* 1988;62(8):2755.

138. Nishimura MI, Stroynowski I, Hood L, Ostrand-Rosenberg S. *J Immunol.* 1988;141:4403.

139. Natali PG, Giacomini P, Bigotti A, Imai K, Nicotra MR, Ng AK, Ferrone S. *Cancer Res.* 1983;43:660.

140. Bernards R, Dessain SK, Weinberg RA. *Cell.* 1986;47:667.

141. Khoury G, Tanaka M, Isselbacher K, Jay G. *Science.* 1985;228:26.

142. Weinstein IB, Gattoni-Celli S, Kirschmeier P, Lambert M, Hsiao WL, Backer J, Jeffrey A. In Levine AJ, eds. *Cancer Cells, The Transformed Phenotype.* Cold Spring Harbor, NY: Cold Spring Harbor Laboratory Press; 1984:229–237.

143. Kolber MA, Walls RM, Hinners ML, Singer DS. *Alcoholism: Clin Exp Res.* 1988;12:295.

144. Lambert M, Garrels JI. In Lambert ME, McDonald JF, Weinstein IB, eds. *Eukaryotic Transposable Elements as Mutagenic Agents; Banbury Report 30.* Cold Spring Harbor, NY: Cold Spring Harbor Laboratory Press; 1988:255–263.

145. Garrels JI, Farrar JT, Burwell IV CB. In Celis J, Bravo R, eds. *Two-Dimensional Electrophoresis of Proteins: Methods and Applications.* New York: Academic Press, Inc.; 1984:38–90.

146. Garrels JI. *J Biol Chem.* 1979;254:7961.

147. Kraemer K, Coon HG, Petinga RA, Barrett SF, Rahe AE, Robbins JH. *Proc Natl Acad Sci (USA).* 1975;72:59.

148. Cleaver J, Charles WC, Hong SH. *Photochem Photobiol.* 1984;40:621.

149. Joe CO, Norman JO, Irvin TR, Busbee DL. *Biochem Biophys Res Commun.* 1985;128:754.

150. Taylor-Papadimitriou J, Purkis JP, Lane EB, McKay IA, Chang SE. *Cell Differ.* 1982;11:169.

151. Rask L, Lindblom JB, Peterson P. *Eur J Immunol.* 1976;6:93.

152. Chen E, Carr RW, Ginder GD. *Mol Cell Biol.* 1987;7:4572.

153. Friedman RL, Stark GR. *Nature (London).* 1985;314:637.

154. Shirayoshi Y, Burke PA, Appela E, Ozato K. *Proc Natl Acad Sci (USA).* 1988;85:5884.

155. Ryals J, Dierks P, Ragg H, Weissman C. *Cell.* 1985;41:497.

156. Baldwin AS, Sharp P. *Proc Natl Acad Sci (USA).* 1988;85:723.

157. Baeuerle PA, Baltimore D. *Science.* 1988;242:540.

158. Korber B, Mermad N, Hood L, Stroynowski I. *Science.* 1988;239:1302.

159. Chiu R, Boyle WJ, Meek J, Smeal T, Hunter T, Karin M. *Cell.* 1988;54:541.

160. Rauscher RJ, Cohen DR, Curran T, Bos TJ, Vogt PK, Bohmann D, Tijan R, Franza RJ. *Science.* 1988;240:1010.

161. Franza BR, Rauscher FJ, Josephs SF, Curran T. *Science.* 1988;239:1150.

162. Eisenbach L, Kushtai G, Plaskin D, Feldman M. *Cancer Rev.* 1986;5:1.

163. Chimini G, Pontarotti P, Nguyen C, Toubert A, Boretto J, Jordan BR. *EMBO.* 1988;7(2):395.

164. Bird A. *Nature (London).* 1986;321:209.

165. Miyazaki J, Appella E, Ozato K. *Proc Natl Acad Sci (USA).* 1986;83:9537.

166. Ehrlich R, McGuire JE, Singer DS. *Mol Cell Biol.* 1988;8:695.

167. Dasgupta JD, Yunis EJ. *J Immunol.* 1987;139:672.

168. Phillips ML, Moule ML, Delovitch TL, Yip CC. *Proc Natl Acad Sci (USA).* 1986;83:3474.

169. Kittur D, Shimizu Y, DeMars R, Edidin M. *Proc Natl Acad Sci (USA).* 1987;84:1351.

170. Fehlmann M, Peyran JR, Samson M, van Obberghen E, Brandenburg D, Brossette N. *Proc Natl Acad Sci (USA).* 1985;82:8634.

136

BASIC IMMUNOLOGICAL CONSIDERATIONS

171. Due C, Simonsen M, Olsson LC. *Proc Natl Acad Sci (USA)*. 1986;83:6007.

172. Schreiber AB, Schlessinger J, Edidin M. *J Cell Biol*. 1984;98:725.

173. Solano AR, Cremaschi G, Sanchez M, Borda E, Sterin-Borda L, Podesta EJ. *Proc Natl Acad Sci (USA)*. 1988;85:5087.

174. Dasgupta JD, Cemach K, Dubey DP, Yunis EJ, Amos DB. *Proc Natl Acad Sci (USA)*. 1987;84:1094.

175. Taylor DS, Nowell PC, Kornbluth J. *Proc Natl Acad Sci (USA)*. 1986;83:4446.

176. Dasgupta JD, Watkins S, Slayter H, Yunis EJ. *J Immunol*. 1988;141:2577.

177. Taylor DS, Nowell PC, Kornbluth J. *J Immunol*. 1987;139:1792.

178. Blue ML, Craig KA, Anderson P, Branton KR, Schlossman SF. *Cell*. 1988;54:413.

CHAPTER 6

Antigen–Antibody Interaction

Chester M. Zmijewski

Professor of Pathology and Laboratory Medicine, University of Pennsylvania Medical Center, 3400 Spruce Street, Philadelphia, PA 19104-4283 USA

In the most global sense antigen–antibody interactions can be considered as occurring in two stages. The first of these consists of the specific binding of antibody molecules to haptenic antigenic determinants which are present on a suitable carrier. This carrier may be a large complex molecule, such as a protein, in which certain amino acid sequences or perhaps carbohydrate side chains form the actual antigenic determinants or epitopes. On the other hand, the carrier may be as large as a bacterial or mammalian cell, in which the antigenic determinants are unique surface structures composed of complex polypeptides and/or polysaccharides, in which the epitopes may consist of both structural and conformational portions of the critical molecules. The second stage consists of a series of events that exert some effect on the carrier and are a direct result of the formation of the initial antigen–antibody complex. Some common effects are precipitation, agglutination, and lysis.

A complication arising from such a global view is that explanations regarding these reactions, which may appear quite simple theoretically at the molecular level, are actually exceedingly complex as they occur in reality. For example, many of the facts and principles to be discussed are derived from experiments using highly specific monoclonal antibodies and antigens that carry but a single epitope. Unfortunately that is not quite the case in the real world. The types of antigens capable of eliciting normal immune responses are complex molecules or entire cells carrying a large number of different epitopes. Furthermore, the response that is elicited is polyclonal, involving the differentiation and multiplication of a large number of cells. As a result, a variety of antibodies are produced whose specificities are directed toward the many different epitopes on the immunizing antigen. Thus under normal circumstances the antigen–antibody reaction observed is an average reactivity of many antibody molecules in a given serum against a myriad of epitopes on a given preparation of antigen. It is very important to keep this in mind when attempting to translate concepts such as those pertaining to the specificity and binding affinity of an antiserum into the events that may be occurring at the molecular level or vice versa.

Primary Antigen–Antibody Binding

As stated previously, the first stage of an antigen–antibody reaction involves the specific binding of an antibody molecule to its epitope. This binding involves the development of noncovalent bonds between various chemical groupings on the epitope with genetically and conformationally determined amino acid sequences in the hypervariable region of the immunoglobulin molecule. It may include hydrogen bonds, electrostatic bonds, van der Waals forces, and hydrophobic bonds. Each of these contributes to the strength of the complex, which collectively is expressed as the binding affinity.[1]

A considerable degree of binding affinity results from the "biochemical fit" of the antibody molecule for its antigen. The ideal antibody in terms of binding affinity has a structure that is totally complementary to its epitope. This type of conformational and structural similarity affords the maximum contact between oppositely charged and chemically suited groups that would offer maximum electrostatic and hydrogen bonds between the two molecules. Practical experience dictates that such an ideal is not always possible. Indeed a normal immune response consists of the proliferation of a large number of different antibodies, each of which may not be totally complimentary to antigen but approximate it as closely as possible. Therefore, the result is the development of a kind of array of cross-reactivities that is known as antibody diversity.[2]

The valence of the antibody, ie, the number of combining sites for antigen, will influence the magnitude of expressed binding affinity. Depending on the physical configuration of epitopes on an antigenic molecule it might be possible for all five antibody-combining sites on a molecule of IgM to react with an antigen. Such an antibody would express a higher binding affinity than an IgG antibody of the same specificity but with only two combining sites or another IgM antibody identical to the first but reactive with an antigen whose epitopes are configured differently. Although this is true in large measure, in in vitro systems such external factors as the composition of the reaction mixture may likewise have an effect. Consequently, the temperature of the reaction mixture, the pH, and the ionic strength can effect the strength and speed of binding.

The antigen–antibody reaction is a reversible reaction that obeys the laws of mass action[3] and can be expressed as follows:

$$K_0 = \frac{[AgAb]}{[Ag][Ab]} \tag{1}$$

The association constant K_0 is a function of the average binding affinity of the antibody. From this expression it should be clear that at a particular value of K_0 the concentration of the reactants, ie, antigen and antibody will favor either the formation or dissociation of antigen–antibody complexes. This can have very important implications in designing and carrying out in vitro assays for either antigen or antibody. The implications in in vivo reactions may be even more serious since under some conditions the formation of complexes can lead to the development of pathologic conditions.

The first stage of antigen–antibody reactions, which involves only binding, can be detected and measured in a number of different ways, including the Farr technique,[4] equilibrium dialysis,[5] or direct visualization using labeled antibody methods, such as a radioimmunoassay (RIA)[6] and enzyme-linked immunosorbance (ELISA).[7]

The Farr technique makes use of the differential solubilities of free antigen and antigen–antibody complexes in 50% saturated ammonium sulfate. Free antigen, such as bovine serum albumin, is soluble in this solution; however, immunoglobulin and therefore antigen–antibody complexes are not. The measurement of antigen in supernatants and sediments can give a measure of antibody binding.

In equilibrium dialysis the antibody is placed in a dialysis sac, which is impermeable to antibody molecules but allows antigen-bearing molecules to diffuse freely. The sac is placed in a fluid containing the antigen and dialysis is allowed to take place until the antigen concentration in the bath remains constant. At this point, equilibrium is achieved and the amount of bound antigen is equal to the concentration of antigen in the bath less the amount of free antigen in the sac.

The RIA procedure is based on the competition of the antigen to be assayed with a radioactively labeled counterpart for binding to a limited and standard amount of antibody. In practice, a standard quantity of radiolabeled antigen is reacted with antibody in the presence of varying amounts of unlabeled antigen in order to establish a standard curve that depicts the amounts of radioactive antigen that remain bound to antibody at different concentrations of cold antigen. In a parallel reaction the unknown antigen is substituted as the cold antigen and its concentration is estimated from the standard curve.

In the ELISA method, the antibody is chemically coupled to an enzyme that has the ability to break down a substrate with the formation of a colored product. Typical enzymes include alkaline phosphatase and horseradish peroxidase. When such a labeled antibody reacts with its antigen the enzyme becomes bound. The addition of a suitable substrate results in the formation of a visible color whose intensity is proportional to the amount of enzyme present and therefore to the amount of bound antibody.

Enzyme-linked antibodies can also be used to visualize directly the location of antigens present in tissue section and are widely used in histochemical procedures. Other methods used for visualizing antigens directly involve the coupling of antibodies to fluorescent compounds, such as a fluoresceine diisothiocyanate or rhodamine.[8] Antigens can also be localized in cellular ultrastructures in electron micrographs by coupling antibodies to electron-dense compounds, such as ferritin.[9]

Secondary Antigen–Antibody Reactions

The second stage of an antigen–antibody reaction occurs as a series of events that result in the destruction or immobilization of the antigen. Although contemporary thinking has reduced antigen–antibody reactions to highly sophisticated biochemical interactions between complementary molecules, the fact remains that the primary biologic function of antibodies is to rid the host of undesirable antigens.

This is accomplished through the second stage and can be manifest in vitro in three major ways. These include precipitation, agglutination, and lysis. A similar series of second-stage events may occur in vivo but to a different degree. These are discussed later (see In Vivo Antigen-Antibody Reactions).

The type of second-stage reaction that is observed in any given antigen–antibody reaction is to a large extent governed by the physical form of the antigen. Thus soluble antigens mixed with antibody usually lead to the formation of a precipitate containing an insoluble complex resulting from a crosslinking of molecules of antigen by molecules of antibody. On the other hand, antigens that form an integral part of a cell wall or those which are attached to a cell wall or large particle will be crosslinked by antibody and form an agglutinate of the cells or particles. This is the usual end product of antigen–antibody reactions involving bacterial antigens or those found on red blood cells. Finally, certain types of antibody molecules when complexed with antigen can cause the activation of complement components, which are found in all normal sera. The activation of this cascade leads to the production of cytolytic enzymes that can cause the lysis of antigen bearing cells as well as the release of pharmacologically active substances that promote phagocytosis of the antibody-coated particles.

Precipitation and agglutination are both reversible reactions that follow the same general laws of mass action as those controlling the first stage. The dynamics of the antigen–antibody reaction as well as the principles that govern both the precipitation and the agglutination reactions can best be described by the quantitative precipitation curve.[10] However, some additional factors, which will be discussed later, enter into the process of agglutination. This curve is derived by plotting the weight of the precipitates formed as a function of varying antigen concentration when the concentration of antibody is kept constant. A typical curve of this type is shown in Figure 6-1. It indicates that as increasing amounts of antigen are added to a given amount of antibody the quantity of precipitate gradually increases until it reaches a maximum and then begins to decrease and eventually disappears.

The curve can be divided into three distinct zones based on an analysis of the precipitate and the supernatant in each. This reveals that the supernatant found in the first zone contains free antibody, the supernatant in the third zone contains free antigen, whereas the supernatant found in the second or central zone contains neither free antigen nor free antibody. Therefore this zone alone can be considered a zone of equivalence in which conditions in terms of the relative proportion of antigen concentration to antibody concentration are optimal for maximum precipitate formation.

One way to explain these findings is to envision a situation in the first zone in which there is so much antibody in relation to the amount of antigen that all available epitopes on the antigenic molecule are saturated with antibody. Therefore, lattice formation cannot take place. By the same token in the third zone there is more antigen relative to antibody and small complexes form composed of antibody saturated with antigen and remain in solution.

A similar conclusion can be reached in a more elegant, although no more truthful manner, from the mass action expression $K_0 = [AgAb]/[Ag][Ab]$. Thus for any

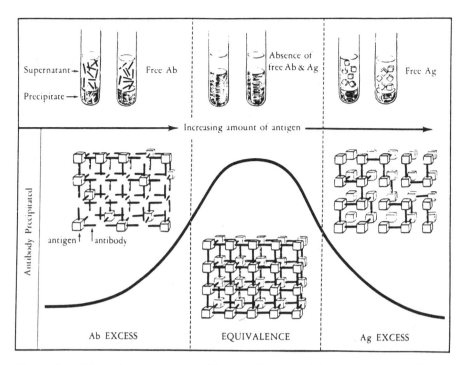

Figure 6-1. Schematic representation of the quantitative precipitation curve. Ab, antibody; Ag, antigen. (Reproduced from Ref 11 with the authors' permission.)

given value of the association constant, K_0, if the concentration of either Ag or Ab falls, the concentration of the AgAb complex must fall as well.

Serologic Applications of Antigen–Antibody Reactions

The fact that maximum precipitate occurs at optimal proportions of antigen and antibody and can dissolve in antigen excess has been used to develop a number of useful in vitro serologic methods. When the precipitation reaction is carried out in a semisolid medium such as agar and the antigen and antibody are allowed to diffuse toward one another a precipitation band will form at some point between them. This will be located at the point at which the two reactants are present in optimal proportions and will depend on their initial concentrations as well as their diffusion constant. Since different antigenic molecules have different diffusion constants because of their size and composition, the technique can be used to differentiate antigens and to identify them. In addition, since the point of optimal proportions depends on the initial concentration of antigen, the method can be used as an analytical tool to quantitate antigen.

The most widely used of these methods is based on a technique developed by Ouchterlony.[12] In this method two adjacent wells are formed in a layer of agar. The antigen-containing mixture is placed in one, the antibody in the other, and the two

Optimal proportions

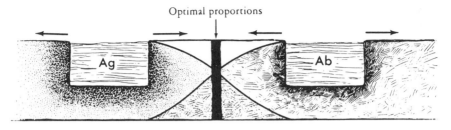

Figure 6-2. Schematic representation of a cross-section of the Ouchterlony double diffusion. Ab, antibody; Ag, antigen. (Reproduced from Ref 11 with the authors' permission.)

reactants are allowed to diffuse against each other. As shown in the cross-sectional diagram depicted in Figure 6-2, during the process of diffusion a concentration gradient forms in the agar and at the point of optimal proportion of the antigen with its specific antibody a line of precipitate forms. If the mixture in the antigen well contains two different molecules that diffuse at different rates but carry the same epitope, then two lines of precipitate form, each at its own region of optimal proportions.

When viewed from the top, these reactions appear as a line of precipitate. These can be manipulated to form patterns that establish antigenic identity, nonidentity, or similarity among various antigen-containing mixtures.

A powerful variation of this technique is immunoelectrophoresis.[13] In this technique a complex antigen such as whole serum is placed in a well on an agar-coated slide and subjected to electrophoresis. A longitudinal slit is then made in the agar parallel to the electrophoretic run and filled with an antiserum containing antibodies to one or more serum protein. Each antigen–antibody reaction creates a precipitation arc in its own region of optimal proportions. These arcs, by their shape, position, and comparison with standards, can be used to identify, quantify, and otherwise characterize individual components of the complex antigen-carrying mixture.

In radial immunodiffusion, antibody is incorporated into the agar. A measured amount of the antigen to be quantitated is placed in a well and allowed to diffuse outward. A precipitation ring forms around the well whose diameter is proportional to the concentration of antigen.

A variation of this is known as electroimmunodiffusion or rocket electrophoresis. It is another method that has been developed based on the precipitation reaction in semisolid medium. In this technique an antiserum is first incorporated at a constant concentration into the agar layer. An antigen is applied in a well and an electric current is used to draw the antigen into the antibody-containing agar layer. Since the concentration of antigen varies with its initial concentration and along its electrophoretic path an arc forms in a shape resembling a rocket standing on a launch pad. The length of the arc is proportional to the starting concentration of antigen.

Not all second-stage reactions have the same sensitivity. Table 6-1 lists the amount of antibody that is detectable by various serologic tests. In view of the fact that the soluble antigens that participate in precipitation reactions are small, consid-

Table 6-1. Sensitivity of Quantitative Tests Measuring Antibody Nitrogen

Tests	mgAb (N/mL)
Precipitation reactions	3–20
Immunoelectrophoresis	3–20
Double diffusion in agar	0.2–1.0
Complement fixation	0.01–0.1
Radial immunodiffusion	0.008–0.025
Bacterial agglutination	0.01
Hemolysis	0.001–0.03
Passive hemagglutination	0.05
RIA	0.0001–0.001
ELISA	0.0001–0.001

Source: adapted from Ref 11.

erable amounts must be aggregated by antibody before a visible precipitate is formed. As a result this type of reaction is not very sensitive. Agglutination, on the other hand, involves the use of relatively large antigen-bearing cells or particles. Consequently much fewer numbers of these need to be aggregated by considerably fewer antibody molecules in order to achieve a visible aggregate. This results in greater sensitivity. Quite frequently it is possible to take advantage of this increase in sensitivity by artificially coupling a soluble antigen to a large insoluble particle, effectively converting a precipitation reaction to agglutination. This technique is called passive agglutination and can be carried out using any of a number of different types of particles ranging from bentonite and polystyrene latex to bacterial cells and red blood cells from a wide range of species. Human, bovine, sheep, and even alligator cells have been used. In practice, the antigen can be adsorbed onto the surface of the particle (eg, polysaccharides have a natural affinity for red blood cell surfaces) or chemically coupled via compounds such as chromic chloride or by other means.

The agglutination reaction follows the same dynamics as the precipitation reaction with the exception that the second stage, aggregate formation, is governed by yet another set of physicochemical conditions. This stems from the fact that the large particles used in agglutination are electrostatically charged when in suspension in a solution of electrolytes. Therefore their behavior is governed by a number of laws that apply to charged particles in suspension.

Most large particles such as red blood cells have a net negative surface charge when suspended in isoosmotic aqueous media due to the ionization of amino acids and certain carbohydrates that are part of the cell wall. Therefore, because like charges repel, these particles tend to stay apart from each other a given distance, which is governed by their net surface charge density. Furthermore, when the solution is an electrolyte, the ions in solution orient themselves around the particle to form an ionic cloud. The orientation of ions within this cloud is such that they tend to be very concentrated near the surface of the particle and more diffuse as the distance from the surface increases. The outer perimeter of the cloud forms a surface of shear since as the particle moves through the solution the cloud moves along with it. There is a difference in electrostatic potential between the charge at the surface and that found at the surface of shear, which is called the zeta potential. The magnitude of this potential is governed by the actual net surface charge density of the particle as well as the dielectric constant and ionic strength of the suspending medium. The zeta potential constitutes an additional electrostatic force that exerts further repulsive effects on the particles.[14]

During the second stage of agglutination, bound antibody molecules must crosslink antigenic determinants on adjacent cells in order to form an agglutinated aggregate. Therefore, the gap between two adjacent antigen-bearing particles being held apart by electrostatic forces must be successfully bridged by antibody molecules. In some cases, because of either the effective length of the antibody molecule (the distance between any two combining sites) and/or the specific location of the antigenic determinant on the cell, such as a long polysaccharide or polypeptide that extends from the surface, electrostatic forces do not result in the creation of unbridgeable distances. In other cases, if the antigen is buried in a surface crypt or the effective length of an antibody molecule such as IgG is short, the repulsive distances created by these forces may be too great to allow for spontaneous bridging. In most instances, these repulsive forces can be overcome by subjecting the particles to increased gravitational forces in a centrifuge, thereby counteracting the repulsive effects and forcing the particles closer together. However, there may be cases in which even these efforts fail and agglutination can be accomplished only by altering the electrostatic effects or employing a second antibody.

Repulsive electrostatic effects on particles in suspension can be overcome in a number of ways. First of all since part of this effect is due to the zeta potential steps can be taken to decrease it. As mentioned previously, the zeta potential depends on the net surface charge density, the dielectric constant of the medium, and the ionic strength. Therefore alterations in any of these parameters will alter the zeta. One of the most common methods and one that has been used successfully in blood group work employing red cells is to substitute isoosmotic macromolecular colloidal solutions for electrolytes as suspending media.[15] Such solutions have higher dielectric constants and lower ionic strengths and therefore decrease zeta, thereby reducing the electrostatic repulsive effects and allowing the particles to approach each other more closely.

Another approach that has been used successfully in a number of applications involving red blood cells is to lower the net surface charge density of the particle by pretreatment with enzymes that remove sialic acids, thereby lowering the net negative charge.[16]

The conditions for each of these procedures must be carefully established for each antigen–antibody system since it is possible to create circumstances that will produce nonspecific aggregation. In addition, methods used to alter surface charge densities directly, such as the example cited previously, often call for the use of proteolytic or other types of enzymes that can lead to denaturation or removal of antigenic groups. Therefore, these techniques must be approached with caution and with the use of appropriate controls.

A useful method that can be used to enhance second-stage agglutination is the use of a second antibody.[17] The primary antibody bound to its antigenic determinant on the surface of the particles is itself an antigen since it is an immunoglobulin of a given isotype from a particular species. If the species of the antibody producer is known then an antibody from a different species, usually a rabbit, can be produced against such an immunoglobulin. This antibody then reacts with the primary antibodies already bound to their respective antigens on each particle and form a bridge. Such bridging results in lattice formation and a visible agglutinate.

Second antibodies of this type are most useful and quite common in various in vitro systems apart from agglutination for antigen detection. As mentioned previously, they can be coupled with various external labels, which then can be used to directly visualize and/or measure bound antibody molecules.

Complement Binding

As a direct consequence of certain antigen–antibody reactions, a series of proteins and inactive enzymes present in normal human serum and collectively referred to as complement can be complexed and activated. Once activated, this series of proteins yields products that can have a number of different biological and pharmological effects varying from the lysis of cells to the release of vasoactive and chemotactic substances.[18]

Complement activation via the classical pathway is initiated through specific amino acid groupings found on the Fc portion of certain immunoglobulin molecules. These are carried by all IgM antibodies and are found on IgG1, 2, and 3 but not on IgG4, IgA, or IgE. The actual process of activation requires the presence of two such Fc groupings held in close proximity as a direct result of a reaction with antigen. Therefore, this criterion can be satisfied by a minimum of one molecule of IgM with its five integral Fc portions, whereas two molecules of IgG are required. Thus, IgM is twice as effective as IgG in complement activation. In point of fact, it may be even more efficient than that since the requirement is for the two Fc portions to be in close proximity. In some instances antigenic determinants, especially on cell surfaces, may be located far enough apart to prevent this positioning from taking place. In such cases the addition of a second antibody regardless of its specificity will provide the required Fc portions.

Complement consists of a complex system of serum proteins some of which exist as inactive enzymes. The initial combination of one of these components with antibody molecules complexed to antigen results in the formation of a chemically active compound that then proceeds to convert a second component, and so forth, in cascade fashion, until the final product is activated. This product can act to form a hole in a cell membrane, which leads to lysis.

Eleven major components of complement have been identified whose properties and activities are listed in Table 6-2. As stated previously, this is for the most part an interactive enzymatic system in which each component is activated by the preceding one. It is regulated by the presence of activators and inactivators, some of which are shared with the coagulation system. Thus, there is a direct relationship between complement activation and blood clotting. In addition, complement activa-

Table 6-2. The Complement Components

Component	Serum Concentration (g/mL)	Description and Function
C1		Subunits held together by Ca^{2+}
C1q (1 mol)	180	Reacts with Fc fragment of bound antibody
C1r (2 mol)	100	Enzymatic activity for C4 and C2
C1s (4 mol)	80	
C4	450	Cleaved by C1s
C4a		Remains in plasma; smooth muscle contraction, increase of vascular permeability
C4b		Cell bound
C2	25	Attaches to cell-bound C4b in presence of Mg^{2+}; cleaved by C1s
C2a		Remains with C4b to form C4b2a (C3 convertase)
C2b		Released to plasma
C3	1500	Cleaved by C3 convertase (C4b2a)
C3a		Anaphylatoxin; remains in plasma; smooth muscle contraction, increase of vascular permeability, degranulation of mast cells and basophils with release of histamine, degranulation of eosinophils, aggregation of platelets
C3b		Cell bound, adjacent to C4b2a to form C4b2a3b; opsonization of particles and solubilizaiton of immune complexes with subsequent facilitation of phagocytosis; acted on by C3 inactivator, factor 1, to form C3c and C3d
C3d		Cell bound, biologically inactive
C5	75	Cleaved by C4b2a3b, last enzymatic step
C5a		Anaphylatoxin; remains in plasma; smooth muscle contraction; increase of vascular permeability, degranulation of mast cells and basophils with release of histamine, degranulation of eosinophils, aggregation of platelets, chemotaxis of basophils, eosinophils, neutrophils, and monocytes; release of hydrolytic enzymes from neutrophils
C5a-des-Arg		Chemotaxis of neutrophils; release of hydrolytic enzymes from neutrophils
C5b		Cell bound to C4b2a3b5b complex
C6	60	Binds to C4b2a3b5b
C7	60	Binds to C5b6 (C5b67) complex; can move to new membrane site
C8	80	Binds to C5b67 complex
C9	150	Binds to C8 (up to 6 molecules) to form final lytic factor

Source: adapted from Refs 11 and 19.

tion acts as an amplifier of antigen–antibody reactions. In view of the fact that each enzyme formed has the potential of activating many molecules of the next component, a single antigen–antibody reaction can result in the exponential activation of complement.

Although the principle role of the complement system is to produce lysis, many of the components and/or their byproducts along the activation pathway have many varied biological functions. For example, C3a and C5a are anaphylotoxins that can cause vasodilitation and vascular permeability. In addition, some of the factors are chemotactic and still others promote phagocytosis.

In general, complement activation is an in vivo mechanism for dealing with foreign antigens. However, a number of in vitro serologic procedures make use of this system. The complement fixation test is a classic reaction used to quantitate antigen or antibody in systems that neither precipitate nor agglutinate.[20] In these cases the ability of an antigen–antibody complex to "fix" or use up complement is employed to detect such a complex. The initial reaction of antigen plus suspected antibody is allowed to take place in the presence of a standard amount of complement, which is adjusted so that it is the minimal amount needed to lyse a suspension of sheep red blood cells coated with anti-sheep red blood cell antibody. If the suspected antibody in the primary reaction is present, it will combine with its antigen and use up some of the complement. When the coated red blood cell suspension is added there will be insufficient complement remaining in the system to lyse the cells and they will remain intact. On the other hand, if the suspected antibody of the appropriate antigen is lacking, then no primary reaction will take place, and adequate complement will be present to lyse the antibody coated red cells added in the second step.

Another serologic test that makes use of complement is the lymphocytotoxicity reaction commonly used for human histocompatibility testing.[21] In this reaction, living lymphocytes are first incubated with alloantibody to antigens suspected of being on their cell surface. If indeed the appropriate antigens are present, the antibody is bound and can activate complement in the form of normal rabbit serum that subsequently is added to the mixture. If allowed to go to completion, the activated complement could cause the eventual lysis of the cell. In practice however, the reaction is stopped shortly before this occurs by the addition of formalin. Fortunately lymphocytes do not lyse as readily as some other cell types and what is normally observed is cell death resulting from complement-mediated damage to the nuclear membrane.

The alloantibodies used for histocompatibility testing are most often IgG, and the antigens against which they are directed are freely imbedded in the lipid bilayer of the cell wall, allowing them to move. Consequently this situation is an example of a condition in which the requirement for twin Fc portions of the antibody molecule needed for complement activation may not always be fulfilled. To overcome this problem, advantage is taken of the presence of minute amounts of heteroantibody in the animal serum used as a complement source. This antibody can combine with species-specific antigens located on the cell membrane and provide the extra Fc portions necessary.

Monoclonal antibodies to human histocompatibility antigens are most frequently IgM and therefore do not require the synergistic effects provided by rabbit anti-human antibodies for complement activation. As a matter of fact, the presence of such antibodies under these conditions could lead to nonspecific complement activation, premature cell death, and false-positive results. Consequently, the rabbit serum used as a complement source for use with monoclonal antibodies must be carefully selected so as to contain low levels of heteroantibody. Serum from younger animals is usually best for this purpose.

In Vivo Antigen–Antibody Reactions

Antigen–antibody reactions that occur in vivo are governed by the same physicochemical laws of mass action that control their interaction in vitro. However, their manifestations and function may be quite different. For example, no reaction takes place if there is insufficient antibody and, by the same token, soluble complexes can be formed in antigen excess. However, since the primary biological purpose of the humoral immune system of which antibodies are a part is the protection of the host, the most common secondary reactions operative in vivo are designed either to remove directly or facilitate the removal of the offending antigen.

By far the most efficient removal mechanism is through the phagocytic action of macrophages.[22] This type of activity can occur in the absence of antibody; however, it is greatly increased and more efficient when specific antibodies complex with antigen. There are several reasons for this. First of all, phagocytic cells carry on their surface receptors for the Fc portion of antibody molecules as well as for certain complement components. Therefore, antigen-bearing cells or particles complexed with antibody become attached to phagocytic cells via these receptors, greatly increasing the opportunity for phagocytosis. If the antigen antibody reaction has activated complement, not only is a further point of attachment provided but the products of complement activation are chemotactic and attract phagocytic cells.

Second, cells primarily phagocytize insoluble particles. The precipitating or agglutinating properties of antibody molecules help to particulate and otherwise immobilize antigens in preparation for phagocytosis. In addition, activation of the complement cascade can trigger the coagulation pathway, resulting in fibrin deposition, which tends to wall off and further immobilize the offending antigens.[23]

Under normal physiologic conditions agglutination and/or precipitation do not take place in vivo to the same degree as in vitro systems. However, they can occur under some conditions and lead to harmful consequences. This can happen in the hyperimmunized individual who has produced a large amount of antibody when challenged with a massive dose of antigen. However, the most common harmful effects of antigen–antibody reactions can result from the formation and deposition of soluble antigen–antibody complexes in certain tissues, such as the glomerular basement membrane, vascular endothelia, and synovial spaces. These complexes can lead to complement activation and the subsequent release of chemotactic and vasoactive substances that lead to inflammation. Although inflammation has beneficial effects in terms of fighting off foreign microbial organisms, it can be destructive of normal healthy tissue and lead to the development of pathologic conditions, such as glomerular nephritis, vasculitis, and certain forms of arthritis.[24]

Toxin neutralization is a highly specialized in vitro antigen–antibody reaction in which an antibody is formed to a specific toxic group present on an antigenic molecule and then reacts with this group, rendering the substance nontoxic. Typical examples of such antibodies are tetanus antitoxin and diphtheria antitoxin. These antibodies are formed as the result of deliberate immunization with appropriate toxoid (chemically inactivated toxins) containing vaccines or as a result of actual infection and subsequent recovery. The antibody acts by neutralizing the toxin through its combination with toxic groups. The resultant complexes are removed through normal metabolism. However, sometimes insoluble complexes are formed, which are then disposed of through phagocytic processes.

The second most common in vivo reaction is complement-mediated lysis. On occasion this type of reaction can be harmful to the host. This can occur when the lysis is so brisk that intracellular materials are liberated in quantities too large to be handled by metabolic means. One such condition is endotoxic shock resulting from the rapid elimination of gram-negative pathogens. Such rapid lytic events can also lead to pathologic conditions by the concomitant depletion of inhibitors, which are common to the coagulation pathway and critical to maintaining hemostasis. This can lead to a potentially life-threatening condition known as disseminated intravascular coagulation in which the coagulation pathway rages in an uncontrolled cascade.[25] This results in the formation of many tiny useless clots and ironically leads to hemorrhaging into extravascular spaces.

There is one particular antigen–antibody reaction that occurs only in vivo. This is the anaphylactic reaction, which takes place as the result of the specific complexing of an antibody molecule of the IgE isotype with its antigen.

Antibodies of this type are usually produced in response to exposure to certain types of compounds known as allergens. This class of material is composed of a wide variety of natural substances, including pollen, animal dander, and foodstuffs, which are either inhaled or ingested. The IgE immunoglobulin produced, although present in exceedingly small amounts in the serum, primarily remains fixed to tissues in the nasopharynx, the lung, and the gastrointestinal tract. The most common cell type involved in this fixation is the tissue basophil or mast cell.

When antigen combines with such tissue-fixed IgE molecules, crosslinking takes place, with subsequent cell activation. This leads to a degranulation of the mast cells with the resultant release of histamine. This compound causes vasodilitation, which, if generalized, can lead to shock.

In general, in vivo antigen–antibody reactions are a good thing, without which the animal cannot survive. However, under certain conditions, many of which are not yet known, the sequelae of such reactions can lead to pathologic effects.

In vitro reactions are extremely sensitive and highly specific. As a result they lend themselves to many useful applications other than those that are purely diagnostic for a particular infectious disease. By making high-titered pure monoclonal antibodies to a variety of organic molecules, it has been possible to develop systems for the quantitative detection of exceeding small amounts of many substances, including hormones, enzymes, and drugs.

References

1. Karush F. *Adv Immunol.* 1962;2:1.

2. Matsunaga T. Dev Exp Immunol. 1985;9:585.

3. Sell S. Antigen–Antibody Reactions. In *Basic Immunology.* New York: Elsevier; 1987:117–145.

4. Farr RS. *Infect Dis.* 1958;103:239.

5. Eisen HN. Equilibrium dialysis for measurement of antibody hapten affinities. In *Methods in Medical Research,* Eisen HN, ed. Chicago IL: Year Book Medical Publishers; 1964:106.

6. Yalow RS. *Science* 1978;200:1236.

7. Schuurs AHWM, Van Weemen BK. *Clin Chem Acta.* 1977;81;1.

8. Coons AH. *Int Rev Cytol.* 1956;5:1.

9. Fleischmajer R, Gay S, Perlish JS, Cesarini JP. *Invest Dermatol.* 1980;75:189.

10. Kabat EA, Mayer MM. *Experimental Immunochemistry,* 2nd ed. Springfield, IL: Charles C Thomas; 1961.

11. Zmijewski CM, Bellanti JA. Antigen–antibody interactions. In *Immunology,* Vol. III, Bellanti JA, ed. Philadelphia PA: W.B. Saunders; 1985:Chapter 8.

12. Ouchterlony O. *Prog Allergy.* 1962;6:30.

13. Ouchterlony O, Nilsson L-A. Immunodiffusion and immunoelectrophoresis. In *Handbook of Experimental Immunology,* 3rd ed., Weir DM, ed. Oxford: Blackwell Scientific Publishers; 1978:19.1.

14. Pollack W, Hager HJ, Reckel R, Toren DA, Singher HO. *Transfusion.* 1965;5:158.

15. Pollack W, Reckel RP. A reappraisal of the zeta potential model of hemagglutination in human blood groups. In Mohn JF, Plunkett RW, Cunningham RK and Lambert R, eds. *5th International Convocation of Immunologists, 1976.* Basel: Karger; 1977:

16. Pirofsky B, Mangum MEJ. *Proc Soc Exp Biol Med.* 1959;101:49.

17. Coombs RRA, Mourant AE, Race RR. *Br Exp Pathol.* 1945;26:255.

18. Hirsch RL. *Microbiol Rev.* 1982;46:71.

19. Muller-Eberhard HJ, Nilsson UR, Dolmaso AP, Polley MJ, Collcott MA. *Arch Pathol.* 1966;82:205.

20. Rapport MM, Graf L. *Ann NY Acad Sci.* 1957;69:608.

21. Mittal KK, Mickey MR, Singal DP, Terasaki PI. *Transplantation.* 1968;6:913.

22. Nelson DS, ed. *Immunology of the Macrophage.* New York: Academic Press Inc; 1976.

23. Dixon FJ. *J Allergy.* 1954;25:487.

24. Theofilopoulous AN, Dixon FJ. *Adv Immunol.* 1979;28:89.

25. Colman R, Robboy SJ, Minna JD. *Annu Rev Med.* 1979;30:359.

IMMUNOBIOLOGY

CHAPTER 7

Cell-Mediated Immunity (CMI)

Ross Rocklin

Fisons Corporation, Two Preston Court, Bedford, MA 01730 USA

Introduction

The term "delayed hypersensitivity" generally encompasses both the normal and pathologic expressions of cell-mediated immunity (CMI). Its use here is limited to those in vivo manifestations of the cellular immune response that lead to tissue injury. The more inclusive terms "cell-mediated" or "cellular immunity" are used to encompass both normal and pathologic events and include both in vitro and in vivo expressions of specifically sensitized T lymphocytes, as well as those activities carried out by other cellular and humoral components of the immune response.

The cellular reactions involved with this type of immunity are characteristically associated with effector–target cell interactions that result in: (1) acquired host resistance, particularly that associated with facultative intracellular microorganisms; (2) allograft rejection; and (3) tumor surveillance. In each of these reactions, the antigen is either intracellular or sterically inaccessible to humoral host defense mechanisms so that antigen–antibody interactions are relatively inefficient. Reactions mediated by cells, in contrast, appear to be more effective in the elimination of such sterically inaccessible antigens.

Cellular Components
Sensitized T Cells

Development of an immunocompetent population of T lymphocytes proceeds along a well-defined pathway.[1] Initially, a primitive stem cell, which originates during embryogenesis from the fetal yolk sac, liver, and ultimately the bone marrow, has the capability of developing into myeloid, erythroid, or lymphoid lines, depending on its microenvironment. Some of these stem cells migrate to the thymus, where they undergo differentiation, a process that results in the expression of a novel membrane phenotype and new functional capabilities by the eighth week of embryogenesis.[2] Only a small proportion of these thymic lymphocytes reach a stage where they are sufficiently immunocompetent (ie, develop receptors to recognize antigen) to respond in vitro to T-cell stimulants or act as helper cells in the production of antibody by B lymphocytes. This process of intrathymic lymphocyte differentiation is presumably triggered by products of the thymic epithelium, such as thymosin or thymopoietin.

Studies utilizing monoclonal antibodies directed against distinct T-cell antigenic determinants have revealed sequential stages (Table 7-1) of T-cell differentiation within the thymus.[3] It appears that terminal differentiation proceeds along two divergent pathways identified by the appearance of characteristic cell membrane determinants (common determinants or CD): (1) inducer or helper cells bearing the CD T1, T3, and T4 phenotype and (2) suppressor and/or cytotoxic cells expressing the CD T1, T3, T5, or T8 phenotype. These T-cell subsets subsequently populate lymphoid tissues, such as lymph nodes, spleen, blood, and thoracic duct lymph, in varying proportions. In the lymph nodes, T lymphocytes are found in the deep cortical areas, whereas in the spleen they concentrate in the periarteriolar sheaths. At this stage of their differentiation, following encounter with certain antigens, these T cells become activated and are capable of producing the principal expressions of CMI: delayed hypersensitivity, contact hypersensitivity, graft-versus-host response, allograft rejection, immunosurveillance, and eradication of facultative intracellular microorganisms. They also function as potent regulators of the immune response. Once in the periphery, the major subpopulations of T cells recirculate from the blood to lymph and back again.[4] The cells enter lymphoid tissue by traversing the endothelial cells of the postcapillary venules, with which they are thought to share complementary receptors. Such lymphocytes are relatively long lived and presumably are responsible for the persistence of CMI reactivity following sensitization.

It is now recognized that genetically programmed distinct subsets of T lymphocytes (Table 7-2) govern the expression of the various cell-mediated immune functions and that effector functions are regulated by distinct subsets of inducer and

Table 7-1. Maturation of Thymic Lymphocytes[a]

Stage	Surface Marker (Phenotype)
Bone marrow stem cell	None
Early cortical thymocyte	T11
Common thymocyte	T11, T4, T6, T8, T11, T3(Ti), T4, T8
Mature medullary thymocyte	T11, T3(Ti), T4, T12, T1 T11, T3(Ti), T8, T12, T1
Peripheral T lymphocyte in lymphoid organs and blood	T11, T3(Ti), T8, T12, T1 T11, T3(Ti), T4, T12, T1

[a]Stem cells from the bone marrow migrate to the thymic cortex, where they express T-11, a protein that is the receptor for ovine erythrocytes. Later cortical thymocytes express T6, a marker for cortical thymocytes, and T4 (CD4) and T8 (CD8). T4 is the phenotypical marker of cytotoxic-suppressor T cells. However, in the cortex individual thymocytes express both T4 and T8 as well as T3/Ti, the protein complex of the T-cell receptor for antigen. Mature thymocytes in the medulla no longer have T6 but express T1 and T12. The helper-inducer and cytotoxic-suppressor lineages have diverged into two populations with unique phenotypes. These mature T cells then migrate to extrathymic lymphoid organs and the peripheral circulation.

Table 7-2. Human T-Cell Subsets[a]

Cluster Designation	Workshop Antibodies	T-Cell Subset/Function
CD1	T6, Leu-6	Cortical thymocytes
CD2	T11, Leu-5	Pan T cell (E-rosette receptor)
CD3	T3, Leu-4	Mature T cells
CD4	T4, Leu-3	T helper-inducer-DTH subset
CD8	T8, Leu-2	T cytotoxic-suppressor subset

[a]In 1982 the first International Workshop on Human Leukocyte Differentiation Antigens compared different monoclonal antibodies reacting with T-cell surface differentiation antigens. Clusters of monoclonal antibodies reacting with the same antigen were defined. These clusters were designated clusters of differentiation (CD) with the anticipation that CD designation would be used as standard nomenclature instead of individual monoclonal antibody designations.

Note: The L3T4+ and Ly2+3+ T-cell subsets in mice correspond respectively to CD4+ and CD8+ human subsets.

suppressor T lymphocytes.[5] These regulatory cells clearly modulate humoral immunity and appear to control an increasing number of nonimmune responses as well. The concept has emerged that immune responses reflect the net effect of counterbalancing inducer and suppressor populations. It has been shown that inducer T cells regulate macrophage activation, generation of cytotoxic T lymphocytes, differentiation of B lymphocytes, and such diverse activities as hematopoiesis. These regulatory cell populations are part of a complex network that monitors and maintains immune homeostasis. The exact mechanism by which these cells communicate with each other is currently unclear, although a large body of evidence implicates the involvement of soluble factors.[6] Several such factors have been described but those that seem most important are antigen-specific factors that bear idiotypic as well as major histocompatibility complex (MHC) determinants.

Characterization of immunoregulatory subsets of T cells in humans has revealed that suppressor T lymphocytes: (1) bear receptors for the Fc fragment of IgG, (2) bear receptors for histamine of the H_2 variety, (3) are sensitive to 1500–2000 R irradiation and the effects of corticosteroids, and (4) are preferentially activated by the mitogen concanavalin A. Helper or inducer T lymphocytes express a receptor for the Fc fragment of IgM and are relatively resistant to irradiation and corticosteriods. Helper T cells may actually be comprised of two subpopulations; one induces directly a particular immune response, the other engages in activation of suppressor cells with resultant feedback inhibition.[7] Qualitative and/or quantitative abnormalities in these regulatory T cell subsets may account for the immunologic imbalance that may be observed in several pathologic states. For example, defective suppressor T-cell activity may result in excessive production of abnormal antibodies directed against tissue components of possible pathogenetic significance in certain autoimmune diseases. On the other hand, excessive suppressor T-cell activity may be involved in the pathogenesis of immunodeficiency states, such as common variable hypogammaglobulinemia, selective IgA deficiency, and thymoma with agammaglobulinemia.[8]

While it is still useful to subdivide CD4+ helper-inducer T cells and CD8+ cytotoxic-suppressor T cells into functional subsets, it is now clear that T-cell clones of a particular specificity can carry out distinct functional roles, depending on conditions in the local environment.[9,10] Overall, the polyclonal nature of T-cell responses and the potential for multiple functions of individual antigen-specific T-cell clones endows the immune system with enormous adaptability in CMI.

Although the CD4 and CD8 surface antigens differentiate between functional subsets of T cells under normal circumstances, it should be noted that these molecules can be induced in non-T cells. For example, CD4 antigen can be expressed on the surface of activated macrophages or B cells. This accounts for the observation that macrophages and B cells can be infected by the human immunodeficiency virus (HIV), which causes the acquired immunodeficiency syndrome (AIDS), since the virus can enter these cells by virtue of its ability to bind to CD4 as a receptor.

Antigen-Presenting Cells (APC)

Cells of the monocyte–macrophage lineage play a key role in the induction and expression of several types of immune responses[11] by virtue of their ability to: (1) process antigen and present it to T lymphocytes; (2) focus and transport antigen-specific helper and suppressor factors; (3) elaborate soluble factors that facilitate (eg, interleukin 1) or inhibit (eg, prostanoids) T-cell function; and (4) serve as effector cells (ie, engulf microorganisms, kill tumor cells). It seems likely that monocyte–macrophages, like T lymphocytes, are to a certain degree a heterogeneous population.

A system of antigens expressed on APC that is important for the activation of T cells is encoded by the I region (immune response associated) of the major histocompatibility complex (MHC). The products of these genes are class-II MHC antigens, which are also referred to as Ia antigens. They are commonly expressed on B cells, monocytes, and macrophages and subserve cellular interactions in immune responses. The Ia antigens can also be expressed on T cells and, when detected, are a sign of cellular activation.[12,13] Thus, elevated numbers of Ia$^+$ T cells are found in a number of inflammatory diseases, in infections, and in recently immunized normals.[14] In mice the I region of the MHC is divided into the I-A and I-E subregions. The human analogs are HLA-DP, -DQ, and -DR antigens.

Monocyte–macrophage Ia antigens have a limited specificity for binding peptide fragments of antigens. Such fragments are produced by limited intracellular digestion via enzymes.[15,16] The T cell binds complexes of antigen fragment and Ia antigen on the surface of APCs through its receptor, resulting in the antigen–MHC-restricted specificity of T-cell recognition. Dendritic cells in the tissues and Langerhans cells in the skin are highly specialized APCs with high levels of surface Ia antigens. Activation of a wide variety of cell types (endothelial cells, epithelial cells, fibroblasts, astrocytes, etc) by certain stimuli, such as interferon-γ, results in the induction of surface Ia positivity. In most cases this allows such a cell to function as an APC. In some cases, such as thyroid epithelial cells, antigen fragments can be presented to specific T cells but must first be digested by another cell.[17] Expression of Ia antigens on specific tissue cells, such as thyroid epithelial cells, may be important in the development of autoimmunity.[18] Many human diseases are linked to specific MHC haplotypes, such as HLA-DP, -DQ, or -DR Ia antigens. This association may occur because of a specific interaction between a given HLA-D/Ia antigen on an APC and a particular antigen fragment derived from a pathogen or a self-non-MHC molecule, resulting in subsequent T-cell activation and autoreactivity. Recognition of specific antigen and self-MHC is a requirement for delayed-type hypersensitivity (DTH) reactions. This is called dual specificity.

The locus of the MHC class-II specificity requirement of CD4$^+$ T cells in DTH is probably associated with Ia antigens on the surface of macrophage-like APCs. Nearly all responses of inducer T cells are critically dependent upon interaction with the Ia$^+$ subset of these accessory cells. Langerhans cells situated in the epidermis have been shown to function as APCs and to be crucial in the induction of contact-type DTH responses induced by picryl chloride, DNCB, or poison ivy.[19] Langerhans cells take up antigen and migrate to regional lymph nodes, where they induce effector T cells that are relatively resistant to suppression and mediate long-lived DTH. Part of the reason mycobacterial adjuvants induce such strong and long-lived DTH responses depends on their ability to strengthen the antigen-presenting capacity of macrophages.

Antigen-presenting cells are critically important in determining whether DTH is induced, whether it is long-lived, and whether it is resistant to suppression. Although most studies to date have dealt with the role of APCs in the induction of DTH, recent studies indicate that these cells also play an important role in the elicitation of DTH.[20] Therefore, it is likely that antigen associated with Ia determinants on Langerhans cells triggers activation of sensitized CD4$^+$ T cells at the site of an evolving DTH reaction.

Mast Cells and Basophils

Mast cells and basophils function as the principal mediator-releasing cells of immediate hypersensitivity. Furthermore, it has recently been established that mast cells and basophils are involved in in vivo DTH and CMI reactions. This involvement of mediator-releasing mast cells and basophils in delayed-type responses has been shown to have a protective consequence and to confer immune resistance to complex parasites in experimental systems.[21,22]

Mast cells are mediator-containing cells, present in certain tissues (eg, airways and gastrointestinal tract), and produce the symptoms of atopic disease when triggered by allergen. Basophils are similar to mast cells (mediator-containing cells) but circulate in the blood and can be recruited into the tissues during immune responses. In biologically relevant in vivo T-cell-dependent responses, mast cells in the extravascular tissue can initiate an essential response that is necessary for the subsequent arrival into the tissues of late-acting lymphokine-producing T cells of DTH. Thus mast cells can mediate a crucial immediate hypersensitivity-like initiating phase of CMI reactions. This participation of allergic disease mechanisms in biologically relevant immune resistance responses seems to occur as well in at least a limited number of immune tumor resistance model systems.[22]

In contrast to mast cells, basophils are circulating mediator-containing cells that are only one of a number of different kinds of leukocytes that can be recruited to sites of various DTH responses that comprise the infiltrate that is characteristic of these reactions. In the model of resistance to ectoparasitic arthropod ticks cited above, basophils recruited to the site of tick feeding undergo immediate, anaphylactic degranulation with release of mediators. This arrival and anaphylactic degranulation of basophils at delayed reactions has been shown to be essential for the mediation of immune resistance to these complex parasites, thus indicating a protective role for basophil recruitment and anaphylactic release of mediators in this model system.[23]

Induction of CMI

Interaction of Antigen with Its Receptor on T Cells

The induction of a T-cell response involves the recognition of an antigen by the receptor present on a clone of T lymphocytes. In all species so far studied, these T-cell receptors are made up of two different chains, called α and β. Alpha chains are more acidic and in humans have a higher molecular weight (47–52 kd) than the neutral or slightly basic β chains.[24–26] Both chains vary in amino acid sequence from one T-cell clone to another. In mice, both chains are 43 kd. [25,27] The two chains are linked by disulfide bonds and thus form a structure similar to the disulfide-bonded immunoglobulin molecule. Although T-cell receptors are not made up of the same genes as immunoglobulins, similar strategies have been employed to generate a large variety of different receptor proteins from a relatively small collection of genes.

Twenty to forty thousand receptor proteins per cell are expressed on mature T cells. These levels do not appear to vary significantly even when the T cell interacts with antigen or is activated by mitogen. Electron microscopy shows that the receptors are uniformally distributed over the surface of the normal cell, but, as in the case of immunoglobulins, T-cell receptors can be capped or patched with the addition of antireceptor antibodies.[28,29] This capping phenomenon has led to the observation that membrane-bound T-cell receptors are closely associated with another collection of proteins known as T3 (also called Leu 4 or CD3).

As mentioned previously, T3 proteins were first recognized in humans by monoclonal antibodies.[30] These antibodies bind to all peripheral T cells and a percentage of human thymocytes. They share a property of antireceptor antibodies; ie, under appropriate circumstances they may either inhibit or mimic the recognition of antigen by human T cells. Thus, they may function to transmit a signal to the inside of the cells.

Proteins of the T3 complex do not appear to contribute to the part of the T-cell receptor that recognizes antigen or polymorphic regions of the MHC specifically, since T3 proteins do not seem to vary in amino acid sequence between T-cell clones of different specificities. However, T3 does seem to be closely associated with the receptor, since the proteins can be cocapped and crosslinking studies show that the proteins of T3 and those of the receptor are very near each other on the cell surface.[31] The T3 complex is made up of at least three different polypeptide subunits (γ, δ, ε), one of which seems to be buried deeply in the membrane of the cell.

It is currently believed that the specific binding of antigen to T cells involves the formation of a trimolecular complex of receptor, antigen, and MHC product (Figure 7-1). Most often the antigen involved seems to be not the intact protein molecule, but a small peptide fragment produced by proteolysis within the antigen-presenting cell.[32–34] It is likely that the binding reaction proceeds by the initial attachment of two of the components to each other, followed by the introduction of the third component and consequent stabilization of the complex. The order of assembly is not known and indeed may vary depending on the individual components.

Two other surface molecules that contribute to the interaction of T cells with antigen are the CD4 and CD8 molecules. The former is usually found on class-II-restricted, and CD8 on class-I-restricted T cells.[35] There is evidence that these molecules bind to target structures on antigen-presenting cells and thus increase the overall affinity of the interaction. Another T-cell surface protein that also seems to

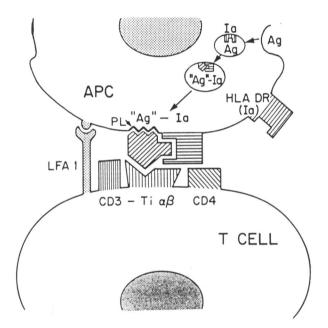

Figure 7-1. Diagram of T-cell surface receptor complex for antigen/self. Native antigen (Ag) is taken up by antigen-presenting cells (APCs), which are characterized by surface expression of Ia (immune-associated) antigens. After uptake, enzymatic cleavage (probably in endosomes) results in antigen fragments (''Ag'') that bind to HLA-D–Ia molecules and form a complex that is then displayed on APC surface. Binding of ''Ag'' on APC surface is stabilized by interaction of hydrophobic ''Ag'' on APC determinants with membrane phospholipids (PL). Complex of ''Ag'' and self-Ia class-II molecule interacts with T-cell antigen/self (T9), which is a two-chain heterodimer of α and β chains. Each α and β chain has constant portions that traverse cell membrane and variable portions that bind ''Ag''–Ia complex. The trimolecular interaction complex of ''Ag''–Ia and Tia is stabilized by binding of T-cell surface CD4 molecules to Ia, and/or binding of CD4 to Tia, and by binding of other accessory adhesion molecules (such as LFA 1) to appropriate ligand and APC surfaces.

promote interactions with the APC include lymphocyte functional antigen 1 (LFA-1), which is related to a similar molecule on macrophages (Mac 1) and granulocytes.

Accumulated evidence indicates that antigen-specific suppressor T cells do not employ the receptor genes of MHC-restricted T cells to bind antigen. Thus, suppressor T cells bind free antigen or the idiotype of the antibody they are destined to suppress.[36,37] Their receptors have immunoglobulin-related and MHC-related determinants. They also secrete antigen-specific suppressor factors following activation by these stimulants.

Requirements for Induction

Experimental studies have generally concluded that CMI responses are best induced by peptides or chemical determinants conjugated to proteins. Although the chemical may be quite simple (hapten), the antigenic specificity of the delayed hypersensitivity response is generally directed against a complex that includes part of the protein "carrier." By contrast, a concomitant antibody response is directed against hapten as well as carrier determinants.

The route of introduction of the antigen is also important in the induction of CMI. Small amounts of particulate or adjuvant-associated antigen introduced into an area with appropriate lymphatic drainage is followed by cellular sensitization and development of CMI at the site and/or draining lymph nodes. By contrast, intravenous injection of a large amount of soluble antigen not only generally fails to induce CMI but may also temporarily block the capacity to subsequently induce CMI to the same antigen by otherwise successful means. Such blockade may induce a process of clonal deletion and/or activation of suppressor cells. In a similar way, hapten-derivatized cells induce CMI reactions when administered subcutaneously and a state of unresponsiveness when administered intravenously.[38,39] This process may involve suppressor T-cell populations and their factors as mentioned above.[40]

The Langerhans cell, a macrophage-like cell found in the epidermis, is currently thought to ingest locally deposited antigen and then transport it to the draining lymph node.[41] When antigen is not processed by APC, suppressor T cells are preferentially activated and a state of specific unresponsiveness is induced. These approaches are currently being applied to experimental models of autoimmune disease and may one day be exploited as therapeutic strategies for the regulation of unwanted immune responses in human disease.

Carbohydrates generally raise vigorous antibody responses, while immunization with proteins leads to strong DTH responses. Chemical modification of antigens can determine whether strong DTH or antibody responses ensue.[42] In animals immunized with complete Freunds adjuvant, DTH reactions are long lived and are accompanied by marked antibody responses. Animals immunized either with antigen emulsified with incomplete Freunds adjuvant (no mycobacteria), with soluble antigens without adjuvant, or with erythrocytes administered intravenously have DTH reactions that are evanescent and are replaced by antibody-mediated reactions.[43]

Repeated skin testing with protein antigens in humans leads to a loss of DTH reactivity and the onset of antibody-mediated wheal and flare reactions.[44]

Expression of CMI

While CMI reactivity may be expressed through a variety of manifestations, the DTH reaction will be considered first since it has been the most extensively studied expression of CMI. It should be emphasized initially that a state of delayed hypersensitivity is a systemic form of altered reactivity. Thus, the intravenous injection of endotoxin-free antigen into an appropriately sensitized host will result in a characteristic febrile response, possibly as a result of leukocytic pyrogen being released following contact of antigen with primed T lymphocytes. Systemic DTH responses may be responsible for at least part of the fever and myalgia that occurs during certain infections and during adverse reactions to drugs and immunizations.

The traditional way of measuring of delayed hypersensitivity is the elicitation of a delayed-type (DTH) skin test response. Characteristically the intradermal injection of a soluble antigen into a sensitized individual is followed after several hours by the onset of an erythematous and indurated reaction, which peaks at 48–72 h (depending on the species) and resolves after several additional days. If the reaction is pronounced, central pallor and a nodule with an erythematous halo may result; necrosis is sometimes observed in very intense reactions. The exact appearance that a particular reaction may take is determined by several characteristics of the antigen itself, in addition to the sensitivity of the host. These include the physicochemical nature of the antigen, its charge, and its size.

The physical charge of the antigen may also determine the pattern and degree of the DTH response elicited and is probably related to the ability of the antigen to bind to the tissue. The bulk of intradermally injected antigen has been shown to leave the skin within 24 h; the residual amounts subsequently leave at different rates, depending on the antigen employed. Whether there is increased residual antigen in positive DTH sites reacting with sensitized cells has not been satisfactorily answered. However, it is likely that studies employing soluble, readily diffusible antigens do not reflect the clinical situation, in which DTH responses are directed against readily ingested particulate antigens that persist at the site for at least several days.

It has been shown that the kinetics and both the gross and histologic appearance of DTH skin test responses are determined in part by the site into which antigen is introduced. For example, the histopathology of DTH responses to the same antigen differs not only between species but also with regard to the particular lymphoid tissues involved or the level at which antigen is introduced into the skin (topical or intradermal).

The primary features (induration and erythema) of the DTH skin test that are usually measured clinically appear to result from a combination of vascular, intracellular inflammatory responses.[45] The application of more sophisticated technology has permitted further understanding of the histological picture of such reactions.[46] In the dermis of most species, a superficial venular plexus lies at the junction of the capillary (upper) dermis and reticular (deeper) dermis. Superficial capillary venules are vascular loops in the capillary dermis that connect arteriolar and venular branches of the superficial vascular plexus. Within hours after the intradermal injection of antigen into a sensitized subject, gaps form between endothelial cells of the superficial capillary venules. This event is followed by increased vascular permeability. The endothelial cells exhibit active DNA synthesis; they swell and this results in narrowing of the vascular lumen. Associated with this may be the subsequent deposition of fibrin in a loose meshwork between the dermal collagen bundles. The collagen bundles retain water and this results in collagen swelling. Such fibrin deposition is considered to be the major component responsible for the induration in DTH skin reactions.

Both the quality and the quantity of inflammatory cells in DTH reaction sites vary somewhat, depending on the host species and the sensitizing antigen. Previous studies of DTH skin test responses to microbial antigens in animals identified cellular components that were initially similar to those found in the peripheral blood (mostly granulocytes), followed by mononuclear cell predominance at the peak of gross reactivity 24–36 h later. In humans, granulocytes are unusual at any time. Thus, some investigators believe that the presence of granulocytes at a DTH site represents an irritant and/or a concomitant Arthus-type reaction to the same antigen. Ultramicroscopic studies have shown antigen in only a small number of macrophages (associated with lysosomal-type structures) and apparently not bound to the surface of lymphocytes.[46] Studies of the histologic evolution of the DTH response as it resolves over days to weeks demonstrate the presence of epithelioid and giant cells and small lymphocytes in perivascular areas of the deep dermis.

Cellular surface markers associated with different functional programs described previously have allowed determination of the phenotype of T cells in CMI reactions in vivo. At sites of human DTH reactions to tuberculin purified protein derivative (PPD), a progressive expression of activation antigens (Ia) by these cells has been demonstrated.[47] In cutaneous infiltrates recorded by biopsy sites in patients with leprosy, a good correlation was found between the T-cell phenotype and the clinical status. In tuberculoid patients with effective CMI resistance to *M. leprae* CD4+ T cells predominated, whereas CD8+ T cells predominated in lepromatous patients who lacked effective CMI to the microorganism.[48] Ultrastructural study of these lesions confirmed that CD4+ tuberculoid lesions contained activated T cells and macrophages, whereas CD8+ lepromatous lesions did not, perhaps because of the suppressive influence.[49]

Effector Mechanisms

Activated T-helper (T_H) cells elaborate lymphokines, some of which activate macrophages and also recruit other lymphocytes and monocytes. The latter cells produce monokines, some of which are necessary for T-cell activation and the induction of inflammation. Thus, a reaction that initially involves a small number of sensitized T cells, can be amplified and expanded to include a large number of cells that are not specifically sensitized to the antigen that initiated the reaction.[50] A list of these effector molecules is shown in Table 7-3.

Macrophages liberate interleukin-1 (IL-1), a monokine that seems identical to leukocyte pyrogen (the cause of febrile reactions) and is required for activation of T_H lymphocytes. The latter cells elaborate T-cell growth factor (interleukin-2 or IL-2), and, together with IL-1, bring about the differentiation of the CD4$^+$ T cells.[51] The CD4$^+$ T cell activated by antigen and IL-1 then releases a series of molecules that can enhance the function of macrophages. One such factor(s) is macrophage activation factor (MAF); this may in fact be an activity involving multiple molecules, one of which seems to be interferon-γ. Once the macrophages are activated, they secrete not only interleukin-1, but also a series of enzymes (neutral proteases, eg, collagenase and elastase) that can digest connective tissue. They also elaborate procoagulant molecules (tissue factor and factor VII) that can cause local coagulation via the extrinsic coagulation pathway, and they release a plasminogen activator. This last enzyme converts plasminogen to plasmin, and plasmin will digest fibrin, thereby slowly reversing clot formation and the induration of DTH sites. As mentioned above, fibrin is deposited at sites of DTH and its intermediate degradation produces "fibrinoid," which is found in increased amounts in connective tissue diseases.

Release of other lymphokines, such as macrophage chemotactic factor (CF), can

Table 7-3. Lymphokines and Their Target Cells

Target cell	Lymphokine
Macrophages or monocytes	Migration inhibitor factor
	Macrophage-activating, factors, including interferon-γ and granulocyte–monocyte colony-stimulating factor
	Macrophage chemotactic factor
Lymphocytes	Interleukin-2
	B-cell-stimulating factor 1
	B-cell-stimulating factor 2
	B-cell growth factor II
	Interleukin-4
	Transfer factor
Polymorphonuclear leukocytes	Neutrophil, basophil, and eosinophil chemotactic factors
	Leukocyte inhibitory factor
	Eosinophil stimulation promoter
	Histamine-releasing factor
	Interleukin-5
Other cells	Interleukin-3 (multicolony-stimulating factor)
	Interferon-γ
	Collagen-producing factor
	Procoagulant (tissue factor)
	Tumor necrosis factor α and β (lymphotoxin)

recruit blood monocytes to the site of reaction, while migration inhibition factor (MIF) immobilizes macrophages and tends to localize them to the vicinity of the immune reaction. Release of another factor, a macrophage aggregation factor (MAggF), facilitates their adherence to one another. The latter factor appears to be fibronectin or fragments derived therefrom. Interleukin-2 is required for the proliferation of certain subpopulations of T lymphocytes. The IL-2 released by the T_H cell interacts with an IL-2 receptor on T-suppressor (T_S) cells (T8$^+$) and, in conjunction with IL-1, activates them. As mentioned previously, the T_S cell regulates both T- and B-cell functions, usually by means of suppressor factors that block the activity of T_H cells and the differentiation of B-cells into plasma cells.

Many deficiencies in CMI now appear to be explained by various defects in this system of interleukin receptors. For instance, patients with active tuberculosis have cutaneous DTH anergy (described below), depressed in vitro T-cell proliferation to PPD, defective production of IL-2, and defective generation of IL-2 receptors.[52] In addition, increased production of IL-1 by activated monocyte–macrophages, which can lead to augmented production of PGE$_2$, may also contribute to anergy in tuberculosis and sarcoidosis by inhibition of T-cell function.[53,54] Similarly, patients with lepromatous leprosy are anergic and have peripheral blood T cells that are not activated to proliferate by lepromin antigen. However, it can be shown that antigen-specific T cells are present in such patients and can be activated by lepromin up to the stage of IL-2 reactivity, but activation proceeds no further.[55] This may result from the production of suppressor factors by monocytes. Thus, the addition of exogenous IL-2 to the in vitro culture reverses the defect. Similarly, mice receiving high doses of mycobacteria have suppressed in vitro lymphocyte function and suppressed DTH. Both of these defects are reversed by the administration of IL-2.[56] These findings raise the possibility that recombinant IL-2 could be used to treat some immunodeficient states. Indeed, preliminary clinical trials of cancer immunotherapy with IL-2 and with effector cells activated ex vivo with IL-2 have shown promising results in some patients.

A summary of the development of a DTH response can be viewed as follows. Recirculating T cells leave the blood and enter the tissues by mechanisms that are not well understood at present. Sensitized mast cells are activated when eliciting antigen binds to their antigen-specific receptors, resulting in release of vasoactive amines. Platelets activated through the release of mast-cell mediators may be another source of vasoactive amines. These vasoactive amines promote the formation of gaps between endothelial cells situated in postcapillary venules. This allows previously sensitized, antigen–MHC class-II-specific CD4$^+$ T cells to enter the tissues. Once in the extravascular tissue space, these T cells can encounter antigen that is probably presented as a digested fragment in association with Ia antigens on the surface of local macrophage-like APCs (Langerhans cells) that are in the skin. Interactions between specific CD3-Ti receptors on the surface of specifically sensitized T cells and antigen fragment–Ia complexes presented by APCs result in activation of T cells for the production of various lymphokine mediators. Some of these substances are chemotactic for nonspecific inflammatory cells (monocytes, polymorphs, basophils, and B cells) that are resident in the circulation. Local vasodilation enhances the diffusion of chemotactic factors into the vessels, attracting more circulating cells to the area. The initial wave of lymphokines released by specifically stimulated T cells also activates endothelial cells and opens gaps in local blood vessels. Thus intravascular, bone-marrow-derived auxiliary cells that have adhered to the local vasculature can then migrate between the interendothelial cell gaps and thereby enter the antigen-containing tissue to produce the full measure of inflammatory infiltrate that characterizes DTH reactions. Other lymphokines, such as MIF, undoubtedly immobilize inflammatory cells once they have arrived, and others, such as macrophage activation factor (MAF) or interferon-γ, may activate these cells for more efficient phagocytosis, greater presentation of receptors for cytophilic antibodies, and augmented ability to kill tumor cells, bacteria, viruses, and parasites. Some evidence suggests that soluble mediators are released that might directly increase vascular permeability and thus further aid the egress of humoral and cellular intravascular components of the immune system to the extravascular local tissue reaction. Furthermore, products of sensitized cells may be released that are mitosis inducing not only for other inflammatory cells (thereby increasing their number), but also for cells of the blood vessels, thereby increasing vascularity and thus facilitating the inflow of protective substances and dispersal of toxic materials.

Role of CMI in Homeostasis

Defense Against Infections

While there is some controversy as to whether DTH responses to microbial antigens are to the overall benefit or detriment of the individual infected with the particular microorganism, there is agreement concerning the following observations:

1. Local resistance to the spread of an infectious focus caused by an organism such a *M. tuberculosis* depends on the presence of sufficient numbers of activated macrophages, whose increased metabolic and enzymatic activities are associated with increased intracellular killing of microorganisms.[57]
2. In a first-exposure infection, DTH skin reactivity to antigens of the infecting organism and enhancement of macrophage reactivity to the organism develop in parallel.
3. Once macrophages are activated by the inciting organisms, they may demonstrate immunologically nonspecific microbicidal activity against certain other pathogens.
4. the capacities for both delayed hypersensitivity and protective immunity can be transferred by subsets of T lymphocytes in an immunologically specific manner.
5. depletion of T lymphocytes in both experimental and clinical situations markedly depresses the capacity to develop this protective immunity.

In clinical CMI immunodeficiency states, there may be increased severity of infection with herpes simplex, cytomegalic inclusion disease, measles, and pox viruses, certain fungi, and other intracellular parasites. Examples of particular associations are: severe combined immunodeficiency disease and progressive vaccinia, Wiskott-Aldrich and herpes simplex, and Hodgkin's disease and herpes zoster. In contrast, the presence of strong DTH reactivity to antigens of the pathogen in some fungal infections is associated with a low incidence of disseminated disease.

Allograft Rejection

Cell-mediated immunity reactions against alloantigens result in rejection of allogeneic skin grafts. The major cell type that is found in the rejected graft in the mouse has the Lyt-1$^+$ (L3T4) phenotype that is characteristic of the T_H cell.[58] However, cytolytic Lyt-2$^+$ T cells may also be present. Passive transfer of allograft hypersensitivity may be achieved with T_H cells alone. The cells recognize differences in the histocompatibility profiles that are encoded by the MHC, as well as by the male antigen (H-Y) that is responsible for rejection of male skin by syngeneic female recipients.[59]

It has been demonstrated that culturing certain tissues in high oxygen tensions allows the subsequent graft of that tissue to have prolonged survival in allogeneic recipients.[60-62] If the transplant recipient is given cells that bear the histocompatibility antigens of the tissue donor, however, the transplanted tissue is rejected. This observation has led to the hypothesis that passenger cells such as leukocytes that bear MHC antigens are largely responsible for the allosensitization that leads to graft rejection.

Contact Sensitivity

This response is induced by applying reactive haptens or salts to the skin. Common examples include the reactivity to pentadecyl catechols in patients with poison ivy[63] and reactions to dyes in clothing and to metals in jewelry. The immune response is directed against the sensitizing chemical, which serves as a hapten after covalent binding to proteins in the skin or serum to create new antigenic determinants. Sensitization is demonstrated by application of a small amount of the sensitizer to the skin of the patient or the pinna of the ear of a rodent; the classical inflammatory response with edema and mononuclear cell infiltration develops over 24–72 h.

Although contact hypersensitivity is considered an expression of CMI, its histological characteristics differ in several respects from other DTH skin reactions that occur primarily in the dermis. Topically applied antigens appear to be processed somewhat differently than antigens administered by other routes. There is antigen binding to skin proteins in some cases, with concentration of such complexes in the epidermis and appendigeal structures. Also, antigens may be processed by the Langerhans cells. Topical challenge of a sensitized subject is followed within 6 h by a perivascular collection of mononuclear cells in the epidermis. Then intercellular edema develops and there occurs a progressive separation of epidermal cells, particularly in the basal layer. In the human, intercellular epidermal edema may lead to vesiculation. A basophilic infiltration is also prominent in these contact reactions.[64] This picture is similar to that observed in the erythematous skin test response which occurs during a transient period after experimental sensitization with small doses of soluble antigen without adjuvant. This reactivity, called Jones-Mote or cutaneous basophil hypersensitivity, can be transferred with lymphoid cells or serum obtained from a sensitized animal.

Granuloma Formation

This immune response occurs in foci of infection with organisms such as mycobacteria and certain parasites that survive after ingestion by phagocytes. Similar responses develop at sites of exposure to such metals as beryllium and zirconium or foreign bodies such as talc. It is believed that persistence of the antigen in the tissues provides the long-term stimulus for the production of granulomas. Histologically, granulomas are composed of macrophages and epithelioid cells with variable numbers of lymphocytes, neutrophils, eosinophils, and plasma cells. The origin of the epithelioid cells is unclear, although there is some evidence that these cells are derived from macrophages. The other cell type that characterizes granulomas is the giant cell, which is believed to be an end stage of differentiation of monocytes and macrophages. Granulomatous reactions in humans occur at sites of persistent antigenic stimulation (tubercles), foreign body deposition, and loci of persistent T-lymphocyte activation, such as sarcoidosis.

Graft-Versus-Host Disease

Graft-versus-host disease occurs when immunocompetent T lymphocytes are administered to recipients that are immunoincompetent and so cannot eliminate the transferred cells. Some examples of recipients that are predisposed to develop graft-versus-host disease include newborn animals (the immune system has not fully developed), F_1 hybrids that do not identify parental cells as foreign while the parental cells react against the alloantigens of the other parent, and animals that have been immunosuppressed (drugs, irradiation).[65,66] The donor cells may react against class-I or class-II antigens of the MHC, as well as minor, non-MHC-determined antigens.

Two general consequences may result because of graft-versus-host disease.[67] One has "stimulatory" features, including lymphoid hyperplasia, hyperimmunoglobulinemia, autoantibody production, and clinical manifestations of autoimmune diseases, such as scleroderma.[68] The other form of graft-versus-host disease is "suppressive" and is expressed as aplastic anemia and hypoplasia of the immune system. The first form of graft-versus-host disease may be mediated by Lyt-1$^+$T lymphocytes that are activated by class-II alloantigens, while the suppressive form may involve recognition of both class-I and class-II alloantigens.

Regulation of CMI

The intensity of the induration in the skin and the expression of virtually all of the effector T-lymphocyte CMI responses are regulated by other T cells with either inducer-helper or suppressor functions and by drugs or treatments that affect either the number of helper or suppressor cells, or their activities. Most experimental data indicate that the regulatory contribution of suppressor cells is dominant over the effects of T_H cells. These T_S cells are usually antigen specific and apparently different from the suppressor cells that regulate antibody synthesis.

Regulation of CMI reactivity is accomplished by several mechanisms including: T_S lymphocytes and their soluble factors; products of monocytes and macrophages; genetic restriction of the interactions between T_S cells and T_H cells by the I-J subregion of the MHC, and genetic control by genes that are linked to those (Igh) that determine the allotype of immunoglobulin heavy chains.

Studies have been carried out to investigate the development and expression of CMI.[69] Lymphoid cells from sensitized donors were transferred to recipients that were disparate at various loci within the MHC. The results have revealed a requirement for identity within the I-A region of chromosome 17 in order to have normal expression of CMI. Other responses, such as granulomatous reactions in the lungs of mice that receive *Bacillus* Calmette-Guerin (BCG) in emulsions, appear to be controlled by loci that are linked to the allotype of the immunoglobulin heavy chain (Igh) on chromosome 12.[70,71] These observations have been extended to the state of diminished DTH responsiveness seen in mice initially immunized with DCG and then subsequently sensitized with sheep erythrocytes (SRBCs). Mice that had the b haplotype at the Igh locus were "anergic" or unresponsive when challenged with SRBCs in the footpads. However, anergy in this model was not associated with a particular H-2 antigen. Another locus that was found to control interaction between helper T cells and suppressor T cells was the I-J region.

Genetic studies of susceptibility to infections with *Mycobacterium lepraemurium* in mice have shown linkage to a gene on chromosome 1 rather than genes within the MHC.[72] In humans, both susceptibility to leprosy and the clinical form of leprosy have been reported to be associated with at least two HLA-linked genes.[73]

Several widely used pharmacological agents may affect the expression of CMI. For example, anticoagulation with heparin inhibits development of induration at the sites of cutaneous DTH reactions due to the loss of the fibrin matrix.[74] Patients with afibrinogenemia develop edema and cellular infiltrates at skin test sites but not induration.[75] Other agents that modulate CMI responses either positively or negatively include indomethacin, amphotericin B, corticosteroids, purine antimetabolites, alkylating agents, histamine type-2 antagonists, and cyclosporin A. Some of these are considered in more detail below.

The intravenous injection of hapten in the form of cell-bound antigen or as a soluble salt may induce either of two suppressor systems. In one, called afferent suppression, *generation* of T_H cells is suppressed. These animals cannot adoptively transfer DTH reactivity to unsensitized recipients. The second mechanism is called efferent suppression because the *activity* of the T_H cells is inhibited by T_S cells.

Suppression of the induction of DTH by suppressor cells is common in antigen-specific regulatory networks that interact through idiotype and anti-idiotype interactions. In these systems, regulatory and effector T cells appear to act by surface- and soluble-antigen receptors with idiotypes that are related antigenically to the idiotypes of immunoglobulins. Also, in these systems there is often a link between these suppressor cells that act at the afferent level and other suppressor cells that act at the efferent phase of DTH. Regulatory-suppressor T cells often are composed of three interacting subsets termed first-order (T_S1), second-order (T_S2), and third-order (T_S3) T_S cells. Each subset has a distinct surface phenotype and a distinct function[76] and often acts via a specific suppressor factor (ie, T_SF1, T_SF2, and T_SF3). The T_SF1 is derived from an Lyl$^+$ I-J$^+$ T cell and is antigen specific and idiotype positive (id$^+$). Its locus of action is on the afferent limb. In addition, T_SF1 acts as a suppressor inducer to initiate a suppressor cascade that suppresses the efferent DTH effector T cells. Thus, T_SF1 causes Ly2$^+$ I-J$^+$ T cells to elaborate T_SF2 that is anti-idiotypic in specificity. The efferent suppressor-effector T_SF3-producing cells are also Ly2$^+$ but are antigen specific and id$^+$ and are induced by immunization. However, they must be activated by the anti-idiotypic T_SF2 to produce their antigen-specific id$^+$ suppressive T_SF3 that acts on the late-acting effector T cells. Both act on the efferent limb and are composed of antigen-specific initiating factors that lead to the generation of nonspecific factors that are responsible for the suppressive effects.

Clinical Assessment of CMI

Measurement of the functions of the CMI system is often undertaken as part of the evaluation of patients with cancer or unusual susceptibility to chronic or recurrent infectious diseases. One clinical observation that should prompt this assessment is the nature of the infections; patients suspected of having defective CMI are usually infected with fungi, such as *Candida albicans;* mycobacteria, including the atypical or nontuberculous mycobacteria; protozoa, such as *Pneumocystis carinii* and *Cryptosporidium* species; or viruses, such as cytomegalovirus, varicella zoster, and other herpesviruses. Opportunistic infections of the skin also suggest impaired CMI. The age of onset of infections may also help discern whether the defect is congenital or hereditary and whether it is caused by impaired maturation of T cells or by other disorders that deplete the cellular components of the lymphoid system or upset homeostatic immunoregulatory processes.

There are currently available methods for both the in vitro and in vivo quantitative assessments of immune functions (Table 7-4). As a screening procedure, clinically relevant information can be obtained from the leukocyte count and differential since the presence of lymphopenia may suggest the diagnosis of a primary immunodeficiency or of a disease process that depletes lymphocytes. Quantitation of T lymphocytes through the measurement of the percentage of cells that form rosettes with sheep erythrocytes has largely been replaced by their quantitation with monoclonal antibodies. These reagents also permit quantitation of the subsets of T cells that have helper/inducer, cytotoxic/suppressor, or accessory functions.[77]

The DTH Skin Test

The most widely used in vivo test for CMI is the intradermal DTH skin test. Selection of appropriate antigens should take into account: (1) prior immunological experiences with vaccines, such as diphtheria, tetanus, or mumps; (2) past illnesses

Table 7-4. Assessment of Cell-Mediated Hypersensitivity

Measurement of components of the T-lymphocyte system
   Leukocyte count and differential
   T cells that form rosettes with sheep erythrocytes (E rosettes)
   T lymphocytes and T-lymphocyte subclasses with monoclonal antibodies
Measurement of T-lymphocyte functions in vivo
   DTH skin tests
   Contact allergy skin test
   Skin graft rejection
Measurement of T-lymphocyte functions in vitro
   Lymphocyte proliferation responses to mitogens and antigens
   Mixed leukocyte reactions
   Production of lymphokines (eg,[a] IL-2, IFN-γ, MIF, chemotactic factors)
Other methods
   Assay for adenosine deaminases and purine nucleoside phosphorylase

[a]IL-2, interleukin-2; IFN, interferon; MIF, macrophage migration inhibitory factor.

(eg, tuberculosis); and (3) infections that are common to the patient's geographic area (eg, histoplasmosis, coccidioidomycosis). Past evaluations employing a panel of antigens that included tetanus toxoid, *C. albicans,* streptococcal proteins, trichophyton, tuberculin (PPD-S), and coccidioidin have revealed that for routine testing, *Candida,* streptococcal proteins, and tetanus toxoid were the most valuable.[78]

The DTH skin tests are performed by injecting an appropriate concentration of antigen into 0.1 mL.[79] The results are read at 24, 48, and 72 h. Zones of induration of 1.0 cm or greater in each diameter are scored as positive. Measurements of between 0.5 and 1.0 cm are considered equivocal, while induration less than 0.5 cm is considered negative. However, any amount of induration may have immunological relevance.

Contact allergic reactions are infrequently used to evaluate immune deficiency but are commonly used in evaluation of persons with suspected allergic skin diseases. The suspected substances are applied to the skin under occlusive dressings that are removed at 48 h. Local reactions appear as eczematoid lesions at 48–72 h. However, for assessment of immune competence, a contact sensitizer, such as 2 mg of dinitrochlorobenzene, may be applied to the skin.[79] Challenge tests with small doses of antigen (50–100 μg) are applied after 10–14 d, and the local reactions are recorded 72 h later. Biopsies of the lesions may reveal an inflammatory response even when the skin test is grossly negative. In most studies, greater than 90% of the normal population can be sensitized by this means.

In Vitro Tests

The in vitro tests that quantify lymphocyte function detect the ability of lymphocytes to proliferate, produce mediators, mount cytotoxic responses, and regulate immune responses.[79,80] Lymphocyte proliferation responses can be evaluated by using nonspecific mitogenic stimulants such a phytohemagglutinin, concanavalin A, or pokeweed mitogen, and by specific stimuli such as soluble or cell-bound antigens. The nonspecific activation of lymphocytes measures both T-cell and B-cell function, although the kinetics of these responses differ (peak T-cell responses, 3 d; peak B-cell responses, 5 d). In contrast, specific antigenic challenge appears to measure only T-cell function. In addition, by using autologous as well as homologous serum in the cultures, one can also determine whether the patient's serum contains factors that may interfere with the proliferative response.

The elaboration of cytokines by lymphocytes and monocytes indicates that these cells are capable of producing factors that are involved in the afferent and efferent limbs of the CMI response. Factors such as interleukin-1 and interleukin-2 are involved in the activation and growth of T cells, while the inflammatory mediators, such as macrophage and neutrophil chemotactic factors (CF), macrophage migration inhibitory factor (MIF), and leukocyte inhibitory factor (LIF), are involved in the expression of CMI. the production of CF, MIF, and LIF have been shown to correlate with in vivo delayed-type skin reactivity,[80] although they do not necessarily measure the function of a particular cell type (T or B cells).

The ability of lymphocytes to act as cytotoxic "killer" cells, in response to either allogeneic target or malignant cells, has clinical relevance in transplant and cancer patients. Moreover, T-cell regulation of immunoglobulin synthesis or antibody production, as well as lymphocyte proliferation, has been found to have clinical application as well. Excessive or diminished regulation of these immune responses can result in disorders in humoral or CMI, or both.

Nowell[81] described in 1960 that phytohemagglutinin, a lectin extracted from kidney beans, nonspecifically transformed small lymphocytes into proliferating lymphoblasts in vitro. Subsequently, in addition to plant lectins, which activate all normal T cells, it was shown that a variety of antigens could also induce proliferation.[82] However, this usually occurred only in those individuals who had positive delayed skin tests to these antigens. Thus, in vitro proliferation to soluble antigens, but not mitogens, was shown to be a good correlate of in vivo DTH.

Even though lymphocytic proliferation correlates with in vivo DTH, its role in the expression of the skin reaction is not clear. Based on what is known about the biological activities of cytokines, these factors appear to be better candidates to serve this function. In fact, when these in vitro tests are correlated with skin testing in normal subjects and in patients with diseases associated with defects in DTH, the measurement of lymphokines more often closely parallels the results of the skin test than does proliferation (Table 7-5).[83]

The antigen-induced inhibition of cell migration has been used as an in vitro correlate of DTH since its original description in 1932. The development of the capillary tube method has greatly facilitated a dissection into its mechanism and the discovery of MIF.[84] It is a protein produced by sensitized lymphocytes upon activation by specific antigens or mitogens. Human MIF exhibits heterogeneity in its molecular weight (MW), isoelectric point, and glycosylation.[85]

That LIF is a mediator distinct from MIF was initially established in studies using molecular sieve chromatography.[86] Supernatants from antigen-stimulated lymphocytes contained a LIF activity that was found to elute with molecules having a MW

Table 7-5. Inhibition of Cell Migration: Correlation Between Skin Test Reactivity
and in Vitro Lymphocyte Function in Patients with Depressed Cellular Immunity

Patient Diagnosis	Skin	MIF	Tritiated Thymidine
Group I (61 patients)	+	+	+
Hodgkin's disease, sarcoid collagen disease			
Group II (70 patients)	−	−	−
Hodgkin's disease, sarcoid collagen disease, chronic candidiasis, DiGeorge's syndrome (22 pts)			
Chronic candidiasis, sarcoid, collagen disease (34 pts)	−	−	+
Hodgkin's disease, collagen disease (14 pts)	−	+	+

of 58,000 and this fraction had no inhibitory effect on macrophage migration. Furthermore, like MIF, its production was shown to be antigen-specific by the lymphocytes of the sensitized donor.

The results of migration inhibition assays correlate well with delayed cutaneous hypersensitivity reactions. One can assess the production of LIF or MIF in response to stimulation with a variety of antigens, such as environmental antigens, tissue antigens, contact allergens, or drugs, either in conjunction with in vivo testing or when in vivo testing is impractical (such as with a patient receiving steroids or anticoagulants). Lack of reactivity provides a useful screening test for immunodeficiency, since diminished lymphokine production can result from: (1) abnormal lymphocyte function, (2) a defect in macrophage accessory cell activity, (3) blocking factors, or (4) a lack of antigen-specific lymphocytes. These assays can also be used to monitor patient immunocompetence during the course of therapy and to detect reactivity to drugs or to antigens that may produce CMI-mediated inflammatory diseases.

Whenever possible, more than one in vitro test of lymphocyte function should be measured, since each assay may detect a distinct subpopulation of cells. Furthermore, the present evidence indicates that lymphocytes are compartmentalized; that is, cells in the blood may be functionally different from those in the lymph nodes, spleen, or other organs. Therefore, sampling of blood lymphocytes alone may not yield representative results. An evaluation, therefore, should include quantitation of the numbers of T cells (and their subsets) and B cells, determination of proliferative responses to mitogens and specific antigens, measurement of at least one lymphokine (MIF, LIF, or CF), and determination of a cytotoxic response. If any of these functions is found to be abnormal, then assessment of suppressor cell activity would be indicated. It should be pointed out that the precise role of suppressor cells in disease is presently an area of active investigation and it is difficult in many instances to determine whether a defect in suppressor cell function (hypo- or hyperresponsive) is primary or secondary to the disease process.

With the advent of recombinant DNA technology a number of lymphokines and cytokines have already been cloned and are being mass produced. In the future, this should lead to the development of radioimmunoassays (RIA) that are more sensitive and specific than the existing bioassays. Thus, the availability of RIA kits will allow more widespread application of in vitro CMI tests to office and clinic settings. This should also permit the systematic investigation of their correlation with a variety of disease states.

Clinical States Affecting CMI

Anergy

The term "anergy" was used initially to describe the transient loss of tuberculin sensitivity seen in patients with measles[87] and was subsequently expanded to imply an absence of the capacity to express DTH skin test reactivity to environmentally encountered antigens (so-called "recall" antigens). Detecting the presence of anergy depends to a large extent on the number and type of antigens employed in the skin test evaluation, the minimum size reaction considered to be positive, and certain technical factors (eg, application of test reagents). Most investigators use an antigen panel and criteria that result in over 90% of normal persons exhibiting at least one positive reaction to the four or five antigens employed. This percentage is understandably lower in normal children because they have had less opportunity for exposure to the microorganisms that normally result in such DTH reactivity.

Relative deficits are more difficult to evaluate and are probably more common than the presence of absolute anergy in the clinical disorders described below. It is also appreciated that in some clinical settings, individuals may exhibit a selective deficit in expressing a DTH reaction to a particular antigen previously encountered, while other recall DTH responses are normally expressed. In addition, reactivity to newly encountered antigens may not develop, while DTH responses to environmental antigens previously established are normal. Some nonimmunologic factors that should be considered when a patient fails to mount positive DTH responses to a panel of antigens are shown in Table 7-6.

In more recent studies, investigators have focused on the cellular basis of anergy. Using the vitro technology described earlier, abnormalities involving several components of the DTH response have been described. Moreover, it has become apparent that other T-cell-dependent functions are frequently impaired. Such deficits may either serve an important role in the pathogenesis of a particular disease or occur as a consequence of that disease. A list of primary and acquired immunologic diseases associated with decreased expression of DTH skin test responses is presented in Table 7-7.

Effect of Age and Nutrition on DTH Responses

It has become evident that certain patient population characteristics may affect the interpretation that a particular disease has on the expression of DTH skin tests. For example, the aging process is accompanied by alterations in CMI. The extent of such changes has been assessed by a number of in vivo and in vitro studies, sometimes with conflicting results. These discrepancies may in part reflect the heterogeneity of the populations under study, the use of different age stratification techniques, and/or

Table 7-6. Nonspecific Factors Involved in Loss or Expression of Cutaneous DTH

1. Technique of skin test application
2. Incorrect choice of antigens
3. Pediatric age group
4. Recurrent or current viral infection (measles, EBV)
5. Recent viral vaccination
6. Hypothyroidism
7. Uremia
8. Protein calorie malnutrition
9. Recent surgery
10. Immediate hypersensitivity reaction at site
11. Scurvey
12. Defect in expression inflammatory response
13. Pregnancy
14. Old age
15. Immunosuppressive drugs
16. Severe burns

differences in the immunologic techniques used to assess these parameters. In addition, such elderly populations, who have already been selected for survival, are usually compared at one point in time with a group of younger individuals. It would be more appropriate to assess the same individuals sequentially over a period of years to determine whether significant changes occur within the same population. Variable responses have been obtained in studies carried out in individuals older than 70 years. These reports describe either diminished or normal recall DTH responses and a diminished capacity for DNCB sensitization.[88,89] Furthermore, numbers of circulating T cells have been shown to decline with age or remain unchanged, whereas in vitro responses to phytohemagglutinin (PHA) generally are depressed, and the incidence of serum autoantibodies is increased. Preliminary analysis in humans of

Table 7-7. Primary and Acquired Diseases Causing Anergy

Primary	Acquired
DiGeorge syndrome	Acquired immunodeficiency disease (AIDS)
Severe combined immunodeficiency	Hodgkin's disease
Wiskott-Aldrich syndrome	Sarcoidosis
Ataxia telongiectasia	Cancer
Thymoma	Primary biliary cirrhosis
Common variable immunodeficiency	Chronic active hepatitis
MHC class I or II deficiency (bare	Intestinal lymphagiectasia
lymphocyte syndrome)	Tuberculosis
Immunodeficiency with partial	Lepromatous leprosy
albinism	Chronic mucocutaneous candidiasis
	Coccidioidomycosis
	Secondary syphilis
	Rheumatologic diseases
	Systemic lupus erythematosis
	Pyoderma gangrenosum

this apparent immunologic imbalance has revealed both an increase and a decrease in the number of, or activity of, suppressor cells.[90,91] Similar discrepant findings have been reported in the mouse, where an age-related decline in T_H-cell function has also been reported.[92] The relationship of aberrant T-cell function to the increased incidence of infections, malignancy, or autoimmunity seen in the elderly is currently unclear.

The nutritional status of the patient is also important. In a review of a number of studies,[93] it was reported that malnourished individuals expressed fewer DTH responses to environmental antigens and were less readily sensitized to DNCB. Variable degrees of altered in vitro lymphocyte reactivity have been reported in different types of protein–calorie malnutrition. Lymphoid tissue depletion is particularly prominent in the paracortical areas where T cells reside. These defects may explain to some degree the increased susceptibility of malnourished patients to infection. A cause and effect relationship is suggested by the return of immune parameters to normal following nutritional repletion.

Depression of CMI by Acute Illness

In considering the transient depression of CMI associated with any single disease entity, it is worthwhile to note that several studies have reported decreased DTH skin reactivity in patients with a wide variety of acute illnesses, including myocardial infarction or pulmonary embolism.[94] Therefore, it is difficult to distinguish between the effects of factors such as fever, vascular integrity, and drugs in such cases. However, because of the return toward normal patterns of DTH skin reactivity in one group of patients that were restudied after hospitalization, one must interpret with caution the results of such evaluations of DTH responses carried out during acute illnesses.

It has been recognized for many years that CMI may be depressed for variable periods, during and after infections with measles, rubella, herpes simplex, influenza, and Epstein-Barr viruses. Reactivity to a DTH skin test can be depressed for weeks to months after natural or vaccine-induced measles. In vitro addition of live or inactivated virus may suppress PHA and antigen-induced lymphocyte proliferation. A direct effect of the virus on the lymphocytes may be at least partially responsible in this case.[95] Decreased DTH skin test reactivity has also been found during the first two weeks of infectious mononucleosis, accompanied by decreased lymphocyte responses to PHA, antigen, and allogeneic cells, as well as transiently altered blood levels of T and B lymphocytes. Increased numbers of cells bearing an activated T_S-cell phenotype (Ia positive) and increased suppressor T-cell activity have been found during the acute phase of infectious mononucleosis, but their relationship to the above abnormalities is not clear.[96,97] By contrast, T_S cells are responsible for the impaired pokeweed mitogen (PWM)-stimulated B-cell responses seen in these patients. Since the Epstein-Barr virus infects B lymphocytes, the appearance of these cells during uncomplicated infectious mononucleosis may represent the host's attempt to retard virus replication and B cell proliferation.

Depression of CMI by Chronic Disease

Anergy secondary to systemic disease has probably been studied most extensively in Hodgkin's disease. A review of some of these studies emphasized the relative, not absolute, nature of depressed delayed hypersensitivity in Hodgkin's disease.[98,99] In a prospective study, 66% of patients reacted on skin testing to at least one of six recall antigens, whereas only 23% responded to two or more. Similar responses were seen in 100% and 66% of normal subjects, respectively. Some studies reported depressed DTH reactivity predominantly in those patients with more advanced disease (stage IV) with lymphopenia, whereas other studies find no such correlations. Anergy is also more common when the lymphocyte-depleted (histiocytic) pattern is present in involved lymphoid tissues. Decreased capacity to be sensitized to DNCB is also observed in this disease. Early in the disease course, such abnormalities can be detected when suboptimal sensitizing doses are employed.

Most investigators have found some decrease in mitogen- and antigen-induced (recall antigens and mixed lymphocyte) proliferative responses in Hodgkin's disease. Decreased reactivity was found mainly in lymphocytes obtained from patients with advanced disease. Some of these defects appear to be secondary to the presence of blood monocytes obtained from Hodgkin's disease patients that elaborate excessive amounts of prostaglandin E (PGE).[100] Removal of these cells or treatment of the cultures with indomethacin restores these responses toward normal levels. It is unknown whether PGE-secreting suppressor monocytes are responsible in part for reduced DTH responses observed in these patients. However, preliminary studies suggest that indomethacin, administered in therapeutic doses, does not restore normal expression of DTH.

Depressed tuberculin PPD DTH skin reactivity has long been noted in the majority of patients with sarcoidosis, sometimes persisting well into remission.[101] Studies employing a panel of recall antigens have shown overall decreases in DTH skin test reactivity. Primary sensitization with DNCB induced positive DTH responses in only about 10–15% of patients with sarcoidosis but in over 90% of normal individuals. In vitro proliferative responses to mitogens and antigens are generally depressed during active disease in most patients with cutaneous anergy, but some patients may have reactive cells. There may be some correlation between decreased PHA responsiveness and the extent (beyond the thoracic area) and/or severity of the disease. Serum factors as well as indomethacin-insensitive adherent suppressor cells have been implicated in the depression of in vitro proliferative responses.[102] Numbers of circulating T cells are reduced in patients with both acute and chronic disease but are normal in remission. Alterations in levels of T cell subsets have been seen as well, with increases in T cells bearing Fc receptors for IgG and decreases in T cells bearing Fc receptors for IgM.[103] Studies of cells obtained by bronchopulmonary lavage have revealed increased numbers of activated T4+ cells that spontaneously produce lymphokines.

Certain chronic infections, particularly those with intracellular facultative microorganisms may be associated with a state of depressed CMI. In some cases, the defective CMI response is selective for antigens of the infecting organism. In others, the defect produces global anergy with progression of the disease. For example, reduced DTH skin test responsiveness to many antigens is often seen in patients with miliary tuberculosis, possibly related to poor nutrition, lymphopenia, or both. The lymphocytes from some of these patients respond normally to tuberculin PPD when cultured in vitro in a medium containing "normal" serum. However, the sera from such patients may inhibit tuberculin-induced lymphocyte proliferation when used in the culture medium.

In studies of patients with mycobacterial infections, at least two mechanisms of immunosuppression have been identified. Some patients with recently diagnosed *Mycobacterium tuberculosis* infections have impaired expression of CMI which is mediated by radiation-resistant, plastic-adherent lymphoid cells from the peripheral blood.[104] A different mechanism of immunosuppression was found to be present in patients with chronic pulmonary infections with *Mycobacterium avium-intracellulare*.[105,106] A soluble suppressor factor was found in the serum, and the immunological abnormality also included poor responses to recall antigens such as *Candida albicans,* as well as to antigens from both *M. tuberculosis* and *M. avium-intracellulare*. In some of these patients, T-cell responses to mitogens such as PHA were also impaired. The observation that CMI functions could be partially or totally corrected in vitro and in vivo by indomethacin[105,106] has led to the suggestion that the immunosuppression is mediated by prostaglandins that have potent immunoregulatory activities.

A small percentage of patients with the fungal infection coccidioidomycosis develop severe disseminated disease and lack of reactivity both in vivo and in vitro to coccidioidin in the presence of normal CMI reactivity to other antigens.[107] Thus, an immune imbalance is suggested by the presence of concomitant elevated serum titer of certain anticoccidioidal antibodies. A similar picture has been reported in extensive or disseminated histoplasmosis. In vitro T-cell proliferative responses to mitogens are frequently depressed in a broad array of disseminated fungal disorders. As in the case of tuberculosis, this deficit may reflect modulation of CMI by a number of nonimmunologic host factors. However, in certain patients depressed proliferative responses are caused by macrophage-dependent T-cell-mediated suppression.[107]

Pharmacologic Modulation of CMI

Corticosteroids

Corticosteroids have long been considered potent suppressors of the DTH response in several species, including humans.[108] Pharmacologic doses of steroids can variably depress DTH skin test responses, generally after days to weeks of therapy. Skin test reactivity returns to pretreatment levels within several weeks after cessation. In highly sensitive subjects, significant depression may not be noted when a single dose of antigen is used, as in the routine evaluation of CMI, but only when suboptimal concentrations of antigen are used. Long-term steroid therapy may result in breakdown of old quiescent infectious foci containing intracellular parasites such as *M. tuberculosis* and certain fungi. This is associated with increased likelihood of dissemination of the infection.

The mechanisms underlying the suppressive effects of steroids are still incompletely understood. Steroid administration to humans is followed by transient increases in levels of blood neutrophils and decreases in numbers of monocytes and lymphocytes, particularly T cells.[108] Extensive animal and some human studies suggest that steroids lead to a redistribution of lymphocytes from blood to bone marrow. The lymphocytes that remain in the blood are less hyporesponsive to concanavalin but respond normally to PHA. Steroids also affect macrophage function, with variable effects on phagocytosis and impaired digestion of ingested materials. Associated with the latter is diminished release of lysosomal enzymes and resultant decrease in the expression of inflammatory responses. Migration of macrophages from blood into inflammatory sites is reduced, primarily by margination of these cells to vascular endothelium with decreased diapedesis through vessel walls. In vitro chemotactic response of monocytes is also depressed. The elaboration of lymphokines by T cells is largely unaffected, while the response of macrophages to preformed lymphokines is reduced.[109]

Purine Antimetabolites (Mercaptopurines, Methotrexate)

Mercaptopurines act at multiple loci in the suppression of purine synthesis by actively replicating cells.[110] Because of this cell-cycle action, effective suppression is achieved much less readily with already developed immune responses than is the case in which a primary sensitization can be anticipated (such as organ transplantation). Azathioprine, the imidazole derivative of 6-mercaptopurine, is most commonly employed in clinical situations. It appears to suppress certain humoral immune responses modestly, but the expression of CMI appears to be suppressed to a much greater degree by these drugs. This suppression is seen mainly in the primary response to new antigens but can even occur to some degree in well-established DTH responses. Blood levels of large lymphocytes and monocytes are reduced more than those of small lymphocytes because of suppressed proliferation of cells in the bone marrow. There is a decrease in the mononuclear cell inflammatory exudate in skin windows of humans receiving these drugs. In contrast, there is only a modest suppression of PHA- or antigen-induced proliferation of blood lymphocytes obtained from patients treated with these drugs. Production of migration inhibition factor may be depressed in some but not all treated subjects.

Methotrexate is a potent antimetabolite that may lead to relatively rapid and sometimes unpredictable immunosuppression or side effects.[111] Although impressive therapeutic results have been reported, use of this agent has been limited, possibly because of concerns about the hazards of progressive hepatic fibrosis and neutropenia. Although study of immune mechanisms in methotrexate-treated humans has been much less extensive, the pattern of effects appears to be similar to that of the mercaptopurines.

Alkylating Agents (Cyclophosphamide, Chlorambucil, Nitrogen Mustard)

Cyclophosphamide has emerged as the agent most widely used in this group. It offers a theoretical advantage over purine antimetabolites in that it acts against both replicating and nonreplicating cells involved in immune responses.[112] Therefore the likelihood exists of a suppressive effect on the immunocompetent cells sensitized by prior exposure to the antigen and now in the resting or slowly dividing state. Cyclophosphamide, particularly at higher doses, has been shown to exert a more profound effect than the purine antimetabolites on immune responses important to the development and expression of CMI. Blood levels of small lymphocytes, particularly T cells, are markedly decreased. In addition, there is less proliferation and lymphokine production induced by mitogen or antigen in those lymphocytes that remain in the blood following cyclophosphamide treatment. This drug also appears to be effective in suppressing secondary and ongoing immune responses. Its use in patients is reserved by most investigators to serious life-threatening situations because of the relatively high incidence of side effects involving not only the bone marrow but also the bladder, nail growth pattern, and reproductive organs.

Cyclosporin A

Cyclosporin A is an agent widely used at present for the control of allograft rejection. The mechanism of action of the drug, at least in part, results from its ability to reduce the production of lymphokines through inhibition of transcription of the genes for interleukin 2 and interferon-γ.[113] The drug interferes with the function of helper-inducer cells and induces the formation of antigen-specific suppressor cells. Cytotoxic T-cell generation is also impaired. It has recently been shown that cyclosporin A binds to calmodulin and can therefore block the transduction of the signal initiated by the binding of antigen with the CD3–Ti–MHC trimolecular complex.[114] Another site of action of potential importance is its ability to inhibit IL-1 production and accessory function of macrophages.[115,116] The drug is a powerful inhibitor of the elicitation of DTH but does not inhibit the generation of DTH effector cells.[117,118] The use of cyclosporin in other disorders is not yet well defined.

In conclusion, pharmacologic modulation of CMI has been mainly directed toward suppression of the adverse expression of this immunity. Although qualitative changes in cellular immune function may occur in the drug-treated subject, much of the in vivo activity appears to be related to a variable reduction in the levels of immunocompetent cells as well as the antiinflammatory action in tissue sites.

References

1. Owen JJT. Ontogeny of the immune system. In *Progress in Immunology*, Vol. II, Brent L, Holborow J, eds.; Amsterdam: North-Holland Publishing Co.; 1974.
2. Raff MC, Cantor H. Subpopulations of thymus cells and thymus derived lymphocytes. In Amos B, ed. *Progress in Immunology*. New York: Academic Press Inc; 1971.

3. Reinherz EL, Schlossman SF. *New Engl J Med.* 1980;303:370.

4. Hall JG. Observations on the migration and localization of lymphoid cells. In Brent L, Holborow J, eds. *Progress in Immunology,* Vol. II. Amsterdam: North-Holland Publishing Co.; 1974; Vol. 3.

5. Cantor H, Gershon RK. *Fed Proc.* 1979;38:2058.

6. Germain RN, Benacerraf, B. *Springer Sem Immunopathol.* 1980;3:93.

7. Thomas Y, Sasman J, Irigoyen O, et al. *J Immunol.* 1980;125:2402.

8. Waldmann TA, Broder RM, Brate S, Krakauer R. *Ann Intern Med.* 1978;88:226.

9. Schwartz, RG. The role of gene products of the major histocompatibility complex in T-cell activation. In Paul WE, ed. *Fundamental Immunology.* New York: Raven Press; 1984.

10. Shigeta M, Takahara S, Knox SJ, et al. *J Immunol.* 1986;136:6.

11. Rosenthal, AS. *New Engl J Med.* 1980;303:1153.

12. Ko HS, Fu SM, Winchester RJ, et al. *J Exp Med.* 1979;150:246.

13. Reinherz EL, Kung PC, Pesando JM, et al. *J Exp Med.* 1979;150:1472.

14. Yu DTY, Wincester RJ, Gibofsky A, et al. *J Exp Med* 1980;151:91.

15. Simonkevitz R, Colon S, Kappler JW, et al. *J Immunol.* 1984;133:2067.

16. Ashwell JD, Schwartz RH. *Nature (London).* 1986;320:176.

17. Londei M, Lamb JR, Bottazzo GF, Feldmann M. *Nature (London).* 1984;312:639.

18. Bottazzo GF, Pujol-Borrell R, Hanafusa T, Feldmann M. *Lancet.* 1983;2:1115.

19. Ptak W, Rozycka D, Askenase PW, and Gershon RK. *J Exp Med.* 1980;131:302.

20. Rheins LA, Nordlund JJ. *J Immunol.* 1986;136:3.

21. Brown SJ, Askenase PW. *J Immunol.* 1985;134:1160.

22. Van Loveren H, Den Otter W, Meade R, et al. *J Immunol.* 1985;134:1292.

23. Brown SJ, Galli SJ, Gleich GJ, Askenase PW. *J Immunol.* 1982;129:790.

24. Marrack P, et al. *J Exp Med.* 1983;158:1635.

25. McIntyre B, Allison J. *Cell.* 1983;34:739.

26. Meuer S, et al. *J Exp Med.* 1983;157:705.

27. Kappler J, et al. *Cell.* 1983;34:295.

28. Farr A, et al. *Cell.* 1985;43:543.

29. Meuer S, et al. *Nature (London).* 1983;303:808.

30. Reinherz EL, et al. *J Immunol.* 1979;123:1312.

31. Brenner MB, Trowbridge IS, Strominger JL. *Cell.* 1985;40:183.

32. Allen PM, et al. *J Immunol.* 1985;135:368.

33. Shimonkevitz R, et al. *J Immunol.* 1984;133:2067.

34. Ziegler K, Unanue E. *Proc Natl Acad Sci (USA).* 1982;79:175.

35. Swain S. *Proc Natl Acad Sci (USA).* 1981;78:7101.

36. Dorf ME, Benacerraf B. *Annu Rev Immunol.* 1984;2:127.

37. Germain R, et al. *J Exp Med.* 1979;149:613.

38. Bach BA, Sherman L, Benacerraf B, Greene MI. *J Immunol.* 1978;127:1460.

39. Claman HN, Miller SD, Suy M, Moorehead JW. *Immunol Rev.* 1980;50:105.

40. Weinberger JZ, Germain RN, Benacerraf B, Dorf ME. *J Exp Med.* 1980;152:161.

41. Silberberg-Sinakin I, Baer R, Thorbecke J. *Prog Allergy.* 1978;24:269.

42. Parish CR. *Eur J Immunol.* 1972;2:143.

43. Askenase PW, Hayden BJ, Gershon RK. *J Immunol.* 1977;119:1830.

44. Askenase PW, Atwood JE. *J Clin Invest.* 1976;58:1145.

45. Dvorak HF, Galli SJ, Dvorak AM. *Int Rev Exp Pathol.* 1980;21:119.

46. Goldberg B, Kantor FS, Benacerraf B. *Br J Exp Pathol.* 1962;43:621.

47. Platt JL, Grant BW, Eddy AA, Michael AF. *J Exp Med.* 1983;158:1227.

48. Van Voorhis WC, Kaplan G, Nunes Sarno E, et al. 1982;307:1593.

49. Kaplan G, Van Voorhis C, Nunes Sarno E, et al. *J Exp Med.* 1983;158:1198.

50. David JR, David RR. *Prog Allergy.* 1972;16:300.

51. Lowenthal JW, Cerottini JC, MacDonald HR. *J Immunol.* 1986;137:1226.

52. Toossi A, Kleinhenz ME, Ellner JJ. *J Exp Med.* 1986;163:1162.

53. Spagnuolo JJ, Ellner JJ, Bouknight R, et al. *J Immunol.* 1980;125:3.

54. Fujiwara H, Kleinhenz ME, Wallis RS, Ellner JJ. *Am Rev Respir Dis.* 1986;133:73.

55. Nath I, Sathish M, Jayaraman T, et al. *Clin Exp Immunol.* 1984;58:522.

56. Colizzi V. *Infect Immun.* 1984;58:531.

57. Patel PJ. *Infect Immun.* 1980;29:59.

58. Loveland BE, et al. *J Exp Med.* 1981;153:1044.

59. Greene MI, Benacerraf B, Dorf ME. *Immunogenetics.* 1980;11:267.

60. Parr EL, Bowen KM, Lafferty KJ. *Transplantation.* 1980;30:135.

61. Talmage DW, Dart GA. *Clin Immunol Immunopathol.* 1980;15:314.

62. Vesole DH, Dart G, Talmage DW. *Proc Natl Acad Sci (USA).* 1982;79:1626.

63. Johnson RA, et al. *J Allergy.* 1972;8:578.

64. Galli SJ, Askenase PW. Cutaneous basophil hypersensitivity. In Abramoff P, Philips SM, eds. *A Comprehensive Treatise,* Vol. 9, *RES and hypersensitivity.* New York: Plenum Press; 1986.

65. Wick MR, et al. *May Clin Proc.* 1983;58:603.

66. Cleichmann E, et al. *Immunol Today.* 1984;5:324.

67. Parkman R, Rappaport J, Rosen F. *J Invest Dermatol.* 1980;74:276.

68. Jaffee BD, Claman HN. *Cell Immunol.* 1983;77:12.

69. Miller JFAP, et al. *Proc Natl Acad Sci (USA).* 1976;73:2486.

70. Allen EM, Moore VL, Stevens JO. *J Immunol.* 1977;119:343.

71. Schrier DJ, et al. *J Immunol.* 1982;128:1466.

72. Adu HO, Curtis J, Turk JL. *Infect Immun.* 1983;40:720.

73. de Vruerm RRP, et al. *Lancet.* 1976;2:1328.

74. Cohen S, et al. *J Immunol.* 1967;98:351.

75. Colvin RB, Moseson MW, Dvorak HW *J Clin Invest.* 1979;63:1302.

76. Greene MI, Nelles MJ, Sy MS, Nisonoff A. *Adv Immunol.* 1982;32:253.

77. Romain PL, Schlossman SF. *J Clin Invest.* 1984;74:1559.

78. Gordon EH, et al. *J Allergy Clin Immunol.* 1983;72:487.

79. Rocklin RE. Cellular Components. In Rose N, Freidman H, Faley J, eds. *Manual of Laboratory Clinical Immunology.* Washington, DC: American Society for Microbiology; 1986:258–326.

80. Bernstein L. *J Allergy Clin Immunol.* 1988;82:487.

81. Nowel PC. *Cancer Res.* 1960;20:462.

82. Oppenheim JJ, Dougherty S, Chan SP, et al. Use of lymphocyte transformation to assess clinical

disorders. In Vyas NN, Stites D, Breacher G, eds. *Laboratory Diagnosis of Immunologic Disorders*. New York: Grune & Stratton; 1975:87.

83. Rocklin RE, Reardon G, Sheffer A, Churchill WH, David JR. Dissociation between two in vitro correlates of delayed hypersensitivity: Absence of migration inhibitory factor (MIF) in the presence of antigen-induced incorporation of 3H-thymidine. In Harris J, ed. *Proceedings of the Fifth Leucocyte Culture Conference*. New York: Academic Press; 1970:639–648.

84. David JR. *Proc Natl Acad Sci (USA)*. 1966;56:72.

85. Weiser WY, Greineder DK, Remold HG, et al. *J Immunol*. 1981;56:1958.

86. Rocklin RE. *J Immunol*. 1974;112:1461.

87. von Pirquet CE. *Arch Intern Med*. 1911;1:383.

88. Roberts-Thomson IC, Whittingham S, Youngchaiyud U, et al. *Lancet*. 1974;1:368.

89. Waldorf DS, Wilkens RF, Decker JL. *JAMA*. 1968;203:83.

90. Cobleigh MA, Braun DP, Harris JE. *Clin Immunol Immunopathol*. 1980;15:162.

91. Hallgren HM, Yunis EJ. *J Immunol*. 1977;118:2004.

92. Makinodan T, Kay MB: *Adv Immunol*. 1980;29:287.

93. Law DK, Dudrick SJ, Abdou NI. *Surg Gynecol Obstet*. 1974;139:257.

94. Grossman J, Baum J, Gluckman J, et al. *J Allergy Clin Immunol*. 1975;55:268.

95. Zweiman B, Miller M. *Int Arch Allergy Appl Immunol*. 1974;46:822.

96. Haynes R, Schooley RT, Payling-Wright CR, et al. *J Immunol*. 1979;123:2095.

97. Tosato G, Magrath I, Koski I, et al. *New Engl J Med*. 1979;301:1133.

98. Rocklin RE. Clinical applications of in vitro lymphocyte tests. In Schwartz RS, ed. *Progress in Clinical Immunology*. New York: Grune & Stratton Inc.; 1974.

99. Fisher RI. *Ann Intern Med*. 1980;92:545.

100. Goodwin JS, Messner RP, Bankhurst AD, et al. *New Engl J Med*. 1977;297:963.

101. Daniele RP, Dauber JH, Rossman MD. *Ann Intern Med*. 1980;92:406.

102. Spagnado PJ, Ellner JJ, Bouknight R, et al. 1980;125:1071.

103. Huddlesone JR, Oldstone MBA. *J Immunol*. 1970;123:1615.

104. Ellner JJ. *J Immunol*. 1978;121:2573.

105. Mason UG, et al. *Cell Immunol*. 1982;71:54.

106. Mason UG, Kirkpatrick CH. *J Clin Immunol*. 1984;4:112.

107. Stobo JD, Sigrun P, Scoy REV, Hermans PE. *J Clin Invest*. 1976;57:319.

108. Fauci AS, Dale DC, Balow JE. *Ann Intern Med*. 1976;84:304.

109. Balow JE, Rosenthal AS. *J Exp Med*. 1973;137:1031.

110. Zweiman B. *Transplant Proc*. 1973;5:1197.

111. Webb DR, Winkelstein A. Immunosuppression and immunopotentiation. In *Basic and Clinical Immunology*, 4th ed. Los Altos, CA: Lange Medical Publishers: 1982.

112. Askenase PW, Hayden BJ, Gershon RK. *J Exp Med*. 1975;141:697.

113. Kronke M, et al. *Proc Natl Acad Sci (USA)*. 1984;81:7922.

114. Bucy RP. *J Immunol*. 1986;137:809.

115. Varey AM, Champion BR, Cooke A. *Immunology*. 1986;57:111.

116. Palay DA, Cluff CW, Wentworth PA, Ziegler HK. *J Immunol*. 1986;136:12.

117. Milon G, Truffa-Bachi P, Shidani B, Marchal G. *Ann Immunol*. 1984;135:237.

118. Schiltknecht E, Ada GL. *Cell Immunol*. 1985;95:340.

CHAPTER 8

Immediate Hypersensitivity

Oscar L. Frick

School of Medicine, University of California, San Francisco, CA 94143 USA

Hypersensitivity or allergy encompasses a wide range of immunologic reactions that generally have adverse consequences involving one or many organ systems of the body. In von Pirquet's 1908 original concept, *allo* (altered) *ergos* (action), or "allergy," referred to any immune reaction that differed from the helpful protective response anticipated from an immunization.[1] Included under this concept of allergy are a positive tuberculin test; poison ivy; a rejected transplanted kidney; a mismatched blood transfusion; an autoimmune disease, such as SLE; coeliac syndrome; and hayfever. In this chapter, the meaning of "allergy" will be restricted to IgE-mediated atopic reactions in man and to similar models in animals. The human atopic diseases are hayfever or seasonal and perennial allergic rhinitis, asthma, atopic dermatitis (eczema), some urticarias and gastrointestinal reactions to foods or chemicals, and anaphylaxis.

At the turn of this century, the recently discovered immunization with denatured diphtheria and tetanus toxins, producing a protective immunity or prophylaxis, caused an intensive search for other vaccines. However, Portier and Richet observed rapid shocklike, even lethal reactions, in dogs repeatedly immunized with a sea anemone toxin—instead of helpful prophylaxis, they observed harmful anti-phylaxis or "anaphylaxis".[2] Hayfever and asthma were quickly recognized as being human diseases similar to anaphylaxis in animals.

Anaphylaxis may potentially occur in any member of an animal species, including man. The first exposure to an antigen—protein, carbohydrate or drug/chemical—attached to these large molecules leads to immunization or sensitization of the individual. Upon a subsequent exposure of such a sensitized individual to that antigen, combination with its antibody attached to mast cells or basophils results in contraction of endothelial cells of blood vessels and smooth muscle cells of bronchi causing extravascular fluid leakage (shock) and narrowed airways (wheezing), respectively. Such anaphylactic reactions proceed rapidly and can result in death from shock or asphyxia within minutes. Common examples are anaphylaxis from stinging insect venoms; drugs, such as penicillin; and foods, such as shrimp and walnut.

Atopy or IgE antibody-mediated allergy, in contrast to anaphylaxis, occurs usually only in a genetically predisposed individual with a positive family background of atopic diseases, such as hayfever, asthma, or atopic dermatitis. Allergies occur in 15% of the general population, with certain races having a higher susceptibility. For example, some Polynesians in the Pacific Islands have a 50% susceptibility. If both parents are allergic, there is a 75% chance of the child developing an allergy—50% within the first 5 years of life. If one parent is allergic, about 50% of offspring develop an allergy; in a large study of 2000 individuals, only 30% of allergic patients had no immediate family history of allergy. What is inherited is the allergic constitution.[3]

The genetic bases for atopy lie in at least three known sites—total IgE production, specific IgE antibody production, and bronchial hyperreactivity. The serum levels of total IgE in identical twins are practically identical, while they may diverge in fraternal twins.[4] Even in identical twins raised in different environments, total IgE levels are the same.[5] Specific IgE antibodies to particular antigens or allergens have correlated with certain HLA haplotypes, especially within families. In several large population studies, Marsh et al observed particular HLA associations with certain allergic epitopes or antigenic determinants in pollen extracts; eg, Ra5 of ragweed (HLA-D2, B7), Rye I of ryegrass (HLA-B8, D3, A1).[6] Relatives of asthmatics have increased bronchial hyperreactivity to methacholine, which suggests a genetic association of this additional parameter of allergy. Environmental factors superimposed upon the genetic makeup of an individual probably eventually determines whether clinical allergy will develop; there are identical twins with identical IgE levels, yet only one manifests allergic symptoms.

Allergic reactions in a sensitized individual can affect most, if not all, organ systems. The respiratory and gastrointestinal tracts and skin are most frequently affected in man. Clinically, these present as seasonal hayfever, perennial allergic rhinitis or asthma from exposure to particular pollens, animal danders, or mites. Reactions to foods commonly cause abdominal discomfort, vomiting, and/or diarrhea or in skin—urticaria or flares of atopic dermatitis (eczema). Beyond these "classic" allergic syndromes, there is great current interest but inconclusive research results in allergic vasculitis and synovitis, that could account for clinical reports of allergens, such as dusts and foods, that exacerbate headaches, mood changes, memory, cardiac arrythmia, and arthritis.

Mechanisms of the Allergic Response

A thorough understanding of this mechanism is essential to the successful management of allergies in patients, for there are a number of points for therapeutic attack on this mechanism (Figure 8-1). There is first an immunologic trigger for such reactions to release a variety of diverse mediators, some of which have direct pharmacologic actions and others recruit other inflammatory cells that cause sustained tissue damage. Both an immediate and an early-phase response is commonly, but not always, followed by a late-phase inflammatory response. Some individuals have only an early response, while others have only a late response. An example of a dual response (Figure 8-2) shows an immediate bronchospastic response (fall in FEV_1) to a provocative challenge inhalation of a house dust mite extract in a mite-

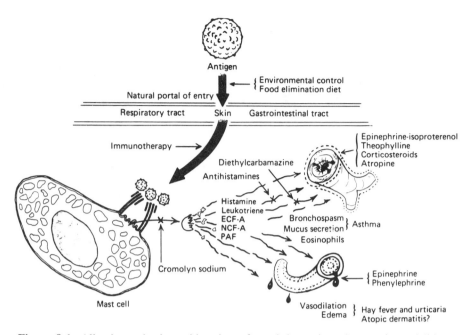

Figure 8-1. Allergic mechanism with points of attack by various therapeutic modalities. (Reprinted, with permission, from Frick OL, Immediate hypersensitivity. In DP Stites, JD Stobo, JV Wells, eds. *Basic and Clinical Immunology.* Norwalk, CT: Appleton & Lange; 1987:197.)

sensitive asthmatic patient. This early response peaks in 10 min and lasts about an hour, with FEV_1 returning toward baseline. This is followed by a second more profound and sustained fall in FEV_1 (bronchospastic late-phase response) peaking at 6 h and gradually resolving over 2–3 days. Bronchoalveolar lavage at 8 h shows the bronchial fluid containing a marked increase in inflammatory cells—neutrophils, eosinophils and mononuclear cells. During this late-phase response, there is a markedly enhanced bronchospastic response to nonimmunologic mildly irritant stimuli, such as ozone, smog, exercise, cold air, and such chemicals as methacholine, and histamine.

Immunologic Components of an Allergic Response

Allergens

These are proteins, carbohydrates, or drugs that are inhaled or ingested that generally are harmless and do not elicit a harmful immunologic response. In genetically susceptible individuals, these allergens, which are usually glycoproteins or peptides of 10–70 kd, activate the IgE-producing B lymphocytes to produce specific IgE antibodies to the allergen under the regulatory guidance of T_H or T_S lymphocytes. Only minute amounts of allergen are required to stimulate the IgE antibody system, while larger amounts appear to stimulate preferentially IgG and IgM (or possibly

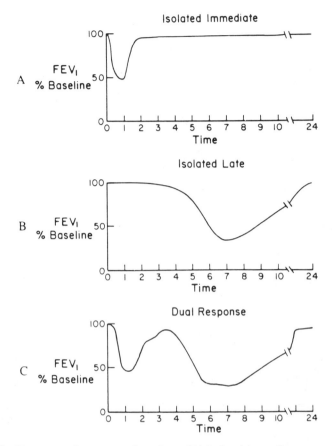

Figure 8-2. Airway reaction patterns in asthma. (A) Isolated immediate response; (B) isolated late-phase response; (C) dual response.

IgA) blocking antibodies; this latter is the basis for immunotherapy in allergy. Some success has been attained by mildly denaturing the allergens with formalin or glutaraldehyde (allergoid) to cause polymerization that results in reduction in "allergenicity" with increased antigenicity, ie, reduced IgE but increased IgG antibody production.

IgE Antibodies

The passive transfer of allergic "reaginic" reactivity from an allergic to a non-allergic individual by blood transfusion or with serum injected in the skin was recognized in the 1920s (Prausnitz-Kustner reaction).[7] However, development of new protein fractionation techniques in the 1960s enabled the discovery, isolation, and characterization in allergic sera by the Ishizakas and by Johanssen and Bennich of a new immunoglobulin E (IgE) that was responsible for this passive transfer of allergy.[8,9] Immunoglobin E occurs only in ng mL^{-1} amounts in plasma of normal and allergic individuals. In nonallergic adults, serum IgE levels have a mean of about 200 ng or 90 U mL^{-1} (1 U IgE = 2.3 ng) ± 40–700 ng (29–80 U). Allergic individuals usually have elevated IgE levels, ranging from 200 to 2000 U mL^{-1} for allergic asthmatics and rhinitis patients and up to 10,000–20,000 U mL in patients with atopic dermatitis. Although most allergic patients have elevated IgE levels, some individuals may have normal IgE levels but with most of that IgE committed to antibody to one or two allergens, especially in hayfever.[10] Patients with helminthic parasites or allergic bronchopulmonary aspergillosis have IgE levels in the 5,000–50,000 U mL^{-1} range, while patients with hyper IgE syndrome may reach 200,000–500,000 U mL^{-1}.

Immunoglobin E-staining lymphocytes are already apparent in 11-week-old human fetuses; however, cord blood IgE levels are normally less than 0.5 U mL^{-1} (μ = 0.24) and rise slowly during childhood, reaching adult levels by 7 years.[11] Elevated cord blood IgE (< 0.9 U mL^{-1}) is a good predictor for the subsequent development of allergy with and without an allergic family history. In Croner's study, elevated cord blood IgE was a better predictor than positive family history.[12] Rapidly rising total IgE in young children can also predict subsequent development of allergy; Orgel et al found that 11 out of 34 positive family history infants had IgE > 20 U mL^{-1} at age 12 mo; 10 of 11 developed allergic symptoms by age 2 years.[13]

Occurring as a 196,000-kd (8S) monomer with typical immunoglobulin structure, IgE consists of two light chains and two E-heavy chains linked by disulfide bonds (Figure 8-3). The 550-amino acid E-heavy chain has five domains with an intra-domain disulfide bond each—VE1, CE1, CE2, CE3, CE4—it has a structure similar to monomeric IgM but is 19 amino acids shorter at the C terminus. The IgE molecule is rich in carbohydrates, 12%. An IgE antibody, Fab, binds allergen with very high affinity ($K_A \sim 10^{-11}$, compared to 10^{-7} for IgG or 10^{-8} for IgM).

Immunoglobin E antibodies bind to various effector cells, especially to tissue mast cells and circulating basophils, by a high-affinity receptor $F_{CE}R_I$ ($K_A \sim 1 \times 10^9$ M^{-1}) and to lymphocytes, monocytes, and eosinophils by a low-affinity receptor $F_{CE}R_{II}$ ($K_A \sim 1 \times 10^7$ M^{-1}). These receptors are described subsequently. There are conflicting data about which E-heavy chain domains are involved in binding to IgE receptors. Synthetic peptides are used to block binding of radio-labeled IgE to mast cells $F_{CE}R_I$. The main binding occurred by the C_{E2} and C_{E3} domains.[14] Heating the IgE molecule at 56°C for 2 h or reducing it with 2-mercaptoethanol alters the E-heavy chain so that it no longer binds to $F_{CE}R_I$ on mast cells and basophils. Because IgE-Fc has no binding site for the placenta, it does not pass from the mother's plasma to her fetus as the IgG does.

Immunoglobin E resembles IgA in that it fails to fix complement except in high concentrations in aggregated form, and it occurs primarily on internal body surfaces, such as the mucosa of the respiratory, gastrointestinal, and urinary tracts; they both appear to function in the secretory immune system. Immunoglobin E differs from IgA in that it occurs only as a monomer and has no association with IgA-secretory component. Immunoglobins E and A appear to have arisen late in immunoglobulin evolution for they share penultimate and last positions (' 3P), respectively, on the immunoglobulin heavy-chain genome.

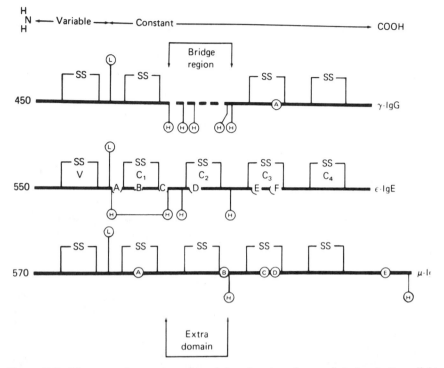

Figure 8-3. Diagrammatic representation of domains, inter-heavy-chain bonds (L = light chain, H = heavy chain), and carbohydrate units (A, B, C, etc). Deletion of a counterpart to the $C_\epsilon 2$ and $C_\mu 2$ domains is one possible explanation of the structure of the general structure of the bridge region of the γ chain. (Reproduced, with permission, from Bennich H. *Prog Immunol.* 1974;2:49.

The normal physiologic function of IgE antibodies is not fully comprehended. In tropical countries with endemic helminth parasitism, most individuals have high plasma levels of IgE, much of which, but not all, is antibody directed against these parasites. When such parasitized individuals move from rural to urban environments with better sanitation and get rid of their parasite load, their IgE levels fall dramatically, but often they also develop allergies. Similarly, in the United States, children born into immigrant parasite-free families from parasite-endemic regions have high IgE levels. United States-born Filipino children have three times the IgE level of United States Caucasian or Black children and they often have the most severe asthma or atopic dermatitis.[15] It has been suggested that in the tropics, the IgE system is devoted to defense against parasites and when this IgE is no longer needed for this purpose, IgE is available to react with allergens.

Immunoglobin E antibodies may also be involved in deposition of immune complexes as part of the body's normal inflammatory defense mechanism. The IgE antibodies fixed to mast cells or basophils react with circulating antigens to cause histamine release; histamine then causes contraction of endothelial cells, which leak plasma containing IgG and IgM antibodies into the tissues and facilitate diapedesis of inflammatory cells into the tissues. Treatment of animals and man with antihistamine and antiserotonin agents prevented the deposition of immune complexes of IgG and IgM.[16]

Measurement of IgE Antibodies to Allergens

The classic, simple, inexpensive, and exquisitely sensitive method for assessing specific allergies is the immediate wheal and flare skin test. For this, the skin of the patient's forearm or back is pricked through a drop of concentrated allergen. If the patient is sensitive to that allergen, his skin will become red within a few minutes (erythema and itching occur) followed within minutes by a central wheal as fluid leaks from the dermal capillaries and venules. This wheal gets surrounded by a red flare. In a strong skin test, the wheal becomes irregular in shape, sometimes in the form of a red streak, as lymphatics take up allergens enroute to the regional lymph nodes. The skin test can be made quantitative by using serial dilutions of allergen to determine the endpoint dilution for a minimal positive wheal–flare response. In asthmatics, the endpoint titration allergen dose correlates well with threshold concentration of allergen needed to cause bronchospasm (fall in FEV_1) upon challenge inhalation with the same allergen.

Immunoassay for IgE

Total IgE and IgE antibodies to specific allergens are also measured by immunoassays using monoclonal and polyclonal animal-origin anti-human IgE antibodies labeled with radioisotopes (^{125}I), enzymes (horseradish peroxidase or avidin-biotin), or fluorescein, as in the RAST (Figure 8-4), ELISA, or FAST methods, respectively. For specific IgE antibodies, protein allergen is coupled to cyanogen

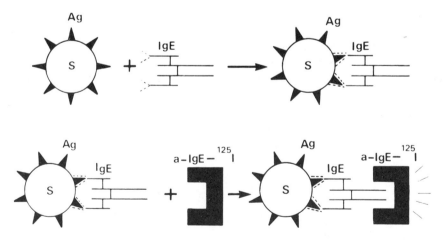

Figure 8-4. Schematic diagram of the radioallergosorbent test (RAST). S is sorbent, with antigenic determinants (Ag). Human IgE attaches to the antigen and is detected with radiolabeled anti-IgE. (Reprinted, with permission, from Frick OL, Immediate hypersensitivity. In DP Stites, JD Stobo, JV Wells, eds. *Basic and Clinical Immunology*. Norwalk, CT: Appleton & Lange; 1987:197.)

bromide-activated cellulose or filter paper disks or adsorbed to wells of polystyrene or polyvinyl microtiter plates. Excess protein is then washed off. After incubation with HSA or BSA to block further absorption and after washing, the patient's serum is added. His antibodies react with the allergen immobilized on the solid matrix. After further washing, labeled polyclonal rabbit or goat or monoclonal mouse IgG anti-human IgE is added and after further incubation and washing, the label is quantified (by counting in a gamma counter for ^{125}I or reading the enzyme–substrate color intensity in a spectrophotometer or the fluorescence intensity in a fluorometer). The intensity of the label is a direct measurement of the amount of IgE antibody directed against the allergen. In an allergic individual, the IgE, RAST and ELISA results correlate well with the skin test endpoint dilution result and with the clinical degree of allergy as determined by an inhalation provocation test.

Regulation of IgE Antibody Production

Immunoglobin E production by IgE-bearing B-lymphocytes is under exquisite regulatory control by T_H and T_S lymphocytes and appears to be independent of T-regulatory cell controls for IgG, IgM, and IgA antibody production. Katz has proposed the "allergic breakthrough mechanism of IgE-antibody regulation" (Figure 8-5).[17] Because of the extremely potent pharmacologic and physiologic effects of mast cell mediators initiated by minute amounts of IgE antibodies attached to mast cells, it is critically important to keep IgE production under very tight control; this is a function of T_S lymphocytes or a "damping mechanism." It has been thought that SJL inbred mice are genetically IgE nonresponders because they do not make any IgE antibodies to antigens in immunization regimes used in other IgE responder mouse strains (CBA, AKR, etc). However, Chiorazzi et al have shown that if SJL mice are subjected to either low-dose irradiation, cyclophosphamide or anti-lymphocyte serum 10 d before antigen injection, these procedures preferentially destroy T_S lymphocytes and spare T_H lymphocytes.[18] Such pretreated nonresponder SJL mice become good IgE responders with high levels of IgE antibody within 1–2 weeks after immunization. Intravenous injection of normal spleen cells containing T_S lymphocytes from other nonimmunized SJL mice to IgE-producing SJL mice, will promptly

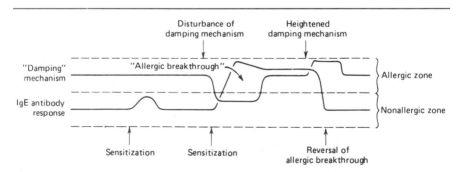

Figure 8-5. Possible pathogenesis of "allergic breakthrough." (Reprinted, with permission, from Katz DH et al. *J Immunol.* 1979;122:219.)

abrogate their IgE antibody within 2 h, thereby returning them to their "nonresponder" state. Katz[19] has reasoned that the potent IgE antibody system and its inflammatory mediators are held in check by the "damping" effect of T_S lymphocytes.

All individuals are potentially IgE responders but response is held in check by T_S cells in the nonallergenic zone. Any event or treatment that temporarily or permanently impairs the T_S lymphocytes permits the escape from damping of the T_H lymphocytes. Upon stimulation with an antigen, these T_H lymphocytes make IgE antibodies, putting the individual into the allergic zone. Such "allergic breakthrough" events may be caused by certain drugs, eg, cyclophosphamide, or natural events, eg, certain viral infections. Restoration of the damping effect of T_S lymphocytes by allergen immunotherapy or by drugs (such as corticosteroids) abrogates the IgE antibody production and returns the individual to the nonallergic zone. Therefore, there is a fine-tuned regulatory balance between T_H and T_S cells for production of IgE antibody by B cells and subsequent development of allergy.

Recent attention has turned to lymphokine products of activated T_H and T_S lymphocytes that act as nonspecific and antigen-specific regulatory substances. Complete Freunds adjuvant (CFA) along with an antigen is a good adjuvant for IgG and IgM antibody production. Katz has shown that mice given CFA with antigen fail to make IgE antibody and their serum contains a factor that suppresses IgE antibody formation in other immunized mice; this is called suppressor factor of allergy or SFA.[19] He has also subsequently isolated an enhancing factor of allergy (EFA) from sera of immunized IgE-producing mice. Both these factors (SFA and EFA) are present concomitantly in immunized mice and can be absorbed selectively on lectin-affinity columns (concanavalin A lectin for EFA and lentil lectin for SFA) and desorbed with the appropriate sugar in excess (mannose for EFA and galactose for SFA).

Ishizaka showed that resting T lymphocytes can be activated by macrophages presenting antigen or by IgE itself.[20] Such activated T lymphocytes expressed an $F_{CE}R$ for the Fc portion of the IgE molecule (Figure 8-6). These activated T lymphocytes produced IgE-regulatory factors (IgE-binding factors), which instruct B lymphocytes whether or not to produce IgE antibodies. Ishizaka called these IgE-potentiating and IgE-suppressing factors, which appear to be identical or similar to Katz's EFA and SFA, respectively. Furthermore, these activated T lymphocytes were under further regulatory control of other T lymphocytes. In the mouse and rat, on the one hand, antigen-stimulated Lyt-1 lymphocytes produced a protease, glycosylation-enhancing factor (GEF), that glycosylates IgE binding factor; this has an IgE potentiation activity that signals B lymphocytes to make IgE antibodies. On the other hand, antigen-stimulated Lyt 2^+ lymphocytes produced a fragment of phosphorylated lipomodulin or glycosylation-inhibiting factor (GIF), which inhibits glycosylation of IgE binding factor; this has an IgE suppressive activity and signals the B cells not to make IgE antibody. Thus, the nature and biologic activation of IgE binding factors produced by the same activated T lymphocytes that instruct the B cells to start or not make IgE antibodies is under the delicately balanced control of GEF and GIF produced by other T lymphocytes.

Some of the potentiation and suppressive factors are nonspecific for all IgE

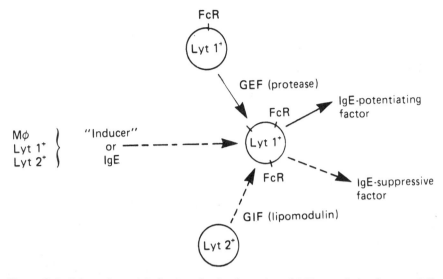

Figure 8-6. Schematic models for the selective formation of IgE-potentiating factor or IgE-suppressive factor. In the presence of GEF, FcR+ Lyt 1+ T-cells form IgE-potentiating factor, but the same cells form IgE suppressive factor in the presence of GIF. (Reprinted, with permission, from Ishizaka K. *Annu Rev Immunol.* 1984;2:159.)

production, and some are specific for IgE antibody response only to a specific antigen. Currently, there is great effort to isolate and make hybridomas of activated murine and human T lymphocytes that produce large amounts of these IgE regulatory factors in culture. The ultimate goal is to produce large amounts of IgE suppressive factor or GIF to prevent or turn off IgE antibody production to specific allergens without affecting the general IgE antibody system, which may have a useful physiological role, such as destroying parasites.

Target Cells in Allergy

Tissue mast cells are the chief targets for IgE antibody-mediated reactions. They are "sentinal cells," abundant on body surfaces such as skin and mucosa and around blood vessels, especially venules. They were first described by Ehrlich who thought they had a "feeding" or "mast" function, whereas Selye called them an "emergency kit" to start an inflammatory reaction against invaders—therefore, a "sentinal function." Mast cells have many metachromatic granules that store powerful inflammatory agents, such as chemotactants for other cells, proteases that hold acid heparin and basic histamine or serotonin in ionic combination, and degradation and repair materials, such as chymase and hyaluronic acid involved in ground substance formation. Activation of mast cell membranes causes arachidonic acid formation and its cleavage into platelet activating factor (PAF), lipoxygenase products (5 and 15 HETE's and leukotrienes B4, C4, D4, and E4) and cyclooxygenase products (prostaglandins, prostacycline, and thromboxanes). Mast cells are, therefore, the first line of defense, exquisitely sensitive to minute stimuli that cause release of their inflammatory mediators. Histamine (and serotonin in mice and rats) causes marked vasodilatation and contraction of endothelial cells, which permits rapid passage of plasma containing antibodies and complement into tissues and facilitates diapedesis of phagocytes and lymphocytes into the invaded area. Such cells have been called in by chemotactants, such as eosinophil chemotactic factor allergy (ECF-A) and high molecular weight–neutrophil chemotactic factor (HMW-NCF).

Mast-cell heterogeneity has recently gained attention.[21] Typical connective mast cells are located near blood vessels. These are large cells (>20 μm) with many granules and high histamine content (>15 pg cell^{-1}). Heparin and histamine are bound to a highly sulfonated proteoglycan. They have both tryptase and chymase. In the skin they are concentrated in areas of frequent trauma, such as in foot pads and in mouth-muzzle areas of animals. They are readily degranulated by immunologic signals, especially those mediated by IgE and by nonspecific agents, such as polymyxin and opiates. Mediator release is prevented by cromolyn sodium, ketotifen, and theophylline.

Atypical mast cells that are smaller (<10 μm), with fewer granules and lower histamine content (~2 pg cell^{-1}) and present in rat gastrointestinal mucosa are described by Enerback;[22] these have also been termed "mucosal mast cells" or "globule leukocytes." These cells are lysed by the usual formalin tissue fixation methods and so are frequently missed. They can easily be seen by fixation in basic lead acetate and staining with 1% alcian blue and 0.1% eosin. They contain a low-sulfonated proteoglycan that binds histamine without heparin and have only tryptase, not chymase. Atypical mast cells are abundant in mucosal surfaces of lung and intestine, where they proliferate profusely in response to parasitic infection. They are relatively stable to polymyxin and opiates. Their degranulation is not blocked by cromolyn or theophylline, although doxantrolzole and the flavinoid quercitin appear to block it.[21]

Atypical mast cells are extremely T cell dependent, either arising from T cells or dependent upon a T-cell lymphokine, IL-3. In tissue culture, T-cell precursors with IL-3 differentiate into mucosal-type tryptase-staining mast cells, which upon further growth with IL-3 further differentiate into typical mast cells, staining with tryptase and chymase. Kobayashi et al have observed the reverse differentiation back to atypical mast cell in mouse mast-cell cultures, but not in humans.[23]

Basophils are 0.5–2% of circulating leukocytes. They are intermediate in size (5–7 μm), with many granules, and have low histamine content. Although they resemble mast cells, their granules on EM are different. Basophils do not contain PGD_2 and their mediator release is not blocked by cromolyn. They appear to accumulate in late-phase reactions in the nose of allergic subjects after allergen inhalation tests.

Allergic Mediators

Generally allergic mediators are synonymous with the potent pharmacologic agents released by mast cells. However, with recent recognition of the late-phase reaction and other cell types contributing to allergic inflammation, the agents released by these other cells can also be considered as allergic mediators, some of which further degranulate mast cells in a circular process.

Defense against parasitic nematode and trematode infection involves IgE antibody reactions that cause mast cells to release their mediators, causing vasodilatation and permitting leaked IgG and IgM antibodies to attack the parasite. Furthermore, they call in eosinophils that attach to the parasitic surface, line their granules onto that surface, and discharge their highly basic proteases that dissolve the parasite's skin into fragments. In animals, IgE anti-parasite antibodies protect them against subsequent infection by that parasite, "the self-cure phenomenon."

The allergic mediators from mast cells may be classified as: (1) the preformed mediators, which are released in pharmacologically active form within seconds after the stimulus; such are histamine, serotonin, ECF-A, NCF-A; and (2) those which are formed from arachidonic acid activation from membrane phospholipids; leukotrienes, prostaglandins, and thromboxanes.

Histamine

Histamine is a 111 mol wt basic amine that is formed from histidine and stored in mast cell granules. Although on a molar basis it is less active than some other mediators, because of its abundance in mast cell granules, it is recognized as the important allergic mediator. It contracts smooth muscle cells and endothelial cells causing bronchospasm and vascular leakage, respectively. It also stimulates mucus secretion. Histamine is an important mediator in anaphylaxis, acute asthma, urticaria, and nasal congestion in allergic humans.

Serotonin

Serotonin or 5-hydroxytryptamine is a 176-mol wt amine preformed from tryptophane and stored in platelets and in murine mast cells. It acts similarly to histamine in mice and rats, where it is the chief allergic mediator, but apparently not in humans or other animals.

High Molecular Weight–Neutrophil Chemotactic Factor

The HMW-NCF is a 750-kd mol wt glycoprotein released from an allergen-induced reaction that is chemotactic for neutrophils. It has not been isolated or well characterized but it is released into circulation and tissues immediately after a stimulus, including cold urticaria.

Eosinophil Chemotactic Factor A

The ECF-A polypeptides range from 300 to 5000 mol wt and are probably preformed and released by an allergic stimulus. Two catabolic tetrapeptides, val-gly-ser-glu and ala-gly-ser-glu, are strongly chemotactic for eosinophils.

Neutral Proteases

Neutral proteases account for 70–80% of proteins in mast cells and hold the amines and proteoglycans in the granules.[24] Tryptase is a 144-kd mol wt tetrameric protein present in all mast cells and contains active serine and histidine but is not inhibited by trypsin inhibitors. It is released simultaneously with histamine and is measured spectrophotometrically by using TAME (tosyl-L-arginine methyl ester). It cleaves C3 into C3a and C3b and further degrades C3a into smaller inactive peptides; thus it modulates C3 activity. Atypical mucosal mast cells contain only tryptase, whereas typical skin mast cells also contain chymase. Enzyme-labeled anti-chymase and anti-tryptase serum provides a simple means of localizing and differentiating the two types of mast cells.[25]

Chymase

Chymase in rat typical mast cells is also known as rat mast-cell protease I. It is a 26–29 kd single-chain protein that is measured spectrophotometrically by BTEE (N-benzoyl-L-tyrosine ethyl ester). Naturally released chymase hydrolyzes type-IV collagen of basement membrane, fibronectin, fibrinogen, neurotensin, but upon release from mast cell granules, chymase remains complexed with heparin and has a lower activity.

Rat Mast-Cell Protease II

Rat mast-cell protease II (RMCP II) is distinct from chymase and is found in rat mucosal mast cells and can help activate lymphocytes. A similar protease in human atypical mast cell is being sought.

Carboxypeptidase

Carboxypeptidases are associated with mast-cell tryptase. In rat typical mast cells, carboxypeptidase A is a 35-kd single-chain protein that hydrolyzes peptide and ester bonds on the amino end of C-terminal tyrosine and phenylalanine. It also remains complexed with heparin and chymase upon dissolution of mast-cell granules.

Acid Hydrolases

Mast-cell granules also contain acid hydrolases, such as β-hexosaminidase, β-glucuronidase, and β-D-galactosidase, which releases sugars from carbohydrate side chains, and alkyl sulfatase, which cleaves sulfated esters, possibly leukotriene C4.

Proteoglycans

Proteoglycans have a protein core with carbohydrate side chains that form part of the ground substance and are also present in cartilage and bone. Heparin is the proteoglycan of typical connective tissue mast cells; it has an alternating serine–glycine core with each second or third serine branching off an amino sugar side chain—glycosaminoglycan (GAG) or disaccharides of glucosamine linked to glucuronic or iduronic acid that is sulfonated. Rat serosal mast-cell heparin has 750-kd mol wt, while smaller human heparin is ~60 kd. Heparin stores the other amine mediators in mast-cell granules in inactive forms. Upon release of the granules, histamine and acid hydrolases are released from heparin in exchange for Na^+ from the extracellular fluid. Heparin has multiple biological activities, such as anticoagulation and fibrinolysis, anticomplement, modulation of neutral proteases, and inhibiting eosinophil cytotoxicity in late-phase reactions.

Chondroitin Sulfate E

Chondroitin sulfate E is the proteoglycan of the atypical mucosal mast cell in the mouse and human with a structure similar to heparin but with a unique GAG. In the maturation and differentiation of mast cells in the mouse, the mucosal mast-cell chondroitin sulfate E adds xyl-ser to become heparin as the mast cell becomes the typical larger mast cell. A similar change occurs with human mast cell in tissue culture.

Arachidonic Acid Metabolite Mediators

Arachidonic acid metabolite mediators are newly formed from plasma membrane phospholipids upon activation of the mast cell by an immunological reaction.[26] Activated phospholipase A_2 (PLA_2) acts on membrane phospholipid to split out arachidonic acid, which in turn is metabolized by three pathways: by either cyclooxygenase, 3 lipoxygenases, or PLA_2 to form prostacyclines, eicosanoids, and platelet activating factor (PAF), respectively (Figure 8-7).

Cyclooxygenase adds a molecular oxygen to arachidonic acid to form unstable cyclic endoperoxides, PGG_2 and PGH_2, which are further converted by non-enzymatic or enzymatic means to slightly more stable prostaglandins, prostacycline, and thromboxanes. The principal prostaglandin of the mast cell is PGD_2 which occurs in about ⅕ to ⅒ the amount of histamine present. Released PGD_2 causes vascular leakage and smooth muscle contraction. From pure mast cells, small amounts of PGE_2, PGF_{2a}, 6-keto-PGF_{1a}, and TXB_2 are released, whereas from a chopped human lung preparation, immunologic stimulus results in release of abundant PGF_{2a} and TXB_2. This suggests that other cells, such as macrophages, contribute major amounts of prostanoids. Such prostanoids as PGF_{2a} and 6-keto-PGF_{1a} in allergic reactions contribute to bronchospasm and increased vascular permeability, while PGE_2 causes an opposite effect to modulate the response.

The thromboxane TXB_2 appears to help the release of the mediators from inflammatory cells because the inhibition of its formation by a thromboxane synthetase inhibitor (OKY-048) prevents the release of the cells' granular contents and inhibits the bronchial hyperreactivity of a late-phase reaction.[27] It also has a powerful action favoring platelet aggregation, while PGI_2 causes platelet disaggregation; TXB_2 thus participates in a counterbalanced modulatory control in blood clotting.

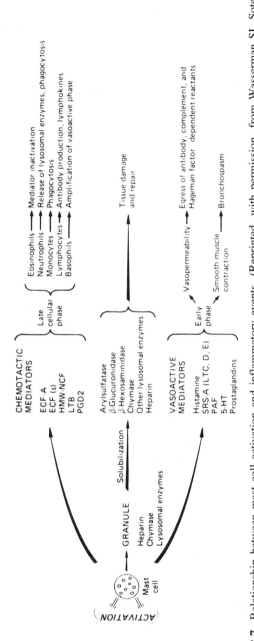
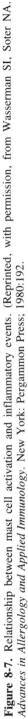

Figure 8-7. Relationship between mast cell activation and inflammatory events. (Reprinted, with permission, from Wasserman SI, Soter NA. *Advances in Allergology and Applied Immunology.* New York: Pergammon Press; 1980:192.

Lipoxygenases metabolize arachidonic acid at three carbon atom pairs, resulting in an unstable hydroperoxieicosatetranoic acids (HPETES) which are converted to slightly more stable hydroxyeicostetranoic acid (HETES) at the 5-OH, 15-OH, and 12-OH positions in different cell types.[26] The 5-lipoxygenase products predominate in mast cells, neutrophils, and macrophages, whereas, 12-lipoxygenase occur in platelets, and 15-lipoxygenase di- and tri-HETES occur in eosinophils and in surface cells such as endothelial, bronchial epithelial cells, and keratinocytes. The 5-lipoxygenase converts 5-HETE to a transitory leukotriene LTA_4, which reacts with glutathione that donates sulfonated methionine by an S-transferase enzyme to form leukotriene, LTC_4. This is metabolized further by cleavage of glutamic acid to form LTD_4 and then cleavage of glycine to form LTE_4. These three leukotrienes are potent smooth muscle constrictors and vasodilators and are known as slow-reacting substances of anaphylaxis (SRS-A). Acted upon by epoxide hydrolase, LTA_4 forms a 5.12-diHETE, LTB_4, which is a potent chemotactic agent for other inflammatory cells, especially neutrophils, and promotes their adherence to endothelial cells and their degranulation.

Platelet-Activating Factor

Platelet-activating factor (PAF) is a parallel metabolite of immune-activated cell membranes from mast cells, eosinophils, neutrophils, macrophages, and other cells.[28] PLA_2 hydrolyzes membrane phosphorylcholine to form an ether link in a sn-1 glycerin backbone and acyl substitution occurs at sn-2 to form 1-alkyl-2 lyso-sn glycero-3-phosphocholine (lyso PAF); this latter is acylated by acyltransferase enzyme from acetyl-CoA to form 1-alkyl-2-acyl ether-glycero-3 phosphocholine (known as AGEPC in the United States or as PAF-acether in Europe).

Platelet-activating factor was first identified as a product released from sensitized rabbit basophils. It causes aggregation and activation of rabbit platelets, which released their histamine and PF_4. In the allergic late-phase reactions PAF appears to be a major mediator of inflammation. Dramatic protection has been affording asthmatics by blocking PAF action with ginkolides.

Biochemical Events in Mast Cells for Release of Allergic Mediators

This involves a complex cascade of events that starts with an allergen reacting with IgE on a mast cell surface and culminates with the release of various mediators that affect adjacent tissues and cells, such as smooth muscle, vascular endothelial, and inflammatory cells.

The IgE high-affinity receptor ($F_{CE}R_I$) on mast cells and basophils is a glycoprotein complex of three dipeptides comprised of two each of a, β and δ chains (Figure 8-8). The K_A for the IgE monomer is $2–8 \times 10^9$ mol^{-1}. An extra membrane portion consisting of a carbohydrate-rich a1 and a2 (mol wt $\sim$ 50 kd) binds the Fc portion of IgE antibody. These a monomers are coupled to an intramembranous β1 chain (mol wt $\sim$ 20 kd) complexed to β2 (mol wt $\sim$ 10 kd) exposed on cytoplasmic side along

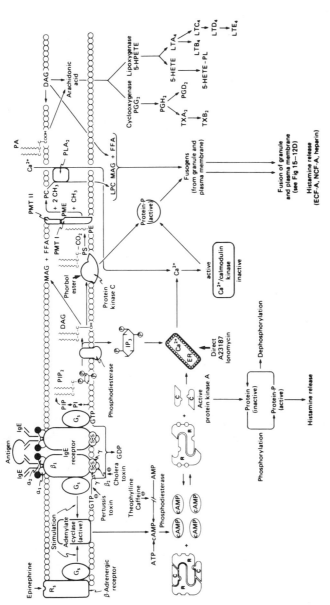

Figure 8-8. After binding of antigen to IgE to IgE receptor, activation of phosphoinositol pathways from PIP_2 to form IP_3 to mobilize intracellular Ca^{2+} from endoplasmic reticulum and diacylglycerol (DAG) from membrane to form fusogens that fuse mast cell granules with plasma membrane and release of allergic mediators. (Reprinted, with permission, from Frick OL: Immediate hypersensitivity. Stites DP, Stobo JD, Wells JV, eds. *Basic and Clinical Immunology.* Norwalk CT: Appleton & Lange; 1987:197; and Berridge MJ. *Annu Rev Biochem.* 1987;56:159.)

with a dimer of a second δ chain (mol wt $\sim$ 9 kd) joined by disulfide bonds. The β and δ chains activate the biochemical events involved in degranulation.

A second IgE low-affinity receptor ($F_{CE}R_{II}$) is present on surfaces of eosinophils, platelets, monocyte, macrophages, and lymphocytes. It has a K_A for IgE of $\sim 10^5$ to 10^8 mol^{-1} or it is about 100 to 10,000 times less avid for IgE than $F_{CE}R_I$ in mast cells and basophils. Direct activation by antigen of the IgE-sensitized alveolar macrophages and subsequently the eosinophils via this $F_{CE}R_{II}$ has been postulated to be of great importance in late-phase asthmatic reactions. The study of the structure of the $F_{CE}R_{II}$ is currently underway.

In an allergic reaction, multivalent allergen binds to two IgE molecules by their Fab portions with high avidity. These two crosslinked IgE monomers bind to two adjacent $F_{CE}R_I$ high-affinity receptors, which pulls them together from the lipid sea of the plasma membrane. This binding of crosslinked IgE antibody, creating an approximation of the two IgE receptors, initiates the complex enzyme cascade. Two IgE receptors can also be approximated by anti-IgE serum or rabbit anti-IgE receptor antibody. Crosslinking of IgE receptors is crucial, because binding of just one receptor by either a monovalent hapten, the Fab' fragment of anti-IgE, or the Fab' of anti-IgE receptor fails to initiate a response and inhibits the subsequent addition of a divalent reagent.

There are at least three enzyme cascades activated by crosslinking IgE receptors ($F_{CE}R_I$), but the order in which they are activated is still not clear. The order is different in various models studied—rat peritoneal mast cells, bone marrow-derived mouse mucosal mast cells, rat basophil leukemia cells, human basophils, and human bronchial lavage mast cells.

A group of GTP-dependent membrane proteins, G Proteins, transduce signals from external receptors across the plasma membrane to the cell's interior.[29] The IgE receptor, like most other receptors, probably acts through a membrane G protein; although the type of G protein is still uncertain. Resting G proteins (mol wt $\sim$ 40 kd) are trimers of a, β, δ chains (Figure 8-9). Agonist or hormone binds to its receptor, which in the presence of GTP causes dissociation of the $G_{\beta'''\delta}$ chains from the activated G_a chain bound to GTP; this converts a precursor to active product for effector action in our IgE-R model of mediator release. As effector product (E) builds up, some E* is bound to form the G_aGTPE*, which in the presence of water undergoes moderately slow catalysis and releases one inorganic phosphate to form G_aGDP-E. The energy lost releases effector, and the free G_a then reassociates slowly with $G_{\beta'''\delta}$ to reconstitute the inactive resting trimer, $G_{a,\beta'''\delta}$.

In the adenylate cyclase activation systems, binding of G-stimulating protein (Gs) to adenylate cyclase activates the breakdown of ATP to cyclic AMP, and binding to protein kinase A is thus activated. *Vibrio cholera* toxin can stimulate this Gs protein, whereas *Bordella pertussis* toxin inhibits the Gs protein. Under different circumstances, binding of G-inhibitory (Gi) protein occurs, ATP breakdown to cyclic AMP is inhibited, and there is no activation of protein kinase A.

In a similar manner, the receptor's signal binding stimulates a different G protein to activate phospholipase C to split PIP_2 into IP_3, which causes the mobilization of intracellular Ca^{2+}, and 1,2-diacylglycerol (DAG), which causes the activation of

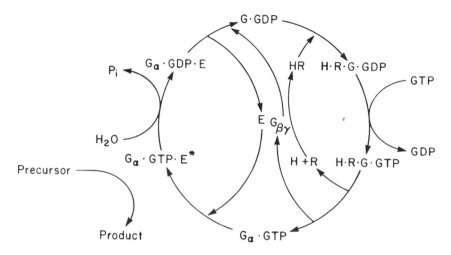

Figure 8-9. Interactions of receptor, G protein, GTP, and effector. (Reprinted, with permission, from Gilman AG. *Annu Rev Biochem.* 1987;56:615.)

the membrane protein kinase C.[30] Receptor signal binding also stimulates another G protein to activate a different phospholipase C to cause phosphatidylcholine to release phosphocholine (PC) and a third G protein activates phospholipase D to release phosphotidic acid (PA) from phosphatidylcholine.

In human basophils, binding of concanavalin A, compound 48/80, thrombin, and N-formyl-L-methionyl-L-leucyl-L-phenylalanine stimulates a G_{sa} protein and histamine release; this activity is blocked by *B. pertussis* toxin. However, after binding IgE receptors by anti-IgE, Saito et al have reported that histamine release is not blocked by *B. pertussis* toxin.[31] They have concluded that IgE-independent stimuli, such as Con A, involve binding of a Gs or Gi protein, but that this G protein is not involved in transducing signals by bridging IgE receptors. It is still conceivable that a different G protein, not susceptible to *B. pertussis* toxin inhibition, may be involved in activation of IgE receptor bridging. Cholera toxin activates Gs for adenylate cyclase but inhibits the G protein that activates IP formation. There appear to be several types of G proteins involved in these activations.

The first enzyme cascade after the G-protein activation is the mobilization of intracellular calcium (Ca^{2+}) from the endoplasmic reticulum. This is the earliest event in the initiation of histamine release in rat mast cells, mouse mucosal mast cells, and human basophils.[30] This is measured by Quin-2 uptake within 10–15 s and is followed by histamine release in 30–120 s. Ethylenonglycoltetraacetate (EGTA) blocks the influx of extracellular Ca^{2+} through the Ca^{2+} channel. In rat mast cells with EGTA Quin-2 rise and histamine release occur, showing that Ca^{2+} is mobilized from within the cell, whereas in mouse mucosal mast cells and human basophils, EGTA blocks both Quin-2 rise and histamine release. In these last two IgE-sensitized cells, Ca^{2+} enters from outside the cell, emphasizing species and cell maturation differences in calcium mobilization.

Calcium enters the cells by two channels (Figure 8-10). First, a potential (or

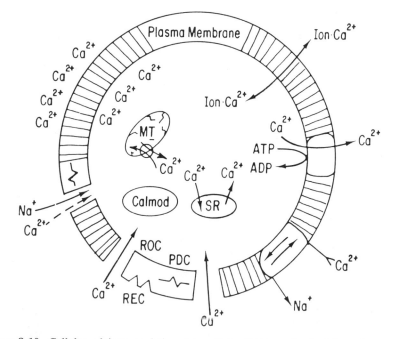

Figure 8-10. Cellular calcium regulation. Intracellular Ca^{2+}, maintained in resting state at 10^{-7} mol mL^{-1}; ionized Ca^{2+} is bound to the internal membrane surface and sequestered within sarcoplasmic reticulum (SR) and mitochondria (MI) via active uptake processes. The intracellular Ca^{2+} binding protein (Ca^{2+} receptor) is shown as calmodulin (Calmod). Calmodulin may be membrane or cytosol associated. Exit of Ca^{2+} can occur through a plasma membrane ATPase-driven Ca^{2+} pump and by a Na^{+}–Ca^{2+} exchange mechanism. The latter can operate in both directions, and with high intracellular Na^{+} can serve as an entry mechanism for Ca^{2+}. Additional entry routes for Ca^{2+} are shown as the recptor-operated (ROC) and potential-dependent (PDC) Ca^{2+} channels and (as a minor component) through the fast Na^{+} channel. A nonphysiological bypass mechanism is shown as ionophore-mediated Ca^{2+} entry (Ion = ionophore A23187, ionomycin). (Reprinted, with permission, from Triggle DJ. *Allergy.* 1983;38:1.)

voltage)-dependent channel (PDC) is activated by K^{+} depolarization, which opens a plasma membrane channel, permitting influx of Ca^{2+}. Such PDC channels in cardiac muscle and vascular smooth muscle are blocked by verapamil and nifedepine. Second is a receptor-operated channel (ROC), which opens upon binding of hormones or agonists to membrane receptors that are not blocked by verapamil and nifedipine. The ROC channels appear in mast cells and basophils so these drugs are not effective in alleviating asthma. However, cromolyn sodium may bind close to and block this ROC gate, for rat basophil leukemia cells have a specific cromolyn receptor for cromolyn that blocks Ca^{2+} influx.[32]

Phosphatidyl inositol turnover (Figure 8-8) is involved in signal transduction from IgE and crosslinking of IgE receptors, which activates membrane phospholipase C and initiates phosphorylation of inositol (I) to phosphoinositol (IP) to isositol 4,5-diphosphate (PIP$_2$). In turn, PIP$_2$ is cleaved by phospholipase C into isositol triphosphate (IP3), which enters the cytosol and to 1,2-diacylglycerol (DAG), which remains in the membranes. Then IP3 approaches the endoplasmic reticulum and mitochondrial membrane to phosphorylate (activate) a calmodulin-dependent protein kinase that releases to the cytosol, CA^{2+} bound to these organelles. Calmodulin is an intracellular Ca^{2+}-binding receptor in the cell sol or on a membrane.

In the plasma membrane, DAG, the remaining cleavage product from PIP_2, activates protein kinase C, which rises abruptly to peak in 30 s after antigen–IgE reaction and precedes histamine release by about 60 s. Activation of phospholipase C and DAG lipase causes release of free arachidonic acid and its metabolites prostacycline, eicosanoids, and AGEPC. Furthermore, DAG, monoacylglycerol (MAG), and lipohosphotidic acid (LPA) are all fusogens that fuse small mast-cell granules into a large granule sac, which then fuses with the plasma membrane and discharges its granule contents to the cell's exterior milieux.

A second enzyme cascade activated by crosslinking of IgE receptors involves a rapid (< 15 s) activation of a serine esterase and adenylate cyclase and a rise in intracellular cyclic AMP. Adenosine added immediately after the antigen signal enhances both rise in cyclic AMP and mediator release, while adenosine added before the antigen blocks both. Theophylline in low dose (10^{-8} mol mL^{-1}) prevents the adenosine-augmented rise of cyclic AMP and histamine release.[33] Therefore, adenosine and theophylline affect mast-cell adenylate cyclase activation and subsequent mediator release.

Formation of phophatidylcholine on the outer membrane by activation of methyltransferases is a third enzyme system (Figure 8-8) activated by IgE receptor crosslinking on mast cells and basophils.[34] The resultant phosphokinase C activation decarboxylates phosphatidyl serine on the inner surface of the plasma membrane to phophatidyl ethanolamine. This in turn is methylated once by methyltransferase I and two additional methyl groups are added by methyltransferase II in the other membrane which forms trimethylated phosphatidtyl choline into lysophosphatidyl choline and arachidonic acid. This opens a calcium channel to permit influx of extracellular Ca^{2+} into the cell. These methylations immediately precede by 15 s the rise in cyclic AMP.

Therefore, there are multichanneled enzyme cascades that lead to the release of allergic mediators from mast cells and basophils and other inflammatory cells that offer multiple points whereby drugs may interfere with this release process and help relieve or prevent allergic symptoms.

Management of Allergic Conditions

Environmental and Dietary Control

The most important duty of the physician managing an allergic patient is to determine by a comprehensive medical history and confirm by in vivo or in vitro laboratory tests when and where symptoms are occurring and what is causing them. Seasonal symptoms suggest a pollen or mold inhalant or seasonal food, whereas

IMMUNOBIOLOGY

perennial symptoms suggest house dust, animal dander, occupational sources, or daily ingested food as possible causes. Elimination of the offending allergen is the single most effective method of treatment. This can be accomplished in the home either by removing the offending animal source or by house dust- and mold-control measures.

Foods causing the reactions may be determined by history and by positive prick skin tests or RAST. Proof, however, comes from abstaining from the suspect food group and observing for possible improvement, or more importantly, from open or, especially, double-blinded food ingestion challenge. Removal of the food allergen should lead to relief of symptoms.

Immunotherapy

The ubiquitous nature of such allergens as pollens, molds, and house dust mites makes them difficult to avoid. If symptoms are severe, immunotherapy may alter the patient's immunologic perception and reaction to the allergenic pollen, mold, mites, or insect venom. Starting with an extremely weak concentration (eg, $1:10^{-6}-10^{-4}$ wt vol^{-1}) or a mixture of the offending allergen extracts specific for that patient; once or twice weekly subcutaneous injection of gradually increasing concentration of the extract mixture (up to the limit the patient can tolerate without systemic or large local reactions) are given. These injections are maintained on a fortnightly or monthly basis for several years until significant symptom improvement occurs, or for at least one year. Immunotherapy causes a rapid increase in IgG-blocking antibodies that intercept and neutralize the offending allergen before it can reach the sensitized mast cells. Over time there is also a decrease in specific IgE antibodies to the allergen. Both reactions usually occur with clinical improvement.

Pharmacologic Agents

Cromolyn Sodium and Cromones

The next point of interruption of the allergic pathway is by stabilization of the mast cell membrane by preventing release of its granules. The exact mechanism is not known, but cromolyn appears to prevent an opening of the receptor-operated calcium channels (ROC), perhaps by affecting phospholipase A_2 or phosphokinase C. Several cromolyn analogs appear to have diverse effects on heterogeneous mast cells; eg, ketotifen appears to act strongly on typical skin mast cells, but less effectively on lung mucosal mast cells in man. Both the immediate edematous early-phase and the inflammatory late-phase reactions appear to be blocked by cromolyn-like reagents.

Competition of drugs for the end-organ receptors for the allergic mediator have wide therapeutic use.

Antihistamines

These are usually the first medication used and often are the only agent required for simple allergic rhinitis or urticaria. There are seven main categories of antihistamines, many of which have additional actions, such as anticholinergic or anesthetic properties. The leading groups of such agents are chlorpheniramine, diphenhydrazine, ethlyenediamine, hydroxyzine, and piperazine, all of which have sedation as a bothersome side effect. Currently, several nonsedating antihistamines, such as terfenadine and astemizole, are coming into popular use; they do not cross the blood–brain barrier as readily.

A new antihistamine, azelastine, has also a cromone-like structure that appears to have both antihistamine and cromolyn-like therapeutic activities.

Anti-Eicosanoids

Several agents are under development as competitors for leukotriene receptors; as agents for managing asthma, piriprost and FPL55712 and L-649,923 look promising.

Agents that block the cyclooxygense pathway of arachidonic acid metabolism, such as aspirin, indomethacin, and ibuprofen, have been useful in an occasional asthmatic patient, presumably by blocking formation of bronchoconstrictive PGD_2 and PGF_{2a}, but also possibly by preventing release of irritant products from activated neutrophils and eosinophils in late-phase inflammatory responses.

These agents, however, are more likely to cause severe, even life-threatening asthma in patients who are sensitive to aspirin, perhaps by making more arachidonic acid available for PAF or leukotriene formations.

PAF Antagonists

Platelet-activating factor antagonists are being avidly sought to block the PAF receptor. Ginkolides from ginko trees (BN52021) and triazobenzodiazepan (WEB2086) appear to act quite dramatically in preventing acute and late-phase asthmatic reactions in allergen-challenge models.

Therapeutic Agents

Finally, there are a number of classic therapeutic agents that counteract the effects of an allergic response.

Epinephrine constricts the blood vessels dilated by the action of histamine and other mediators and it also causes bronchial smooth muscle relaxation. Other more selective β_2-adrenergic stimulating bronchodilators in widespread use for treating asthma are albuterol, terbutaline, and metaproterenol. These act on adenylate cyclase to stimulate breakdown of ATP to form cyclic AMP, which relaxes the smooth muscles and inhibits the release of mediators from mast cells.

Theophylline in a synergistic action with β-adrenergic agonists prevents phosphodiesterase from metabolizing cyclic AMP, thereby, in effect also raising th cyclic AMP level. Often, small ineffective doses alone of β-agonist or theophyllir when used together synergistically are effective in bronchodilation and prevent of mediators release. In addition, theophylline in smaller doses antagonizes nosine, which has a role in blocking G proteins. This may, in fact, be the main therapeutic effect of theophylline.

Atropine or its longer-acting derivative ipratropium bromide, given by inhalation, blocks the cholinergic response of airways to allergens and other irritants. Although it may be useful in individual patients with asthma, it has found wider use in managing chronic cough in chronic obstructive pulmonary disease.

Corticosteroids have a major antiinflammatory role in many types of diseases. Since the recognition of the inflammatory late-phase reactions in asthma, atopic dermatitis, chronic rhinitis, the rational for using corticosteroids has been clarified. They are not particularly effective in blocking immediate allergic reactions but have a major impact in preventing or alleviating the consequences of inflammation, especially the damage caused by neutrophil and eosinophil degranulation, and probably the products of macrophages, the monokines, and, for lymphocytes, the lymphokines. The roles of these latter substances in allergic inflammations are currently under study.

Summary

Allergic reactions to allergens are generally IgE antibody mediated and are caused by the release of many inflammatory mediators that can affect any tissue of the body. Most commonly affected are the bronchi, causing asthma; the nose, causing hayfever; the skin, causing urticaria and atopic dermatitis; and the gastrointestinal tract. There are two phases of the reaction: the immediate and the late phase. The immediate or early phase, manifested by edema and smooth muscle contraction, is helped by antihistamines, β-adrenergic agents, and theophylline. The late-phase inflammatory reaction with resultant hyperirritability of the organ involved is helped by antiinflammatory corticosteroids. Cromolyn sodium and immunotherapy act on both phases of the allergic response.

References

1. von Pirquet C. *Deutsche Med Wochnschr.* 1908;34:1297.

2. Portier P, Richet C. *Compt Rend Soc Biol.* 1902;54:170.

3. Cooke RA, VanderVeer A. *J Immunol.* 1916;1:201.

4. Bazarel M, Orgel HA, Hamburger RN. *J Allergy Clin Immunol.* 1974;54:288.

5. Hozouri K, Hanson B, Roitman-Johnson B, Walsh G, Blumenthal MN. *J Allergy Clin Immunol.* 1982;69:121.

   rsh DG, Meyers DA, Bias WB. *New Engl J Med.* 1981;305:1551.

   itz C, Kustner H. *Zentralb Bakteriol.* 1921;86:160.

   , Ishizaka T. *J Immunol.* 1967;99:1187.

   O, Bennich H. Studies on a new class of human immunoglobulin. I. Immunologic *mma Globulins: Structure and Control of Biosynthesis,* Nobel Symposium No. 3, kholm: Almqvist and Wiksell; 1967.

   . *Int Arch Allergy Appl Immunol.* 1969;36:220.

   Greillier P, Robinet-Levy M, Coulomb Y. *J Allergy Clin Immunol.*

12. Croner S, Kjellman NIM, Eriksson B, Roth A. *Arch Dis Child.* 1982;57:364–368.

13. Orgel HA, Hamburger RN, Bazarel M, Gorrin H, Groshong T, Lenoir M, Miller JR, Wallach W. *J Allergy Clin Immunol.* 1975;56:296.

14. Perez-Montfost R, Metzger H. *Mol Immunol.* 1982;19:1113.

15. Orgel HA, Lenoir MA, Bazarel M. *J Allergy Clin Immunol.* 1976;53:213.

16. Knicker WT, Cochrane CG. *J Exp Med.* 1965;122:83.

17. Katz DH. *Immunol Rev.* 1978;41:77.

18. Chiorazzi N, Fox DA, Katz DH. *J Immunol.* 1977;118:48.

19. Katz DH, Bargatze RF, Bogowitz CA, Katz LR. *J Immunol.* 1980;124:819.

20. Ishizaka K. *Annu Rev Immunol.* 1988;6:513.

21. Bienenstock J. *J Allergy Clin Immunol.* 1988;81:763.

22. Enerback L. *Acta Pathol Microbiol Scand.* 1966;66:289; *Int Arch Allergy Appl Immunol.* 1987;82:249.

23. Kobayashi T, Nakano T, Nakahata T, Asai H, Yagi Y, Komiyama A, Akabane T, Kojima S, Kitamura Y. *J Immunol.* 1986;136:1378.

24. Schwartz LB, Austen KF. The mast cell and mediators of immediate hypersensitivity. In Samter M, ed. *Immunological Diseases,* 4th ed. Boston: Little Brown and Co; 1988:157.

25. Irani AA, Schechter NM, Craig SS, De Bliss G, Schwartz LB. *Proc Natl Acad Sci (USA).* 1986;83:4464.

26. Parker CW. *Annu Rev Immunol.* 1987;5:65.

27. Chung KF, Aizawa H, Becker AB, Frick OL, Gold WM, Nadel JA. *Am Rev Respir Dis.* 1986;134:258.

28. Barnes P. *J Allergy Clin Immunol.* 1988;81:919–934.

29. Gilman AG. *Annu Rev Biochem.* 1987;56:615–649.

30. Ishizaka T, White JR, Saito H. *Int Arch Allergy Appl Immunol.* 1987;82:327.

31. Saito H, Okajima F, Molski T, Sha'afi RI, Ui M, Ishizaka T. *J Immunol.* 1987;138:3927.

32. Mazurek N, Schindler H, Schurholz T, Pecht I. *Proc Natl Acad Sci (USA).* 1986;81:6841.

33. Holgate ST, Lewis RA, Maguire JF, Roberts LT, Oates JA, Austin KF. *J Immunol.* 1980;125:1367.

34. Ishizaka T, Hirata F, Ishizaka K, Axelrod J. *Proc Natl Acad Sci (USA).* 1980;77:1903.

35. Triggle DJ. *Allergy.* 1983;38:1.

CHAPTER 9

Transplant Immunology

Olivia Martinez and Marvin R. Garovoy

Immunogenetics and Transplantation Laboratory, University of California Medical Center, San Francisco, CA 94143 USA

Introduction

The successful replacement of damaged or nonfunctional tissues and organs by transplantation has been a long-standing goal of clinical medicine. Early attempts at transfer of solid tissues and organs initiated in the 19th century were plagued by limitations in surgical technique and the control of septic complications. Progress in the field of surgery in the early 20th century overcame these difficulties, only to reveal the most formidable barrier of all to successful clinical transplantation—the immune system.

This chapter discusses (1) the immunological basis, including the antigen systems that operate, for determining graft outcome; (2) tissue-typing procedures utilized to identify suitable donor–recipient pairs; (3) specific types of clinical transplantation; (4) immunosuppressive therapies utilized to minimize or control rejection episodes; and (5) current areas of interest in experimental transplantation immunology.

History of Immunocompatibility

The practice of blood transfusion, also a form of transplantation, provided the first indication that genetic disparity between donor and recipient contributes to graft failure. The deleterious effects observed in noncompatible blood transfusions in the 17th century were explained by the work of Landsteiner in the 19th century, who elucidated the role of the blood group antigens ABO in determining the outcome of transfusion. Consequently, blood transfusions have become the most common and successful form of tissue transfer. In contrast, the humoral and cellular mechanisms governing the outcome of solid organ transplantation are not fully understood.

Current understanding of histocompatibility stems directly from the work of tumor biologists at the beginning of the century who were attempting to maintain the growth of specific tumors for study by passaging them successively from one mouse to the next. The results of these transfers were frequently unsuccessful until Jensen[1] and Loeb[2] independently utilized inbred stocks of mice to propagate the tumors indefinitely. These observations suggested that the relatedness of the individuals had some influence on the outcome of the tissue transfer. More extensive genetic studies on mice by Tyzzer[3] led Little[4] to postulate the existence of multiple genes that controlled the outcome of tumor transplantation. These genes are now known to be the histocompatibility genes. Further studies of these genes were made possible by the work of Snell,[5] who developed congenic mouse strains.

Gorer's[6] studies on inbred mice in the 1930s confirmed the genetic relationship between alloantigens and the growth of transferred tumor. Furthermore, Gorer demonstrated that these alloantigens were capable of eliciting the production of specific antibodies. Thus, the basis was established for performing the classical experiments of Medawar[7] and colleagues in the 1940s, which lay the groundwork for modern transplantation immunology. In these experiments, skin grafts were performed on strains of inbred mice. The outcome of grafts between mice of genetically different strains was compared to the outcome of grafts from one location to another on the same mouse. For periods up to 1 week no difference can be distinguished as both types of grafts become vascularized and display no visible pathology. However, after the first week, in the case of grafts between genetically disparate animals, a rejection response becomes evident. Rejection is characterized by discoloration, inflammation, and the eventual sloughing off of the grafted skin to be replaced by host tissue.

Four basic types of grafts can be defined in transplantation depending on the relationship of donor and recipient (Table 9-1). Autografts are made from the recipients own tissue; allografts refer to transfers between genetically disparate individuals of the same species; isografts are made between genetically identical individuals; and xenografts are made between members of different species. Evidence for the role of the immune system in rejection responses is supported by the infiltration at the graft site of mononuclear cells, including lymphocytes and monocytes. As is discussed later (see Allorecognition), T cells are the primary mediators of graft rejection. In addition, transplantation of normal skin displays two very fundamental characteristics of the immune system—specificity and memory. As described in the experiments of Medawar,[7] an allograft results in a first-set rejection response, when the strain-A recipient has not previously been exposed to allogeneic donor tissue of strain B (Figure 9-1). If, however, a second graft from the donor strain is subsequently performed on the same recipient, the rejection is more rapid and vigorous, thus generating a second-set rejection. This is due to immunologic memory which ensues from previous exposure to donor antigens resulting in a

Table 9-1. Types of Transplants

Term	Type	Outcome
Autograft	On the same individual	Accepted
Isograft	Between genetically identical members of the same species	Accepted
Allograft	Between genetically different members of the same species	Rejected
Xenograft	Between members of different species	Rejected

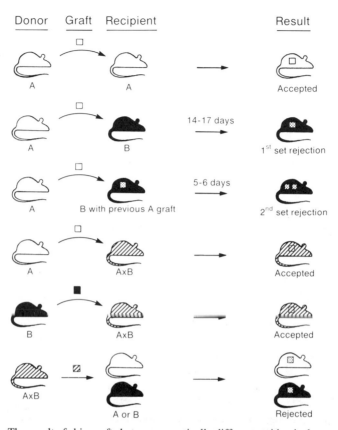

Figure 9-1. The result of skin grafts between genetically different or identical mouse strains. When grafts are transferred from one member of strain A to another they are accepted. Grafts between two distinct strains A and B are rejected within 14–17 d. If the strain-B mouse had previously been grafted with strain-A skin the rejection of a second graft is accelerated (5–6 d). Grafts from either parental strain A or B into an F_1 A × B are accepted. Grafts from an F_1 A × B into either parent A or B are rejected.

primed population of immunologically responsive cells in the recipient. Furthermore, the response is specific in that a graft from a strain-C mouse onto the strain-A recipient will display first-set rejection characteristics. Specificity, memory, and the cellular basis of rejection can also be demonstrated by injecting lymphocytes from an animal of strain A previously grafted with strain-B skin into an immunologically naive animal of strain A. Transplant of a B graft onto the adoptively transferred animal will yield a second-set rejection response, and transplant of strain-C tissue yields a first-set rejection.

Codominant expression of genes governing these responses is apparent when grafts from either parental strain are transplanted to an F_1 hybrid animal. Offspring animals accept grafts from either parent equally well. These observations lead to one of the basic riddles of immunology: How does the immune system distinguish self from nonself? It is clear that histocompatibility genes provide the recognition elements for this process. How the response is learned and regulated is not clear. These questions provide the framework for much of the focus of experimental immunology.

Using F_1 animals it is possible to demonstrate experimentally a unique form of a rejection response termed graft vs. host disease (GVH). In this response, donor cells attack host tissue. Immunocompetent cells from a parental strain A are injected into the F_1 offspring A $\times$ B. The F_1 animal "sees" the A antigens as self since parental types are codominately expressed in the offspring. The immunocompetent cells of A, however, view the B antigens expressed by the F_1 animal as foreign, or nonself. Such a GVH response can result in a "wasting" syndrome and ultimately in death of the host. When the host is immunocompromised or immunoincompetent GVH can also occur. It is of particular concern in clinical bone marrow transplantation.

In some types of transplants, such as corneal, it is possible to observe prolonged graft survival in genetically dissimilar animals. The classical interpretation of this phenomenon is that the site of transplant is immunologically privileged because it is nonvascularized or sequestered from the lymphatic system and so is not accessible to a rejection response as mediated by the immune system. Alternative explanations involving active suppression of the immune system are the focus of current research. In other tissues, such as liver, the organ itself may be immunologically privileged in that it does not evoke a vigorous immune response. This can also be related to the extent of expression of the histocompatibility genes by the allograft.

Histocompatibility Genes

Multiple genetic loci controlling allogeneic responses and tissue compatibility have been demonstrated in all mammalian species studied. The majority of these loci are categorized as minor histocompatibility regions in that they play a lesser, although important, role in the outcome of graft transplantation.[8] In contrast, the genes comprising the major histocompatibility complex (MHC) have been studied extensively and are known to play a dominant role in determining graft outcome. Genetic differences at a single minor histocompatibility locus produce rejection responses much more slowly than those due to differences at the MHC. However, differences at multiple minor histocompatibility loci can lead to a rejection response comparable in severity to that of an MHC-type rejection. In humans the MHC is composed of a region termed human leukocyte antigen (HLA) (Figure 9-2). The HLA is a cluster of closely linked genes on the small arm of chromosome 6 which encode an extremely polymorphic array of proteins. Every individual expresses two complete sets of HLA antigens, one from each parent. "Haplotype" is the term used to identify a single inherited set of HLA antigens. Major histocompatibility complex gene clusters were originally identified and defined for the predominant role they play in graft outcome between genetically different individuals.[9] However, with advances in modern immunology has come the realization that the proteins encoded by these genes play a complex and extensive role in recognition and regulation of the immune response in a variety of ways.[10] This will become clear as specific HLA genes are discussed.

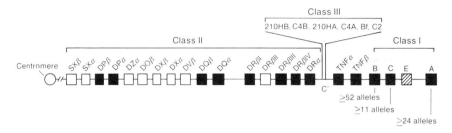

Figure 9-2. The human major histocompatibility complex is the HLA region of chromosome 6 and contains Class-I, -II, and -III genes. The products of these gene clusters are distinguished by their structural characteristics, their cellular distribution, and their role in cell–cell recognition in the immune response. Dark squares designate loci that are expressed. Serological techniques have identified multiple allelic forms of HLA-A, -B, and -C. A new class-I locus HLA-E (hatched square) has recently been described. An allele of this locus, 6.2, was sequenced and showed extensive homology to HLA-A, -B, and -C.

Using structural and functional features it is possible to identify three basic groups of genes within the HLA: classes I, II, and III. The human class-I genes A, B, and C encode the ubiquitous proteins expressed on the membranes of nucleated cells and platelets. These proteins are the classical histocompatibility antigens and are designated HLA-A, HLA-B, and HLA-C. Class-I molecules are the target of recognition by CD8[+] lymphocytes, including cytotoxic T cells, which are key mediators of cellular graft rejection.

The human class-I molecules are an array of highly polymorphic glycoproteins of 44 kd (heavy chain) which are expressed as integral membrane proteins in association with a 12-kd invariant protein termed β-2-microglobulin. Thus the heavy chain carries the HLA-A, -B, and -C polymorphism which has been defined serologically. The extracellular region of the heavy chain consists of three domains: $\alpha 1$, $\alpha 2$, and $\alpha 3$, each encoded by separate exons.[11] Additional domains provide the transmembrane and cytoplasmic regions. Recently, x-ray crystallographic studies have elucidated the three-dimensional structure of the human class-I protein HLA-A2.[12] The results show the $\alpha 1$ and $\alpha 2$ domains of the heavy chain to be situated furthermost from the membrane and folded into two α helices, which form a cleft atop a β-pleated sheet comprising the base of the cleft. The $\alpha 3$ domain and β-2-microglobulin are associated noncovalently and are situated proximal to the membrane to provide stability. The majority of the polymorphic amino acid residues defining genetic diversity are exposed externally and most accessible to the T-cell receptor (TCR) and/or antigen. Sequencing studies have localized the major portion of the diversity to the carboxy-terminal end of $\alpha 1$ and to the amino-terminal end of $\alpha 2$, whereas $\alpha 3$ is virtually nonpolymorphic.[13]

Prior to amino acid and DNA sequencing information the identification of the products of various HLA class-I alleles has been performed serologically and thus limited by the availability of antibodies to define HLA specificities. To date 24 specificities of A, 52 of B, and 11 of C have been serologically determined. Specificities are identified by using antisera that recognize structural determinants of the membrane expressed antigen. Public specificities recognize epitopes common to locus A, B, or C, for example, whereas private specificities are unique and distinct determinants of various HLA-A, -B, and -C types. The HLA nomenclature identifies these specificities numerically. For example, HLA-A2 refers to the second antiserum identifying the A gene product. The letter w before the numeric designation indicates provisional or "workshop" status. Once the specificity is confirmed as unique by the World Health Organization the w is removed.

The rapid advances being made in techniques of molecular biology have prompted a reevaluation of the approach and interpretation of tissue typing data. Indeed, the most recent workshop, The 10th International Histocompatibility Workshop, was largely devoted to compiling and collating serological, cellular, and molecular data to derive a cohesive picture of the immunogenetics of HLA.

Class-II genes encode the Ia antigens which are expressed predominately on cells of the immune system.[14] These molecules serve as recognition signals to mediate cell–cell communication in antigen-presenting responses.[15] Primarily T_H cells, $CD4^+$ cells recognize soluble antigen in association with self-class-II molecules on monocytes, B cells, dendritic cells, or other antigen-presenting cells (APC).

The locus on chromosome 6, which include human class II genes is termed HLA-D.[16] Earlier HLA nomenclature designated HLA-D-derived surface antigens LD (lymphocyte defined), because they were identified as mediators of in vitro proliferative responses of lymphocytes, such as the mixed-lymphocyte reaction (MLR) and the primed lymphocyte test (PLT). Class-II, like class-I antigens, are capable of eliciting the production of specific alloantibodies or monoclonal antibodies (Mabs).

The HLA-D region contains multiple loci, including pseudogenes and the exons for DR, DQ, and DP. The pseudogenes have sequence homology to normal genes but lack the necessary sequences for expression. Homology studies also suggest that multiple class-I and class-II genes develop by reduplication events.

DR subloci contain the gene for a single DR α chain, which is relatively conserved, and DR β chains I–IV. DR beta I expresses the polymorphism, whereas DR beta II is a pseudogene and DR beta III and IV code for particular DR specificities. The DQ subloci contain one DQ α and one DQ β allele, and are 3′ to DX β and DX α (DQ-like pseudogenes) and DV β, a locus for which the corresponding cell-surface product has not been identified. Two other loci, DZ α and DO β, have also been identified in the absence of cellular products.

Deoxyribonucleic acid and amino acid sequencing studies have been able to identify the membrane distal regions of DR α, DQ β, DP β, and DQ α as the sites of allelic polymorphism.

The products of the DR, DQ, and DP genes are expressed on the cell membrane as a noncovalently associated heterodimer comprised of a 33-kd α and 28-kd β subunit which each span the membrane.[17] Both contain two extracellular domains and, like β-2-microglobulin and the α3 domain of class-I antigens, both share homology with immunoglobulin constant-region sequences in the membrane-proximal region.[17] The N-terminal end of the class-II chains most likely contains the antigen binding region.

Unlike the class-I antigens, the expression of class-II proteins can be nonconstitutive and limited by cell type. Cytokines such as γ-interferon (γ-IFN), interleukin-4 (IL-4), and tumor necrosis factor (TNF) have been shown to induce, enhance, or inhibit the expression of class-II antigens depending on the cell type.[18,19]

Class-III genes are situated between class-II and class-I genes within the MHC and encode a series of complement proteins that are not discussed further here.

Tissue Typing

In order to establish the most suitable donor–recipient relationships, in vitro tissue-typing techniques have been developed. Such methods are designed to determine the HLA types of the transplant participants in order to maximize the likelihood of successful graft outcome by selecting histocompatible donor–recipient combinations. For example, studies on living related recipients of kidney transplants show 87 ± 4% graft survival at 3 years for HLA-identical pairs, versus a 56 ± 10% survival for one-haplotype matched pairs, illustrating the value of HLA matching[20] (Figure 9-3). Graft outcome between histoincompatible individuals can be improved with the use of immunosuppressive therapy (see Immunosuppression).

Current tissue-typing procedures can be divided into three categories: serological, cellular, and molecular.

Serological Tissue Typing

The advent of serological tissue typing was Dausset's study of anti-leukocyte antibodies.[21] Today, serological procedures to identify HLA types depend on the avail-

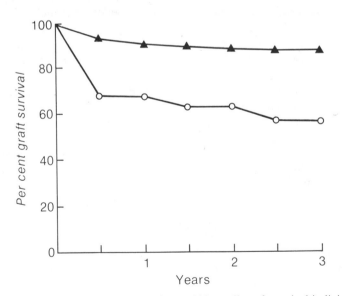

Figure 9-3. The effect of haplotype matching on kidney allograft survival in living related donor–recipient pairs. ▲, HLA identical ($n = 110$); ○, one-haplotype matched ($n = 31$).

ability of specific typing antisera. The most common sources of typing sera are: (1) multiparous women who have been "immunized" with fetal tissue bearing foreign antigens of the father; (2) individuals who have received blood transfusions; and (3) individuals who have received and rejected transplants. All three, in practice, constitute an allogeneic immunization. In most cases, these alloantisera are not monospecific (ie, they have activity against multiple HLA specificities) and so must be tested and characterized fully before use. This can involve absorption on cells of known HLA type. The specificity of the sera can be determined by adding it to panels of homozygous typing cells. Binding of antibody to HLA antigens in the presence of complement causes cell lysis, which can be detected with dyes taken up by damaged cells. Viable cells retain intact membranes and do not take up these dyes. These assays can be performed with a few microliters of antisera and thus are termed microcytotoxicity texts.[22]

Recently Mabs to some HLA specificities have become available. Although it has been difficult, in some cases, to generate a panel of Mabs and correlate their activity with known HLA typing sera, they may ultimately alleviate technical problems presented by limited amounts of weak and polyspecific alloantisera.

In standard HLA tissue typing, microcytotoxicity tests are performed on prospective recipient and donor cells (usually lymphocytes) using a panel of known HLA typing antisera. This is most frequently utilized to identify HLA-A, -B, and -C types. A fully heterozygous individual can express at most six different HLA-A, -B, -C antigens. Because of the limitations of serological techniques detection of a single allele at a given locus may mean (1) the individual is homozygous at that locus or (2) the individual is heterozygous but antisera have not been obtained that identify the allele in question.

Although cell-mediated responses are considered to be of prime importance in graft rejection, there is strong evidence that the presence of preformed antibody to donor antigens in recipients can lead to hyperacute rejection. These antibodies may be present because of any or all of the three means of obtaining alloantisera mentioned above. Consequently, it is critical to screen recipient sera against donor cells or cells bearing donor antigen. A rapid, sensitive "crossmatching" procedure has been described using flow cytometry to identify preformed anti-donor antibodies [23] (Figure 9-4). Using this method it is also possible to distinguish between anti-T and anti-B cell activity. This can be important since there is evidence that some types of anti-B cell activity do not contraindicate transplantation.

A mismatch within the blood group antigens ABO can also lead to hyperacute rejection as mediated by preformed anti-A and anti-B antibodies in recipients lacking these antigens.

Cellular Tissue Typing

Cellular tissue typing most frequently involves the coculture of potential donor and recipient cells.[24] Under appropriate conditions lymphocytes recognize differences in HLA antigens called Lad (lymphocyte activating determinants), which are primarily class-II antigens, and respond by producing lymphokines and monokines.

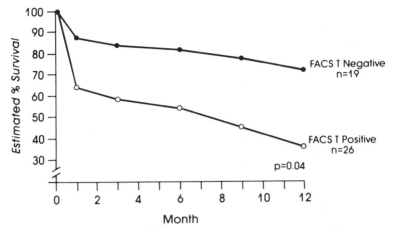

Figure 9-4. The effect of crossmatching on kidney allograft survival. Patients for whom fluorescence-activated cell sorter (FACS) analysis showed a negative T-cell crossmatch (●) against their prospective donor antigens had significantly higher graft survival after 1 year than did those patients who had a positive T-cell crossmatch (○).

This leads to blast transformation, cellular division, and antibody production. Most often the degree of response in the assay is measured by the extent of cellular proliferation as determined by uptake of a radioactive nucleotide. The magnitude of the response is an indication of the extent of genetic dissimilarity. In a one-way MLR one population of cells, for example the donor's, is inactivated by irradiation or mitomycin C treatment. These cells then become inert, target cells to be recognized by the responder or recipient cells. The endpoint of the assay becomes a measure of the extent of foreignness with which recipient "views" donor cells. In a two-way MLR both cell types can respond to each other.

In the PLT, lymphocytes are primed to a particular Lad by homozygous typing cells.[25] These primed lymphocytes are then mixed with test lymphocytes. If the test lymphocytes share the Lad antigen they will induce rapid, vigorous proliferation of the primed cells. The D antigens, of which 26 have been identified, were detected using such cellular assays.

The MLR and PLT assays are useful in detecting differences at the class-II regions; however, one drawback is that the assays take several days to complete and this may not be suitable in some donor–recipient situations due to organ ischemia time.

Molecular Tissue Typing

The most recent and significant advance in tissue typing has come on the heels of breakthroughs in molecular biology. The DNA restriction fragment length polymorphism (RFLP) analysis is a relatively new technique that can be used to complement, enhance, or confirm current serological and cellular tissue-typing techniques.[26] The RFLP analysis involves digestion of genomic DNA with restriction enzymes, electrophoresis of the resulting fragments on agarose gel to resolve them by size, followed by denaturation to obtain single-stranded DNA. Using appropriate radiolabeled class-II-specific cDNA probes to obtain hybridization, allelic differences can be distinguished. This technique is dependent upon identifying restriction enzymes that are sensitive to allelic differences in DNA sequences with extensive sequence homology and the availability of suitable probes (optimally exon specific). Using DNA from homozygous typing cells it is possible to identify hybridization signal patterns unique to particular enzyme–probe combinations. Such profiles may be used to identify genotypes of unknown cells.

Similar to cellular methods of typing, the molecular techniques of sequencing and RFLP are not yet conducive to the time limitations imposed by many clinical requirements in solid organ transplantation. Nevertheless, RFLP has already proved useful in genotype matching of donor–recipient pairs in bone marrow transplantation and will continue to prove useful as a supplement to currently used serological and cellular approaches to HLA tissue typing.[27]

Allorecognition

We have already discussed the immunogenetics of HLA and stated that MHC genes are involved in recognition of self. What are some of the current concepts regarding the manner in which MHC genes operate in distinguishing self from nonself within the immune response?

Class-I antigens function as recognition units or restriction elements for CD8+ cytotoxic T cells (CTL). As originally demonstrated in murine systems, CTL can recognize and lyse virally infected cells only when CTL and target cells share syngeneic MHC class-I antigens. These experiments established that CTL killing is MHC restricted.[28]

In addition, CTL can recognize and kill target cells expressing foreign MHC.[29] The evolution of a mechanism that recognizes foreign tissue has been questioned teleologically. One can rule out the development of such a specific system for the purposes of confounding the transplant physician. The traditional interpretation is that alloantigen "looks" like self plus foreign antigen. Thus, in essence, alloresponses are cross-reactive with self plus antigen responses and overlap with the repertoire of T cells directed at eliminating foreign antigen.

The ability to respond specifically to nonself MHC is termed allorecognition.[30] The process of allorecognition provides the framework for posing questions aimed at elucidating the basic cellular mechanisms underlying allograft rejection as a clinical consequence of histoincompatibility.

Major histocompatability complex restriction also operates for CD4+ T-helper cells, which recognize nominal antigen in association with self-class-II molecules. Experimental evidence suggests that recognition by CD4+ cells is dependent on processing of the antigen by APC.[31] Furthermore, class-II antigens have been shown to bind antigen-derived peptides specifically in solution.[32,33]

Similarly, MHC-restricted killing of virally infected cells by CTL could be duplicated by utilizing peptide fragments of the viral antigen in association with self-class I.[34] Therefore, CD4+ and CD8+ T cells "see" peptide in association with self-MHC molecules and recognize these structures by similar mechanisms. These observations then lead to the question of whether or not allorecognition occurs as a response to peptide plus MHC.

Recently, it has been shown that processed HLA antigen in association with murine self-MHC antigens are suitable targets for murine CTL generated against HLA class I.[35] In other experiments, processed murine alloantigen associated with self-H-2 class-I antigens could reproduce the target specificity of murine CTL generated to allo-class I.[36] Whether or not this mechanism is operative in vivo is not clear.

It has not yet been demonstrated that class-I molecules can physically bind to peptides derived from antigen in solution, as has been shown with class-II molecules. However, cocrystallizing with the HLA-A2 molecules in the cleft containing the majority of the polymorphic residues was a bound peptide suggestive of antigen. Taken collectively, these experiments and others provide intriguing enquiries into the phenomenon of allorecognition.

In most scenarios of graft rejection it is accepted that an interplay of T cells (CD4+ and CD8+), B cells, and monocytes occurs (Figure 9-5). Recipient CD4+ cells may be activated by passenger cells (donor cells transferred with the graft) that bear class-II antigens.[37] In some circumstances CD4+ cells have been shown to be direct mediators of rejection responses. Once activated, CD4+ cells can also release lymphokines such as IFN-γ, IL-2, and IL-4. Production of IL-2 is necessary for clonal expansion of both helper and cytotoxic T cells bearing receptors for donor antigens. Both IFN-γ and IL-4 are known to upregulate expression of class-I and class-II antigens.[18,19] Donor endotheleal tissue can also be a source of stimuli, as it has been shown that class-II antigens can be induced on these cells by IFN-γ.[38] Lymphokine IL-4 provides a critical proliferative signal for B cells. Production of anti-donor specific antibody by B cells can lead to extensive damage to the graft by complement-mediated mechanisms or by antibody-dependent cell-mediated cytotoxicity. Monocytes and macrophages participate by producing IL-1, which is necessary for activation and amplification of the T-cell response. Also involved in this immune cascade is the T-suppressor effector cell that is responsible for downregulating the immune response. Growth and differentiation factors, and the mechanism of recognition by this CD8+ cell are poorly understood. Natural killer cells and eosinophils are also known to infiltrate rejection sites.

Immunosuppression

The use of immunosuppressive therapy is necessary to minimize the immune-mediated response induced by allograft transplantation. In general, the immunosuppressive agents currently in use are nonspecific in their actions and can broadly be classified as radiologic, pharmacologic, and immunologic. Each of these forms of therapy has associated with it potentially harmful and dangerous side effects. Most immunosuppressives function by inhibiting cell division with the aim of preventing development or expansion of anti-donor T-cell responses. Because they are nonspecific, however, the recipient can be left with tissue damage and/or an extremely compromised immune system and ultimately may be more susceptible to infection

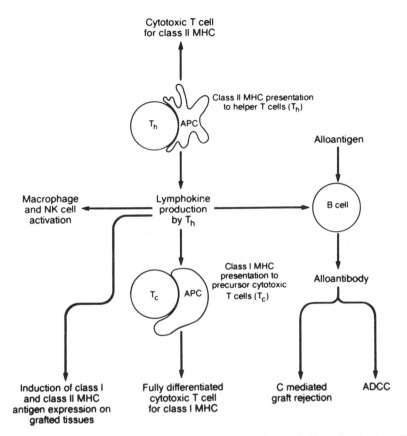

Figure 9-5. The immune response and possible mechanisms of allograft rejection. The introduction of histoincompatible tissue into the host activates humoral and cellular pathways of the immune system, leading to tissue damage by the complement cascade, ADCC, activated cytotoxic T cells, NK cells, and macrophages.

or even malignancy. Consequently, management of immunosuppressive therapy for transplant recipients is complex and not without risks to the patient. The clinician, then, faces the challenge of administering these agents with the goal of maximizing successful graft outcome while minimizing toxic, deleterious effects on the recipient.

Many protocols of immunosuppressive therapy call for simultaneous or sequential administration of multiple drugs. The most frequently utilized agents, their known in vitro mechanism of action, and the types of transplant with which they are effective are discussed here.

Radiation Therapy

The results of early attempts using total body irradiation to achieve immunosuppression and allograft survival were determined to be unacceptable because of irreversible damage to bone marrow tissue, which rendered the patient immunoincompetent.

The approach has given way to total lymphoid irradiation (TLI), which consists of repeated exposure of lymph nodes, spleen, and thymus to radiation while nonlymphoid and bone marrow tissue is shielded.

Studies in rodent systems suggest that TLI not only eliminates mature T cells from the host but produces an immunological setting similar to a fetal or neonatal state where the animal is susceptible to tolerance induction.[39] Tolerance occurred when TLI-treated animals were given allogeneic bone marrow to generate chimeras. Subsequent allografts were accepted in the absence of GVH.

Experimental studies show TLI induces expansion or development of suppressor cells, which can affect cell-mediated and humoral in vitro responses.[40] There is some controversy concerning the phenotype of these cells as it is unclear whether or not they are of the T-cell lineage.

The use of TLI in combination with other immunosuppressive agents has been addressed experimentally. Results show promise but emphasize the importance of radiation dose, form, and interval in achieving optimal allograft outcome.[41]

In some transplant settings TLI is used routinely with clinical bone marrow transplantation. Total lymphoid irradiation has also had some use as an immunosuppressive to enhance kidney transplant survival in high-risk recipients. Difficulties arise in the logistics of treating patients preoperatively who are awaiting cadaveric organ transplant since the exact time of transplant cannot be predetermined. Thus, it is difficult to standardize or optimize TLI administration. In addition, the postoperative immunosuppressive regimens must be evaluated more completely. In many aspects this form of therapy is still considered experimental and is not widely used in solid organ transplantation. Results to date, however, are promising and suggest that further studies are warranted in determining the value of TLI as an immunosuppressive option in solid organ transplantation.

Pharmacological Approaches to Immunosuppression

A wide variety of compounds with immunosuppressive activity have been studied in vitro and in animal systems to identify those which may enhance allograft survival while invoking the fewest harmful side effects.

Current drugs being used most frequently in clinical transplantation include: azathioprine, prednisolone and cyclosporine A (CsA). In many cases triple therapy with these agents is the protocol of choice.

Prednisone and its bioactive derivative prednisolone are corticosteroids used extensively in combination with other compounds as immunosuppressives. In vivo and in vitro studies show that the corticosteroids interfere with the production of the monocyte product IL-1, as well as the T-cell product IL-2. Interleukin-1 is required for the primary activation of T cells, and IL-2 is important as a growth factor for T cells including CTL.

Azathioprine is a cytotoxic agent that is an imidazole derivative of mercaptopurine. Azathioprine is well absorbed and quickly metabolized in vivo to 6-mercaptopurine. 6-Mercaptopurine is an adenine analog and competes intracellularly in the synthesis of adenosine and guanine, thus leading to a decrease in RNA and DNA synthesis. Consequently, dividing cells are most susceptible to the mechanism of action of azathioprine and the outcome can be nonspecific suppression of an active immune response. Deleterious effects include toxicity to non-lymphoid dividing cells and increased incidence of microbial infection.

Azathioprine is often given preoperatively since it appears most effective at preventing development of a rejection response as opposed to controlling an on-going response. In immunosuppressive protocols following heart transplantation, Azathioprine appears to be very effective in combination with CsA at prolonging allograft survival. Similarly, the *Report of the International Pancreas Transplant Registry* showed that over a 4-year period from 1983 to 1987 significantly higher rates of 1-year graft survival were associated with administration of azathioprine with CsA and prednisolone versus various combinations of double therapy or CsA alone.[42]

Cyclosporine A is a product of the soil fungus *Trichoderma polysporum* and is composed of 11 amino acids structured as a cyclic polypeptide. In 1972 Borel was first to demonstrate the potent immunosuppressive properties of this molecule.[43] Subsequent in vitro investigations determined that a primary effect of CsA is to inhibit the production of lymphokines, including IL-2, as well as primary antibody responses to T-dependent antigens.[44] As we have stated IL-2 is required for the generation of helper and cytotoxic T-cell responses at the level of cellular activation. Preactivated T cells are spared by CsA. Significantly, T-suppressor cell activation is less sensitive to the actions of this compound. The sum of these effects, then, is to produce an immunological environment in the host that is more "receptive" to allograft intervention.

Cyclosporine A was approved for clinical use in 1983. Since then CsA has in many ways lived up to its promise as a potent immunosuppressive and is used routinely with kidney, heart, and pancreas transplants to reduce rejection episodes. For example, one study in the United Kingdom reports 5-year cardiac transplant patient survival below 40% using conventional immunosuppressive therapy versus 60% using CsA therapy.[45] Without question CsA has improved allograft acceptance across the board. This has been reported by both multicenter and single center trials. In the case of cadaveric transplantation it has even been argued that CsA overrides the value of HLA-A, -B, -C, and -DR matching. In this way CsA has had an impact on the definition of suitable donor–recipient pairs. These issues are still controversial and not yet resolved, but it is safe to say that CsA has redefined the modern approach to immunosuppressive therapy. Still to consider, however, in addition to the economic impact on the patient who must take CsA is the risk for nephrotoxic and hypertensive consequences. The long-term effect of CsA administration is unclear.

Immunologic Approaches to Immunosuppression

The most common form of immunologically based immunosuppressive therapy relies on administration of immunoglobulin or Mabs directed at lymphocytes or T cells in particular. Heterologous (goat, rabbit, horse) polyclonal antisera preparations specific for lymphocytes (ALG) or thymocytes (ATG) have been used as immunosuppressives with the goal of ablating or inactivating the immunocompetent cells of the host. Difficulty in evaluating the efficacy of these reagents in clinical settings stems from the variation in purity, source, and dosage of the preparations. In some centers, these reagents are used to control active rejection episodes and are not among the prophylactic immunosuppressives of choice. Predictably, the administration of large doses (mg kg^{-1}) of heterologous protein can result in allergic symptoms or serum sickness despite the immunosuppressed state of the recipient.

In an attempt to improve and refine the specificity of immunosuppressive therapy Mabs have been employed. These reagents have the advantages of being fully characterized, monospecific, and less likely to induce side effects from contaminating material. A mouse Mab specific for the T3 complex associated with the TcR present on all mature T cells, OKT3 has been the most often utilized reagent of this class. While OKT3 treatment can lead to elimination of T cells from peripheral blood, the mechanism of action of OKT3 is in question. Clearly, interaction of T3 with OKT3 can induce modulation of the TcR. In addition, OKT3 can potentially mask or "freeze" TcR by binding to T3 and thus modify the function of the T3$^+$ cell. Recent experimental studies in mice suggest that anti-T3 reagents may alter T-cell function or in vivo distribution in a manner that is not clear but that does lead to decreased cell-mediated responses for extended periods.[46] In one published report OKT3 administration produced a significant improvement in cadaveric kidney allograft rescue in cases of rejection that were refractory to other forms of immunosuppression, leading to an overall increase in graft survival at 1 year from 80% to 92%.[47] Monoclonal antibodies have also been used to purge bone marrow ex vivo of mature T cells prior to transplant.

Immunotoxins are hybrid molecules composed of Mabs conjugated to a toxic agent, frequently a toxin fragment.[48] These reagents are a provocative alternative to traditional immunosuppressive therapy. Potentially they offer specificity and potency, but in vivo use has not always fulfilled this promise. The factors at play that determine their efficacy are multiple, complex, and not well understood. In an interesting approach, employing recombinant DNA technology, the gene for the active fragment of diptheria toxin has been cloned and inserted adjacent to the gene for IL-2. The product of these genes is a hybrid protein that can bind to cells expressing the IL-2 receptor (primarily activated T cells) and if internalized can be cytotoxic.[49] This reagent is designed to eliminate actively responding T cells. The IL-2–fragment-A hybrid has been tested in animal models receiving allografts with encouraging results. Certainly immunotoxins are one of the most actively pursued areas in the new wave of immunosuppressive therapy.

Another form of immunomodulatory therapy that can have suppressive effects is donor-specific transfusion (DST).[50] Used primarily in association with living related renal transplantation, DST involves preoperative administration of whole donor blood or packed cells to the recipient. Various protocols are employed depending on the transplant center, but here we discuss results where 200-cc fresh whole blood or packed cell equivalent was given on three separate occasions at 2-week intervals. In one study graft survival in patients who received DST was compared to those who did not but who were HLA identical. The results show a 3-year graft survival of 85% for HLA-identical pairs, and an 84% survival for the DST-treated 0–1 haplotype-matched group.[51] One potential risk of DST is of the recipient's becoming sensitized to donor antigen(s), thereby eliminating the donor as a candidate. This is assessed by crossmatching to test for anti-donor antibody. Sensitization rates of from 10 to 30% have been reported. One approach to minimizing the chance for donor-specific sensitization (anti-donor antibody formation) is to give azathioprine to DST recipients. This appears to be helpful to patients receiving their first transplant who have serum activity against a standard panel of HLA-type cells (PRA) of < 10%.

A statistical model utilizing linear logistic regression has identified six factors that are critical to determining whether a recipient will become sensitized by DST.[52] The factors that weighed toward sensitization were PRA, previous pregnancy, and previous transplant. The factors that decreased the likelihood of sensitization were number of prior transfusions, number of HLA-matched antigens, and the administration of azathioprine.

Often potential transplant recipients have received third-party or multiple transfusions. The transfusion effect is still controversial, with some centers reporting a clearcut benefit from pretransplant transfusion and others reporting no difference in graft outcome in transfused vs. nontransfused recipients. It has been argued that the use of CsA has overcome the benefits of transfusion.

Many mechanisms have been proposed to explain the protective effect of DST. It has been suggested that DST does not alter or modify the immune system of the recipient but only selects for low-responder recipients since those that become sensitized are not transplanted. Evidence for and against this hypothesis exists and selection cannot yet be eliminated as one factor in the DST effect. Mechanisms that involve an active modification of the immune system by DST leading to unresponsiveness can be categorized as humoral or cellular.

A humoral effect has been proposed based on data that describe an "anti-idiotype"-like component in pretransplant sera of transfused recipients.[53] Idiotypes are antigenic determinants within the binding site of an antibody molecule. Anti-idiotype-like activity can be demonstrated in sera of some patients who possess a positive crossmatch to a particular HLA type, which subsequently becomes negative. When mixed with the earlier positive sera the negative sera are shown to specifically inhibit lymphocytotoxicity. Identification of an immunoglobulin-like component in the blocking sera has been interpreted as evidence for formation of an anti-idiotype antibody. The notion that formation of anti-idiotypic antibody can modulate cellular responses leading to unresponsiveness in the DST model awaits experimental confirmation.

A generalized reduction in nonspecific cellular immune assays by PBL of transfused individuals has been reported. It has not yet been possible to identify a suppressor effector in humans to explain these observations. Experimental results in animal models, however, have identified suppressor cells in transfused animals.[54] In one study of transfused animals, a monocyte-like cell was shown to suppress in vitro cellular assays.[55]

Clinical Transplantation

Liver Transplantation

As mentioned previously, the liver constitutes a relatively nonimmunogeneic allograft for transplantation. Most graft losses are not due to rejection episodes. The three most common indications for liver transplantation in adults have been primary biliary cirrhosis, cirrhosis, or sclerosing cholangitis. The use of CsA has had profound impact on survival rates. In one report of 1000 liver transplants 1-year patient survival improved from 32% to 70% when CsA was administered.[56] Because this is a relatively new form of transplant, comparatively few data are available for the effects of HLA matching. Early retrospective data indicate an inverse relationship between HLA matching and graft survival, although the actual number of well-matched grafts was low.[56] The complexity of the immune response in liver transplantation is reflected in the following studies. Experiments where rats receive liver allografts reveal that in certain donor–recipient strain combinations, the liver is able to induce a state of tolerance and can even initiate immune mechanisms that can reverse ongoing rejection episodes at distant sites.[57] This occurs in allogeneic strain combinations where grafting of other organs is rejected in the expected fashion. There is evidence that the tolerant state is partially due to the selective deletion of allospecific clones. These results suggest that the rat model system may be valuable in providing useful information for clinical liver transplantation.

Kidney Transplantation

The largest patient group receiving kidney transplants are sufferers of end-stage renal disease. In most cases well-matched living related donors are not available and patients must undergo dialysis while waiting for a suitable cadaveric donor.

Nevertheless, kidney transplantation has arguably become the most successful form of solid organ transplant performed. The factors most responsible for the improved success rate are a greater understanding of the role of HLA in graft outcome spurred in part by technological advances in the area of tissue typing and the introduction of CsA as an immunosuppressive agent.

The emphasis and understanding of HLA typing in clinical renal transplantation has evolved significantly since the 1960s and continues to change today.

It has been repeatedly shown that kidney grafts between siblings are better tolerated and that this correlates with a high degree of HLA-A, HLA-B matching as compared to poorly matched living related donors.

In contrast, the benefits of HLA-A,B matching for cadaveric donor renal transplants has not been as convincing. This can be interpreted as evidence for the importance and contribution of other untyped histocompatibility loci that are more likely shared between related individuals.

In this regard, the D-region genes have emerged as a focus of increased interest. Initially, D-region typing was done using cellular coculture techniques, such as the MLR, that are not feasible in cadaver-donor situations. More recently, the development of serological reagents to type-B lymphocytes for the DR and DQ gene products as well as advances in molecular biology should generate data that will contribute to identifying the HLA components at play in kidney allograft outcome.

It is evident that deficiencies in HLA typing of cadaveric transplants have been offset or masked by inclusion of CsA in immunosuppressive protocols. The benefits of CsA in living related transplants, however, are equivocal, primarily because traditional immunosuppression with azathioprine and prednisolone have been so effective.

Nevertheless, it is likely that a better understanding of the role of HLA and non-MHC histocompatibility antigen systems in combination with optimization of CsA dose regimens should yield further improvement in the success rate of renal transplants.

Bone Marrow Transplantation

Bone marrow transplantation may be an option in diseases of the blood, including leukemias and other malignancies, such hematopoietic disorders as severe aplastic anemia, and genetic or metabolic diseases. The number of allogeneic bone marrow transplants has increased dramatically in recent years, with over 3000 performed in 1986. Autologous bone marrow transplantation is also increasing in frequency.

Graft versus host reaction is of primary concern in allogeneic bone marrow transplantation, as patients are frequently receiving radiotherapy. A relatively recent approach to avoid GVH has been to purge the bone marrow ex vivo to deplete it of mature T cells. Bone marrow purging has also been used to remove residual malignant cells in autologous transplants. Monoclonal antibodies or cocktails of Mabs have been used to this end. The method of depletion can rely on complement-mediated killing, immunotoxin cytotoxicity, or physical removal with antibody-coated microspheres. Other attempts at purging have employed cytotoxic drugs.

These studies have revealed that total T-cell depletion by purging may not be beneficial to the patient and can be associated with host versus graft reaction or increased relapse rate in some malignancies. Clearly much more work is necessary to determine the optimal conditioning regimen, method of purging, and post-transplant protocols for the specific disease in question.

References

1. Jensen CO. *Centralbl Bakteriol Parasitenk Infektionskrankh.* 1903;34:28.

2. Loeb L. *Z Krebforschung.* 1908;7:80.

3. Tyzzer EE. *J Med Res.* 1909;21:519.

4. Little CC. *Science.* 1914;40:904.

5. Snell GD. *Science.* 1944;100:272.

6. Gorer PA. *J Pathol Bacteriol.* 1938;47:231.

7. Medawar PB. *J Anat.* 1944;78:176.

8. Counce S, Smith P, Barth R, Snell GD. *Ann Surg.* 1956;144:198.

9. Klein J. *Natural History of the Major Histocompatibility Complex.* New York: Wiley-Interscience; 1987.

10. Schwartz RH. *Fundamental Immunology*. New York: Raven; 1984.

11. Malissen M, Malissen B, Jordan BR. *Proc Natl Acad Sci (USA)*. 1982;79:893.

12. Bjorkman P, Saper MA, Samraoui B, Bennett WS, Strominger JL, Wiley DC. *Nature (London)* 1987;329:506.

13. Ways JP, Coppin HL, Parham PJ. *J Biol Chem*. 1985;260:11924.

14. McDevitt HO, Benacerraf B. *Adv Immunol*. 1969;11:31.

15. Benacerraf B. *Science*. 1981;212:1229.

16. Yunis EJ, Amos DB. *Proc Natl Acad Sci (USA)*. 1971;68:3031.

17. Kaufman JF, Auffray C, Korman AJ, Schackelford DA, Strominger JL. *Cell*. 1984;36:1.

18. Chang RJ, Lee SH. *J Immunol*. 1986;137:2853.

19. Paul WE, Ohara J. *Annu Rev Immunol*. 1987;5:429.

20. Salvatierra O, Vincenti F, Amend W, Garovoy M, Iwaki Y, Terasaki P, Potter D, Duca R, Hopper S, Slemmer T, Feduska N. *Trans Proc*. 1983;XV:924.

21. Dausset J, Nenna ACR. *Soc Biol (Paris)*. 1952;146:1539.

22. Terasaki PJ, Vredevoe DL, Porter KA, Mickey MR, Marchioro TL, Faris TD, Hermann TJ. *Transplantation*. 1966;4:688.

23. Garovoy MR, Rheinschmidt MA, Bigos M, Perkins H, Colombe B, Feduska N, Salvatierra O. *Trans Proc*. 1983;XV:1939.

24. Bach FH, Voynow NK. *Science*. 1966;153:545.

25. Sheehy MJ, Sondel PM, Bach ML, et al. *Science*. 1975;188:1308.

26. Bidwell J. *Immunol Today*. 1988;9:18.

27. Andersson M, Bohme J, Andersson G, Moller E, Thorsby E, Rask L, Peterson PA. *Human Immunol*. 1984;11:57.

28. Zinkernagel RM, Dohery PC. *Nature (London)*. 1974;248:701.

29. Lindahl KF, Bach FH. *Nature (London)*. 1975;254:607.

30. Klein J. *Biology of the Mouse Major Histocompatibilty Complex*. New York: Springer Verlag; 1975.

31. Shimonkevitz R, Kappler J, Marrack P, Grey H. *J Exp Med*. 1983;158:303.

32. Babbitt BP, Allen PM, Matsueda G, Haber E, Unanue ER. *Nature (London)*. 1985;317:359.

33. Buus S, Sette A, Colon SM, Jenis DM, Grey H. *Cell*. 1987;47:1071.

34. Townsend ARM, Rothbard J, Gotch FM, Bahadur G, Wraith D, McMichael AJ. *Cell*. 1986;44:959.

35. Maryanski JL, Accolla RS, Jordan B. *J Immunol*. 1986;136:4340.

36. Song ES, Linsk R, Olson CA, McMillan M, Goodenow RS. *Proc Natl Acad Sci (USA)*. 1988;85:1927.

37. Steinman RM. *Transplantation*. 1987;31:151.

38. Pober JS, Gimbrone MA, Cotran RS, Reiss CR, Burakoff SJ, Fiers W, Ault KA. *J Exp Med*. 1983;157:1339.

39. Zan-Bar E, Slavin S, Strober S. *J Immunol*. 1987;121:1400.

40. Slavin S, Weiss L, Moreck S, et al. In Slavin S, ed. *Tolerance in Bone Marrow and Organ Transplantation*. Amsterdam: Elsevier; 1984:105–153.

41. Slavin S. *Immunol Today*. 1987;8:88.

42. Sutherland DER, Moudry KC. In Terasaki P, ed. *Clinical Transplants*. Los Angeles: UCLA Tissue Typing Laboratory; 1987:63–102.

43. Borel JF. *Trans Proc*. 1983;15:2219.

44. Bunjes D, Hardt C, Rollinghoff M, Wager H. *Eur J Immunol.* 1981;11:657.

45. English TAH, Wallwork J. In Terasaki P, ed. *Clinical Transplants.* Los Angeles: UCLA Tissue Typing Laboratory; 1987;13–16.

46. Hirsch R, Eckhaus M, Auchincloss H, Sachs DH, Bluestone JA. *J Immunol.* 1988;14:3766.

47. Stratta RJ, Armbrust MJ, Lorentzen DF, Hoffman RM, D'Alessandro, Sollinger HW, Pirsch JD, Kalayoglu M, Belzer FO. In Terasaki P, ed. *Clinical Transplants.* Los Angeles: UCLA Tissue Typing Laboratory; 1987:183–193.

48. Martinez O, Wofsy L. In Weir DM, ed. *Handbook of Experimental Immunology.* Oxford: Blackwell Scientific; 1986:1–11.

49. Bacha P, Williams DP, Waters C, Williams JM, Murphy JR, Strom TR. *J Exp Med.* 1988;167:612.

50. Salvatierra O, Vincenti F, Amend W, et al. *Ann Surg.* 1980;192:543.

51. Salvatierra O, Melzer J, Vincenti F, Amend W, Tomlanovitch S, Potter D, Husing R, Garovoy M, Feduska NJ. *Trans Proc.* 1987;XIX:160.

52. Colombe BW, Juster RP, Salvatierra O, Garovoy MR. *Transplantation.* 1988;45:101.

53. Singal DP, Fagnilli L, Joseph S. *Trans Proc.* 1983;15:1005.

54. Maki T, Okazaki H, Wood M. *Surg Forum.* 1981;32:396.

55. Wood M, Gottschalk R, Monaco AP. *Transplantation.* 1988;45:930.

56. Gordon RD, Shunzaburo I, Tzakis AG, Esquivel CO, Todo S, Makowka L, Starzl TE. In Terasaki P, ed. *Clinical Transplant.* Los Angeles: UCLA Tissue Typing Laboratory; 1987:43–49.

57. Kamada N, Davies H, Wight D, Culank L, Roser B. *Transplantation* 1983;35:304.

CHAPTER 10

Tumor Immunology

Mark R. Albertini and Paul M. Sondel

The Departments of Human Oncology, Pediatrics, and Genetics, University of Wisconsin, 600 Highland Avenue, Madison, WI 53792 USA

Introduction

The immune system is a multifaceted organization that includes both cells and cellular products involved in the protection of the host from foreign substances (antigens). The immune response comprises the multiple actions of all components of this system. This response can be specific and aimed directly at the foreign antigen. Alternatively, this response may involve cells and cellular products that function in a nonspecific fashion to help protect the host. Neoplasia (Greek, *neos*, new, + *plasis*, a molding) refers to the formation of new tissue or a tumor in an organism. While numerous factors are likely involved in the causation of neoplasia, the development of a neoplasm (potentially a "foreign" tissue) in a previously tumor-free host presents a challenge to the immune system of the host. What allows a tissue that could be considered foreign to develop and escape the protective mechanisms of the host? Once a tumor begins to develop, what prevents the host from recognizing and ultimately controlling this tumor? Are there potential mechanisms that could be utilized to modify the host's immune response and change a previously ineffective response into one that is capable of destroying and ultimately controlling the tumor? This chapter provides a conceptual framework to approach these and other issues in tumor immunology. Basic immunology as directly relevant to immune mechanisms in tumor immunology are briefly reviewed. Immune factors in the etiology of cancer and the issue of immune deficiency and cancer are then discussed. Subsequent sections review the host response to tumor, tumor infiltrating lymphocytes, immunologic effects of cancer itself and of cancer therapy, and the evolution of current modalities for tumor immunotherapy. It concludes with a section that speculates on the future prospects and clinical utility of tumor immunotherapy, focusing on pharmacologic considerations.

Immune Mechanisms in Tumor Immunology
General Principles

The immune system consists of multiple components that may become integrated in the process of generating any one of a number of distinct immune responses.[1] Primary components include T lymphocytes, B lymphocytes, natural killer (NK) cells, macrophages, as well as the secretory products from each of these cells (lymphokines). These components of the immune response interact at several physiologic levels as they collaborate in mediating immune responses. Cellular function describes the cellular reactions mediated by each cell type. Surface phenotype describes the molecular "markers" on the cell surface that are involved in immune function and help identify each of these distinct cell types. The biochemical events that occur during an immune response allow one to predict which types of reactions may be effective in controlling any given foreign antigen. Finally, knowledge of gene rearrangements for antigen-binding molecules allows definition at a molecular level about an immune response and the means by which foreign antigen recognition occurs. Products of these genes are the T- and B-cell receptors, which provide a means to identify foreign antigens, as well as the antibody molecules made by B cells to neutralize foreign pathogens by binding to their foreign antigenic molecules.

T Lymphocytes

T Lymphocytes are primarily involved with the cell-mediated response to foreign antigens.[2] T Lymphocytes are a functionally diverse family and include T-cytotoxic cells, T-helper (T_H) cells, and T-suppressor (T_S) cells. The T-cytotoxic cells are able to lyse specific target cells, including tumor cells.[3] The immunoregulatory T cells (T_H cells, T_S cells) act as helpers or suppressors for interactions among multiple cell types, including T cells, B cells, macrophages, and other cells.[4] T lymphocytes primarily recognize antigens when displayed in the context of self [antigen + self-major histocompatibility complex antigen (HLA in humans)], and by this means are able to recognize "altered self." The immune response to transplanted tissues (allografts) provides a model for this type of reaction by studying strong immune responses directed against foreign (rather than altered self) major histocompatibility complex (MHC) antigens.[5]

Initial T-cell maturation occurs in the thymus and is independent of the presence of antigen. Mature T cells with their antigen receptors are required for an immune response. The T-cell receptor (TCR) structure is composed of an $\alpha-\beta$ chain heterodimer in association with the CD3 molecular complex (γ, δ, and ϵ monomorphic CD3 molecules).[6] The CD3 complex is not involved with antigen recognition but is important for the signalling of activation of T cells. The α and β chains of the TCR are involved with antigen recognition and contain both variable and constant regions. The variable region of the TCR α or β molecule is encoded by noncontiguous gene segments, which recombine in a number of different patterns (a unique pattern for each T-cell precursor) to allow for the tremendous diversity of antigen recognition in the T-cell response. Other T-cell receptors of emerging importance for antigen recognition include the γ chain and the δ chain.[7,8] Other associated molecules exist on the T-cell surface and are also important for functional activities of T cells. The CD4 molecule is a marker of cells with helper activity. These cells secrete a number of lymphoid hormones (lymphokines), such as interleukin-2 (IL-2), which act as a stimulus to other immune cells. The CD8 molecule is a marker of cells with suppressor-cytotoxic function. These CD8 molecules also function as adhesion molecules and facilitate effector to target approximation with subsequent target lysis. Another important adhesion molecule is CD2, which also functions as a putative receptor for activation signals.[9,10] The precise molecular mechanisms by which cytotoxic and immunoregulatory lymphocytes recognize spontaneously arising autologous tumors in humans remain to be adequately described.[11-13]

When T cells come in contact with the appropriate antigen, they become activated to undergo clonal expansion and proliferation. While resting T cells do not bear receptors for IL-2, activated T cells have induced the expression of IL-2 receptors.[14-16] These activated cells can undergo continued proliferation with additional stimulation via this IL-2 hormone receptor system. Thus, IL-2 receptor expression plays an important role in determining the specificity, magnitude, and duration of the T-cell immune response. Important in regulating this response are the activation state of the cell and the level of lymphokines.

This multifaceted activation process results in the generation of effector cells which mediate helper, suppressor, and cytotoxic T-cell function. A lymphocyte population distinct from antigen-specific, MHC-restricted T cells can respond directly to IL-2 and can mediate non-MHC-restricted cytotoxicity. This cell population, the lymphokine-activated killer (LAK) cell, is composed largely of activated natural killer cells (see below) and can preferentially lyse tumor cells to a greater degree than normal tissue.[17,18] Lymphokine-activated killer cells are currently receiving intense investigation for their potential efficacy in tumor immunotherapy (see below).

The in vivo role of T cells in the development of cancer or its treatment is still uncertain. Several modalities employing T cells, as well as strategies for producing appropriate T-cell activation, have been investigated as therapeutic options for cancer patients (see below).

B Lymphocytes

B Lymphocytes are cells of the immune system responsible for immunoglobulin synthesis and the humoral response to foreign antigens. B-cell differentiation occurs in both antigen-independent and antigen-dependent stages.[19] Additional levels of control exist for the production of immunoglobulin molecules, as three separate noncontiguous genes are involved in DNA rearrangement to produce a functional immunoglobulin molecule (variable-, diversity-, and joining-region genes).[20] The complete immunoglobulin molecule consists of two heavy chains and two light chains. The intact immunoglobulin molecule can be divided into two major components, one of which is involved with antigen recognition (variable region) and one of which controls the biologic functions of the molecule (constant region). In addition to immunoglobulin variable-region gene rearrangements, somatic cell mutation for diversity can also occur after gene rearrangement.[21]

There exist several classes and subclasses of immunoglobulin molecules which have varying importance depending on the nature and location of the foreign antigen. When B cells come in contact with antigens they can be induced to become either an antibody-secreting plasma cell or a "memory" cell. This entire process of B-cell activation is very lymphokine dependent, with particular importance for the following lymphokines: B-cell stimulating factor-1, interleukin-1, interferon-γ, and IL-2.[22]

One technique that has had both diagnostic and therapeutic implications for cancer patients is the use of monoclonal antibodies.[23] Monoclonal antibody production results after the fusion of an antibody-secreting plasma cell with a myeloma cell (a monoclonal immunoglobulin protein producing "factory"). The resultant "hybridoma" produces in great quantities a monoclonal population of pure immunoglobulin molecules, all of the same specificity. Intensive screening of different hybridomas has identified certain monoclonal antibodies of great specificity with potential for clinical application. Current and potential uses of monoclonal antibodies are discussed later in this chapter.

Natural Killer Cells

Natural killer cells (NK cells) are large granular lymphoid cells that constitute between 2% and 5% of the lymphocytes in the peripheral blood. These cells do not bear a typical T-cell receptor for antigen recognition but do have some T-cell-associated markers. Other surface antigens are often seen on cells with NK function (such as the Leu-11 and Leu-19 molecules) and help to define these cells. Natural killer cells are able to exhibit spontaneous cytotoxicity against certain cultured tumor target-cell lines without requiring intentional prior sensitization or activation.[24] Cytotoxicity is not specific for a particular target and target recognition is without MHC restriction. Development of NK cells is not dependent on the thymus. The means for NK-mediated recognition of tumor target (or virally infected target) cells is not entirely defined.[25,26] Controversy exists regarding the relative importance of a T-cell-like receptor, recognizing foreign antigen, or a lectin-like receptor that allows binding without immune recognition of a "foreign" antigen. Target reactivity can be augmented with many stimuli, including interferon and IL-2. Interleukin-2-activated NK cells are clearly able to demonstrate LAK activity, with cytotoxicity of otherwise NK-resistant targets.[17] Natural killer cells can also exhibit antibody-dependent cellular cytotoxicity (ADCC) as they bear surface receptors for the Fc portion of IgG. In this reaction, an NK cell can bind to, and destroy, an otherwise "NK-resistant" target if the target is coated with antibody molecules that themselves have an Fc end which is bound by the Fc receptor on NK cells.

Natural killer cells may represent a population of cells playing a tumor preventative role as postulated in the immune surveillance theory.[27] As NK cells can lyse certain tumor targets without prior activation or sensitization, they may constitute a true first-line defense against malignancy. The response of NK cells to established malignancy and their potential role for tumor immunotherapy are discussed later in this chapter.

Macrophages

Monocytes and macrophages are mononuclear phagocytes with multiple potential mechanisms for tumor cell destruction.[28] Phagocytosis of foreign particules was the initial immunologic role attributed to macrophages, and this remains accepted as a vital function for these cells. Macrophages are known to possess at least 40 surface membrane receptors and to produce and secrete over 70 molecules, so their potential diversity of function is tremendous.[29] Equally important is the diffuse distribution of monocytes and macrophages throughout the body.

Two separate mechanisms for macrophage-mediated tumor cell destruction have been described.[30] The first mechanism is antibody-dependent cellular cytotoxicity (ADCC), as seen for NK cells, and requires an initial coating of tumor cells with reactive antibodies prior to macrophage activation and subsequent cytotoxicity of the tumor cell. The second mechanism, antibody-independent tumor cytotoxicity or macrophage-mediated tumor cytotoxicity, involves an initial direct interaction between activated macrophages and tumor targets. For this process to occur, there must exist an initial stimulus causing attraction and proliferation of macrophages near the neoplasm. The macrophage must be able to recognize the tumor, possibly by means of a surface receptor. Macrophage function must then be modulated with subsequent activation of the macrophage, and this activated state must be maintained to allow for effective cell-mediated tumor cytotoxicity. The exact molecules allowing for tumor recognition and the relative importance of antigen-specific surface receptors and adhesion molecules is not known. Included in the 40 separate receptors that have been described (reviewed in reference 29) are several classes of Fc receptors, receptors for complement, receptors for glycoproteins, and potential tumor-cell binding sites. Macrophages must be activated to bind tumor cells efficiently as well as to allow for release of lytic effector substances. A serine protease has been established as one of the lytic molecules with potent tumor cytolytic capabilities. Over 70 additional molecules, including many proteases, tumor necrosis factor, and other cytolytic factors have been identified and may play a large role in macrophage-mediated tumor cytotoxicity.

In addition to direct macrophage-mediated lysis of tumor cells, macrophage-derived lymphokines, such as interleukin-1, are important in facilitating anti-tumor responses mediated by other immune effector cells. This role, as well as their additional functions as antigen-presenting cells and lymphokine-responsive cells, place the macrophages in a critical position in the host's response against neoplasia. Optimal utilization of the macrophage may facilitate the immunotherapy of human tumors.

Lymphokines

Lymphokines, or cytokines, are polypeptide products of activated immune effector cells. They are often recognized via specific receptors and so can be considered the hormones of the immune system. Lymphokines are produced diffusely throughout the body and modulate many aspects of various immune responses. Like antibody, some lymphokines are released by activated immune effector cells in response to antigen, but unlike antibody they function in the response to antigen in a manner that is not uniquely specific for a particular antigen. The effects of lymphokines can be regulatory in both an autocrine and paracrine fashion, and many B- and T-cell responses are dependent on a critical level of surrounding lymphokines. In addition to modulating effector function, lymphokines have regulatory effects on growth and proliferation of many immune cells.

Many seemingly different lymphokines were initially named according to the biologic functions they mediated; however, molecular approaches to these analyses have shown that many diverse biologic reactions can be mediated by the same lymphokine. More recent internationally agreed upon nomenclature has used the term "interleukin" followed by a given number to refer to these distinct molecules.[31] Several lymphokines with well-described biologic functions include the following: interleukins-1, -2, -3, -4, -5, and -6; colony-stimulating factors (CSF), including granulocyte–macrophage CSF, granulocyte CSF, and macrophage CSF; B-cell-stimulating factors; interferons (IFN) -α, -β, and -γ; tumor necrosis factors; as well as other cytokines (see reference 31 for a summary of several biologic properties). In addition to some unique biologic functions, some lymphokines can have multiple functions depending on the receptors expressed by the lymphokine-responsive cells (ie, IL-1, IFN-γ, IL-2). Several lymphokines can also function via different receptors to induce a similar biologic function (ie, IL-2 and IL-4). The interaction of lymphokines on the immune network is critical in determining the final biologic response.

Several lymphokines have been utilized in attempts to modulate the host's immune response to malignancy. The current role for several biologic response modifiers, as well as some exciting potential applications, are described later in this chapter. Potential use of these molecules as pharmacological antitumor therapy requires further understanding of their anatomic and cellular sites of production and action, their catabolism and clearances, and the kinetics of their direct interactions with the desired target tissues.

Immune Factors in the Etiology of Cancer

Overview

The relative importance of immune factors in the genesis of spontaneous malignancies in humans remains controversial. Potential mechanisms can be described for either inadequate surveillance against neoplasia or for an overaggressive immune system resulting in cancer as an autoimmune disease. Current data supporting both theories are discussed after a brief review of the immune surveillance theory.

The Immune Surveillance Theory

The distinction of "self" from "nonself" and the protection of "self" from foreign antigens remains an accepted role for the immune system. The ability of the immune system to differentiate "self" from a spontaneous autologous neoplasm remains less clear. The concept of immune surveillance implies the existence of a population of cells with anti-tumor reactivity able to result in tumor cell destruction. Several cell types have been given this role. As described above, natural killer (NK) cells can exhibit some antitumor reactivity without prior in vitro sensitization. Macrophages are also able to mediate some tumor recognition and cytotoxicity without prior exposure to the tumor target. The T cells may recognize tumor-associated cell-surface antigens and allow for development of protective immunity in the host. The relative in vivo importance for these means of cytotoxicity remain controversial. Also unexplained are reasons for spontaneous tumor growth, which may reflect a failure of immune surveillance. Potential reasons include an initial failure to recognize the tumor, antigenic modulation by the tumor, and the induction of suppressor cells or suppressor factors that deter subsequent immunological responses to the tumor.

Several murine models have been utilized to investigate the relative in vivo importance of immune surveillance (reviewed in reference 27). Murine models utilizing skin carcinogenesis with chemically induced tumors have failed to demonstrate an increased tumor incidence in immunosuppressed animals. Chronic immunosuppression also does not lead to an increased spontaneous tumor incidence in murine models. Some modifications of traditional definitions for immune surveillance appear needed.

Immune Deficiency and Cancer

Immunodeficiency syndromes can either be inherited or acquired and include disorders involving humoral as well as cellular immunity.[32] The primary immunodeficiencies are rare but are clearly associated with certain types of malignancy.[33] B-Cell malignant lymphomas are the most commonly associated malignancies for children with primary immune deficiency.[34] Malignancies seen in patients with the acquired immune deficiency syndrome (AIDS) and renal transplant patients also include B-cell malignant lymphomas, cutaneous squamous cell cancers, Kaposi's sarcoma, and uterine cervical carcinoma.[34,35] Of note is the postulated role for certain viral infections in the etiology of each of these cancers (Kaposi's with cytomegalovirus; malignant B-cell lymphoma with Epstein Barr (EB) virus; squamous cell carcinoma with papilloma virus; uterine cervical carcinoma with herpes simplex virus).[34] The theory that immune surveillance is primarily involved with the immune response to virally induced malignancies has been made and may explain the restricted appearance of these particular malignancies in immune-deficient patients.

Patients receiving cytotoxic chemotherapy exhibit a spectrum of secondary malignancies different from those already listed. These patients have a much higher incidence of secondary leukemias.

Cancer as an Autoimmune Disease

The relationship between the immune system and oncogenesis remains poorly understood. One theory, in direct contrast to the immune surveillance theory, ascribes an autoimmune etiology to several malignancies.[36] Of interest is the association of malignancy with several diseases that have a postulated autoimmune etiology. Such diseases include dermatomyositis, pernicious anemia, and autoimmune thyroiditis.[36,37] Also, the cellular lymphoid aggregates in some rheumatologic conditions have a tumor-like quality. While both specific and nonspecific immune responses may be protective for the host, an uncontrolled immune proliferation may clearly be detrimental. The interface between host and tumor needs additional investigation, as the induced immune network may vary depending on tumor type and host immune status. An improved understanding of this relationship should greatly increase the efficacy of various therapies employing immunomodulation as a therapeutic modality.

Host Responses to Tumor

Overview

The molecular mechanisms by which cytotoxic and immunoregulatory lymphocytes recognize spontaneous autologous tumors in humans remain unclear.[3,11−13] Specific recognition of tumor-associated antigens may be via the classical T-cell receptor complex (disulfide-linked $\alpha-\beta$ heterodimer)[2,38−40] or by the recently described $\gamma-\delta$ receptor.[7,8] Alternatively, antigen specificity may be provided by the B-cell response with subsequent cellular destruction using antibody-dependent cellular cytotoxicity by cells with Fc receptors.[41] Nonspecifically activated T cells may be primarily responsible for the in vivo response to tumors.[42,43] Some animals with experimentally induced tumors have been clearly demonstrated to possess T cells with increased reactivity to tumor-associated antigens.[44] These experimentally induced tumors provide a model system in which the interaction between host immune system and neoplasm can be examined. Similar immunogenic tumor-specific antigens have yet to be adequately defined for most human neoplasms. Many human tumors are known to be infiltrated by T cells, suggesting a T-lymphocyte response.[45] Analysis to date has primarily focused on phenotypic and functional characterization of lymphocyte preparations from these tumor infiltrating lymphocytes.

Animal Models

Highly immunogenic tumors induced in mice have provided an excellent model system to examine the cellular immune response to experimental neoplasms.[46]

These tumors can be induced with various chemicals (ie, methylcholanthrene), oncogenic viruses, and physical agents, such as ultraviolet radiation. Subsequently, various immunization protocols with these tumor cells can then allow induction of lymphocyte subpopulations with increased tumor reactivity. These "immune" lymphocytes can mediate antitumor effects when injected into syngeneic animals. A large number of lymphocytes are often needed to mediate a notable antitumor effect. Elimination of host suppressor factors by providing immunosuppression to the host prior to the transfer of immune cells (such as irradiation or cyclophosphamide therapy) can allow for a greater antitumor effect by the transfused cells.

Cellular immunity induced by immunization with one experimental tumor is not necessarily protective against a different tumor, even if the second tumor is induced by the same agent in a syngeneic animal. The observed cellular response to these immunogenic syngeneic tumors is remarkably similar to the allograft response seen in response to genetically foreign transplanted tissue. Humoral responses are not as important against these cellular antigens.

These experimental tumors are highly mutagenized, and their relevance to spontaneous autologous tumors in humans remains questionable. Most of the spontaneous tumors in humans are minimally antigenic and may not be able to elicit a similar type of immune response. The final immune response may depend on the degree of mutation from normal cells that the neoplasm exhibits.

Tumor-Infiltrating Lymphocytes

The potential importance of tumor-infiltrating lymphocytes (TIL) was first reported in malignant melanoma in 1907 and was subsequently described in many other cancers.[47] The majority of lymphocytes composing the tumor-infiltrating lymphocytes are T cells and some of them are in an activated state.[45] A large population also exists of cells that are small, not activated, and without significant reactivity or cytotoxicity against autologous tumor cells.[48] While many studies have provided useful descriptive data about the cells infiltrating human tumors, most have failed to reveal a lymphocyte subpopulation with increased tumor-specific reactivity.

Tumor-infiltrating lymphocytes cells can be obtained from solid neoplasms by various methods. Most procedures involve a fine mincing of the sample for mechanical disaggregation and a subsequent enzymatic digestion of the sample (as with collagenase, hyaluronidase, and DNAse). Another method involves a thorough mechanical disaggregation of the tumor with a subsequent brief incubation in vitro. The resultant suspension is filtered, allowing separation and characterization of the TIL cells.

Quantitation of precursor cells directed against human tumors has been examined with limiting dilution analysis.[49] The reported phenotype for TIL has been somewhat variable, with some studies reporting a composition similar to peripheral blood lymphocytes and others reporting the majority of TIL to be cytotoxic T-lymphocytes. While TIL have been reported to have the ability to recognize and kill autologous tumor cells,[50] several investigations have failed to demonstrate significant cytotox-icity against autologous tumor cells.[51] Tumor-infiltrating lymphocyte populations show low responsiveness to mitogens.[52] The biological mechanisms accounting for these observations have not been well defined, but the presence of a local suppressive mechanism is possible.

Tumor-infiltrating lymphocytes may represent an attempt by the tumor-bearing host to develop an immunologic attack against a tumor. The infiltrating lympho-cytes appear to represent a heterogeneous population of diverse effector and immu-noregulatory lymphocytes and monocytes. A potential problem with some existing studies about TIL is the presumption of a specific function (ie, tumor-specific cytotoxicity) for this cell population without proof that they mediate such a func-tion. Tumor-reactive lymphocytes, if present, may mediate diverse functions rang-ing from cytotoxicity, helper activity, suppressor activity, or a potential network of effects. Effective dissection of these functions will be facilitated by revealing whether a subpopulation of cells is present in clonally amplified proportions at the tumor site. These studies have been initiated in our and other laboratories. The means by which these cells recognize tumor and the functions they subsequently perform can then be more effectively investigated. Further study of these cells may also offer a means to identify tumor-associated antigens. In vitro expansion and activation of TIL, or of a subpopulation of TIL, may form the basis for subsequent immunotherapeutic trials.

Tumor Markers

Serologically detectable molecules can be identified in some patients with cancer. Two of the better characterized molecules are called oncofetal antigens as they are normally expressed during embryonic development with usual disappearance during postembryonic life.[53]

Carcinoembryonic antigen (CEA) is a glycoprotein that can be detected in the serum of many patients with colon cancer. It can also occasionally be identified in other malignant diseases (pancreatic carcinoma, gastric carcinoma, lung carcinoma, breast carcinoma, prostatic carcinoma, bladder carcinoma, endometrial carcinoma, cervical carcinoma, and ovarian carcinoma) and in certain nonmalignant diseases (emphysema, pancreatitis, alcoholism).[53] α-Fetoprotein (AFP) is another glycopro-tein that is frequently elevated in the serum of patients with several types of germ cell tumors. It can also be elevated in hepatoma and endodermal sinus tumor of the ovary as well as infrequently in other malignant conditions (pancreatic carcinoma, lung carcinoma) and nonmalignant conditions (such as hepatitis and pregnancy).[53] Serial tumor markers may be useful to follow in a patient who has a tumor that expresses the given marker. Other important markers include prostate specific anti-gen (prostatic carcinoma), acid phosphatase (prostatic carcinoma) and β-human chorionic gonadotropin (germ cell tumors). Further investigation may reveal addi-tional markers that are either frequently elevated in patients with a variety of malignancies or are strongly associated with a particular malignancy.

Immunological Effects of Cancer and Cancer Therapy

Pharmacological Considerations

The interrelationship between immunosuppression and the pharmacological management of the cancer patient is a critical and recurrent problem. Well described in many pharmacology texts are the immunosuppressive effects of many forms of chemotherapy. Also well described are the immunosuppressive effects that can accompany major surgery and radiation therapy. Whether the immunosuppressed status of many cancer patients is entirely attributable to the above-mentioned problems, or whether there exists a direct immunosuppressive effect of cancer itself, is an important consideration for cancer patient management. Significant concerns in the management of the cancer patient include the infectious complications that can accompany prolonged immunosuppression. Another consideration is the selection of agents that do not unnecessarily worsen or prolong the patients immunosuppressed status.

There is a current need for the design of treatments that could either lessen the effects of prolonged immunosuppression or that could ''rescue'' the patient from cancer-associated and treatment-related immunosuppression.

Direct Immune Effects of Cancer

Nonspecific measures of immune competence at diagnosis of cancer show a crude relationship to a patient's overall prognosis. Methods utilized for analysis include total peripheral blood lymphocyte count, lymphocyte subpopulation composition, lymphocyte function as assessed by proliferative responses to several mitogens, and serum immunoglobulin levels.[54] Results from these studies generally have a poor correlation with prognosis for the cancer patient.

Local immunosuppression may be induced by the tumor itself and cause decreases in the function of monocytes or lymphocytes in the tumor and surrounding tissues.[4] Postulated mechanisms include the induction of suppressor cells or factors that deter a cytotoxic response against the tumor. Data for local tumor immunosuppression remain inconclusive and in need of additional investigation.

An additional means for tumor immunosuppression would be for widely metastatic cancer to cause bone marrow replacement. The resultant stem cell decrease could be sufficient to result in various degrees of cytopenias with subsequent immunosuppression.

Immunological Effects of Cancer Therapy

Central to the design of effective chemotherapeutic regimens is the selection of agents that not only attack the cancer by different mechanisms but have nonoverlapping toxicities. One potential dose-limiting toxicity is immunosuppression, which can be clinically evaluated by monitoring of various hematological or immunological parameters. Whereas dose reduction to avoid toxicity is sometimes necessary, this may reduce the desired antitumor effects. For several diseases, dose of effective drug delivered can be correlated with response rate to the treatment. The degree of immunosuppression by these treatments may also limit the choice of potentially therapeutic agents.

Several methods to restore immunocompetence in the treated cancer patient are currently being evaluated. Autologous bone marrow transplantation for "rescue" allows for very high doses of immunosuppressive chemotherapy to be given.[55,56] Autologous bone marrow is harvested prior to the administration of marrow toxic chemotherapy. Very high doses of chemotherapy can then be administered, even if total bone marrow ablation occurs as a consequence, in an attempt to eradicate the tumor. The patient can then be given back his own bone marrow to allow reconstitution of his hematopoietic and immune systems. While this treatment regimen is quite demanding, it may effectively allow treatment of patients with selected tumors in which high dose chemotherapy may be curative.

Various colony-stimulating factors are also being evaluated for their ability to improve hematopoiesis in selected patients.[57] Their ultimate role in the management of the cancer patient remains to be defined.

Tumor Immunotherapy

Background

The prospect of intentionally directing cellular or humoral immune responses toward the destruction of human cancer remains an attractive potential clinical modality for therapy. Prior attempts at immunotherapy have met with limited success. Recent progress characterizing the cellular (and possibly molecular) mechanisms by which cytotoxic and immunoregulatory lymphocytes may recognize tumor cells and communicate with one another have enabled newer approaches for the testing of tumor immunotherapy.

There exist several broad categories for tumor immunotherapy.[42] Specific immunotherapy refers to treatment that is directed specifically at the tumor, while nonspecific immunotherapy involves a general stimulation of the immune system with an anticipated increase in antitumor effect. Immunotherapy may also be active or passive. Active immunotherapy involves the immunization of the tumor-bearing host with antigens designed to elicit an endogenous immune response with antitumor effects. Passive immunotherapy refers to the administration of previously sensitized immunologic cells or antibodies to the tumor-bearing host; these immunologic reagents can then mediate a response against the tumor. This section reviews some the many approaches that have been used for the immunotherapy of human cancers.

Nonspecific and Specific Active Immunotherapy

Initial attempts at immunotherapy were largely unsuccessful and primarily involved the nonspecific active stimulation of the host immune system, as with Bacille Calmette-Guérin (BCG) and *Corynebacterium parvum*.[46] Bacille Calmette-Guérin was initially developed as a vaccine against tuberculosis by progressive attenuation of the bovine tubercle bacillus. *Corynebacterium parvum* is a gram-positive microorganism that is used occasionally as an adjuvant with several vaccines. These agents function as vaccines generally to stimulate the activity of the immune system, but this form of general immune activation has not translated into a consistent antitumor response. Bacille calmette-Guérin has also been used for intralesional injection into melanoma lesions. Unfortunately, neither development of systemic immunity nor response of visceral disease has occurred reproducibly with these treatments.[59] A defined role for intralesional injections with localized tumor involvement is currently being investigated in melanoma and other cancers. Localized BCG therapy in localized superficial bladder cancer appears to be effective.[60]

Levamisole, a pharmacologic agent that was originally utilized as an antihelminthic drug, is also known for its immunomodulatory effects and ability to restore cell-mediated immune responses in immunocompromised hosts.[61] Levamisole has been studied for its immunomodulatory effects with several cancers, but there exist conflicting reports as to its efficacy.[62] Factors including dosage of drug and duration of therapy may account for some of the observed variability. Further investigation is needed to determine what role, if any, this form of nonspecific immune stimulation will play in the immunotherapy of human cancer.

Specific active stimulation of the host's immune system has also been attempted with limited success.[1,63] Primary methods have employed both autologous and allogeneic irradiated tumor cells, and various preparations derived from them, as vaccines. Some patients so immunized generate an "antigen-specific" antibody or delayed hypersensitivity response, but this does not necessarily allow for a subsequent clinical antitumor response. To be an effective means of therapy, a "tumor vaccine" must be antigenic as well as induce a reproducible antitumor response. Further investigation is underway to determine whether promising leads with this approach will enable it to become a useful form of immunotherapy.

Interferons

Interferons (IFN) are glycoproteins of cellular origin that have been utilized as biologic response modifiers to mediate antitumor effects. Interferon was characterized in 1957 and was initially described for its antiviral properties, as a virally infected cell will release IFN to help develop a resistant state against infection with a second virus. The interferons were subsequently characterized and found to comprise a whole family of glycoproteins. Initial research production of IFN occurred in cell cultures, but recombinant DNA technology later allowed for production of even larger quantities of purified IFN after the successful cloning of each of the IFN subtypes. There are three major types of IFN, as well as additional subcategories that have been described. Interferon-α is produced by leukocytes; interferon-β is produced by fibroblasts, epithelial cells, macrophages, and lymphoblastoid cells; interferon-γ is primarily produced by T lymphocytes.[58]

Interferons have several in vitro effects that may account for their in vivo action with tumor cells. Viral replication as well as cell transformation by several on-cogenic viruses can be inhibited by interferons.[64] Interferons have antiproliferative effects and can cause a prolongation of all phases of the cell cycle.[65] These anti-proliferative effects result in decreased multiplication of both normal and trans-formed cells. In addition to the direct effects of interferons against tumor cells, interferons have immunomodulatory effects that can result in increased in vitro cytotoxicity mediated by specifically sensitized lymphocytes and by natural killer cells as well as increased antibody-dependent cellular cytotoxicity.[64] Interferons can cause an increase in HLA antigen expression as well as increased expression of tumor-associated antigens by target cells.[65] This effect could potentially increase a tumor's antigenicity and thus render it more susceptible to destruction by immune mechanisms. Important considerations for all of these effects include the dose of interferon to which the tumor cells and lymphocyte effector cells are exposed. Several animal models have also been utilized to demonstrate the importance of drug dosage and schedule for interferon's antitumor effects.

Initial clinical trials were begun in the 1970s and utilized crude α-interferon as prepared by Cantell in Finland.[66] Some initial antitumor responses in patients with advanced breast carcinoma, multiple myeloma, and malignant lymphoma with this partially purified α-interferon lead to much initial optimism for the ultimate role for the interferons as antitumor agents. The subsequent availability of large amounts of both natural and recombinant interferons permitted evaluation of pharmacokinetics and biological effects of interferons in several malignancies.[67] Important considera-tions include the type and subtype of interferon utilized, the preparation of inter-feron (natural vs. recombinant), as well as a possible combination of several types of interferons. As clinical trials to date have involved many types of cancer, these malignancies can be grouped according to their sensitivity to therapy with interferon (see reference 65 for a review of this classification). The most responsive diseases include hairy cell leukemia and some lymphomas, while smaller but measurable responses are seen in melanoma, Kaposi's sarcoma, renal cell carcinoma, and myeloma. Toxicity has been primarily reversible and dose dependent and has in-cluded fatigue, anorexia, weight loss, myelosuppression, mild hepatic toxicity, fever, chills, myalgias, headache, confusion, and gastrointestinal disturbances.

Interferon therapy appears to have fairly defined indications as a single agent for malignant diseases. Many potential applications that utilize interferon's anti-proliferative and immunomodulatory properties as well as its ability to increase tumor antigen expression offer therapeutic promise.

Monoclonal Antibodies

The technology to allow fusion of specific antibody-producing B lymphocytes with selected murine myeloma cells was described by Kohler and Milstein in 1975.[68] Such hybrid cells (hybridomas) can be maintained in culture indefinitely and can produce vast quantities of antibody with defined specificities. Monoclonal anti-bodies can be developed against tumor associated antigens, with more than 100 monoclonal antibodies against human carcinomas currently described.[69] Potential applications, both diagnostically and therapeutically, are tremendous as these monoclonal antibodies provide a means to target the tumor cells selectively. Several considerations are essential when considering applications of these "magic bullets" (see reference 69 for review). While the combining portion of the monoclonal antibody is highly specific, the antigen to which it combines may be present on several different types of neoplasms, may not always be expressed on all tumors of a given histological type, may not be expressed on all cells in a single tumor, and may either be variably expressed or have expression change with time. An additional consideration is the degree of cross-reactivity of these antibodies with normal tissue.

Potential applications of this hybridoma technology for tumor diagnosis and monitoring are numerous and have been discussed elsewhere.[69-71] Therapeutic applications can include both direct antitumor effects of the monoclonal antibodies as well as additional interactions of the antibodies with the immune system. Monoclonal antibodies can also be combined with other tumoricidal agents ("immunoconjugates"). After appropriate in vitro and animal studies, the initial monoclonal antibodies utilized in clinical trials were unconjugated antibodies.[72] The unconjugated antibodies had little direct antitumor effects, but several potential problems with monoclonal antibody therapy were identified (see above and reference 72). Tumors can develop antigenic modulation or can release free antigen into the circulation. The patient can also develop anti-mouse antibodies, which render the administered monoclonal antibodies ineffective. Finally, the inherent lack of significant in vivo cytotoxicity of monoclonal antibodies alone suggested that a combination modality of treatment may be more effective than therapy with monoclonal antibodies alone.

"Immunoconjugates" involving monoclonal antibodies linked to drugs, toxins, or radionuclides are currently being investigated. The theoretical basis for this form of therapy is to allow the monoclonal antibody to provide tumor specificity and thus allow a nonspecific tumoricidal agent to preferentially lyse tumor cells. Many initial questions involving pharmacokinetics, drug dosage, and radiation dosimetry as well as techniques for optimal immunoconjugation are currently being evaluated.

Interleukin-2 and Cellular Immunotherapy

As the cellular immune response is largely responsible for mediating the rejection of allografts and syngeneic immunogenic murine tumors, intense investigation has focused on means of utilizing specifically activated immune cells for the treatment of patients with cancer.[73] Adoptive immunotherapy is the administration of cells with the appropriate inactivity to a tumor-bearing host. Some encouraging results were described in animal models.[46] Highly immunogenic tumors could be utilized to elicit an immune response, with subsequent transfer of these "immune" lymphocytes to syngeneic animals. These adoptively transferred lymphocytes would then mediate an antitumor effect in the tumor-bearing animal. The donor animal would frequently need to be highly immunized, as a large number of cells were needed for a meaningful antitumor response. Several difficulties prevented useful clinical application of this technology. First, it was virtually impossible to document tumor-specific immune cells (even in small quantities) for patients with cancer. Second, in vitro methodology did not allow for the generation of an adequate number of immune cells to effect a clinically meaningful response based on extrapolations from murine models. Clinical trials involving adoptive transfer of haploidentical lymphocytes after in vitro activation with allogeneic antigens did document limited antitumor effects,[74] but larger clinical applications were not feasible.

The description of IL-2 in 1976 and later characterization of lymphokine-activated killer cells (LAK) in 1980 allowed for development of a new form of adoptive immunotherapy.[42] Interleukin-2, originally called T-cell growth factor, is a glycoprotein of 15,000-d molecular weight and is produced by the helper subclass of T lymphocytes after stimulation by mitogens or specific antigenic stimuli. The cloning of the gene for IL-2 in 1983 allowed for subsequent production of large quantities of purified recombinant IL-2.[75]

Lymphokine-activated killer cells result from the incubation of normal lymphocytes in IL-2 and are characterized by their ability to lyse fresh, noncultured, natural killer cell-resistant primary and metastatic tumor cells. Controversy exists regarding the precise nature of the effector cells responsible for the LAK phenomenon,[17,76] but the predominant precursors are felt to be natural killer cells that acquire "LAK activity" after exposure to IL-2. Lymphokine-activated killer cells thus comprise a population of lymphocytes that exhibit a particular activity, rather than a population of cells defined by a given phenotypic marker. The cellular cytotoxicity by LAK cells is mediated without major histocompatibility complex restriction.[77]

Numerous preliminary animal experiments demonstrated a striking antitumor effect for high dose IL-2 or IL-2 therapy combined with LAK cells.[42,78,79] The tumors treated were largely chemically induced or highly mutagenized tumors. Initial human studies involved low doses of IL-2, with subsequently higher doses of recombinant IL-2 administered in later trials. The addition of LAK cells to IL-2 therapy generated tremendous excitement, as antitumor responses generated entirely by immunologic therapy were seen in patients with advanced malignancies.[79,80] The LAK cells were also shown to have a spectrum of activity, with preferential killing of tumor cells but with additional lysis of some normal autologous tissue.[81] The toxicity of high-dose IL-2 and LAK cells is considerable; high fevers, malaise, weight gain, hypotension, pulmonary edema, and renal and hepatic toxicity are observed. Our laboratory and others have been extensively investigating potential means of administration of IL-2 and LAK cells to obtain therapeutic efficacy in a clinically tolerable fashion.[82] While striking immunological changes as well as antitumor effects have been observed with such approaches, clinical responses published to date with all IL-2 regimens remain much less than desired. Additional manipulation of the administration and dosage schedule for IL-2 and LAK cells may allow even greater efficacy. Combination therapy with other forms of immunotherapy offers many theoretical advantages (see below).

Tumor Necrosis Factor and Other Biological Response Modifiers

The utilization of products of the immune system to manipulate immunological responses to tumor cells offers great potential as an additional modality for cancer therapy. Several of the more extensively investigated products have already been discussed. Additional lymphokines, such as tumor necrosis factor (TNF), are likewise being evaluated. Originally called "cachectin," TNF is a polypeptide hormone primarily produced by macrophages.[83] It is known for its ability to produce in vivo hemorrhagic necrosis of several tumors as well as inducing in vitro cytotoxicity against several tumor cell lines. Tumor necrosis factor will normally function in vivo to mediate the lethal activity of endotoxin.[83] The gene for TNF has been cloned to allow large production of recombinant TNF.[84] Clinical trials to date have evaluated TNF as a single agent for several malignancies as well as combinations of TNF with other therapeutic agents.[85,86] While some antitumor effects have been realized, the final role for tumor necrosis factor in the immunotherapy of cancer remains to be defined.

Many immunomodulatory agents are currently being evaluated for antitumor effects. These agents are a heterogeneous group and range from pharmaceutical products to cytokines. Additional research in new drug development as well as elucidating mechanism of action for agents now being evaluated may allow for the successful immunotherapy of cancer. Combination approaches may be needed for optimal therapeutic results.

Future Prospects for Immunotherapy

As we have outlined in this chapter, antitumor effects can be realized by entirely immunological approaches. These antitumor effects have largely been shown in patients with very advanced disease and for whom other potentially effective modalities of therapy were either not available or had failed. The challenge for the tumor immunologist is to translate these "antitumor effects" into potential "cures" for patients with cancer. Several potential approaches may be effective. One approach is to continue refinement of existing biological response modifier therapy by adjusting treatment schedules, doses, and routes of therapy. These therapies could then be evaluated in patients with less advanced disease and in whom immunological intervention may be anticipated to produce a larger response. Use of this immunotherapy in an adjuvant setting could also be evaluated.

The above approach needs to be evaluated, but for a large number of cancer patients it may not be sufficient. Great enthusiasm currently exists for combining forms of immunotherapy with other "standard" therapies. Immunotherapy, if combined in an appropriate fashion with surgery, chemotherapy, or radiation therapy, may allow different antitumor approaches to produce a more effective antitumor response. Different forms of biological response modifier therapy could also be combined and have much theoretical appeal. γ-Interferon could be initially utilized to increase tumor antigen expression, with subsequent therapy with IL-2 (and possibly LAK cell) treatment. Interleukin-2-induced LAK cell activity (induced in vivo or in vitro) could also be combined with monoclonal antibodies, which facilitate antibody-dependent cellular cytotoxicity and potentially greater antitumor effects. The use of monoclonal antibodies as a vehicle to deliver "agents" (radionuclides, chemotherapy, or other toxins) to the tumor has tremendous potential applications. Additional immune mechanisms may then be manipulated to facilitate tumor destruction.

Different effector populations may be utilized in an attempt to increase the specificity of cellular immunotherapy. Clinical trials involving adoptive immunotherapy with tumor-infiltrating lymphocytes are currently in progress.[87] One potential problem with this approach is the heterogeneous nature of cells identified in tumor-infiltrating lymphocytes. If one could identify a cell subpopulation with increased tumor reactivity, that subpopulation could be selectively expanded and utilized for adoptive immunotherapy. This cell population, if present, could also be utilized to help develop monoclonal antibodies that could selectively "target" the tumor and be combined with other forms of therapy.

As can be seen, there are numerous approaches utilizing immune mechanisms that could potentially improve the treatment of many human cancers. Pharmacological considerations including pharmacokinetics, techniques to optimally combine biological reagents, and new product development are of tremendous importance for the success of these approaches of therapy. It is hoped that current investigations will allow the translation of "theoretical appeal" to "clinical efficacy" for the treatment of a significant number of patients with cancer.

Acknowledgments

The authors thank Drs. J. Hank, J. Sosman, P.C. Kohler, G. Hillman, P. Fisch, E.C. Borden, R. Smalley, J. Schiller, and R. Mandell and V. Lam for stimulating discussions, and B. Rayho for preparation of this chapter. This work was supported by NIH grants CA-08397, CA-32685, RR-03186, and American Cancer Society Grant CH-237.

References

1. Sondel PM. The immunology of cancer. In, Kahn B, Love R, Sherman C, Chakravorty R, eds. *Concepts in Cancer Medicine.* 1982:187–200.

2. Royer D, Reinherz E. *New Engl J Med.* 1987;317(18):1136–1142.

3. Lanier L, Phillips J. *Immunol Today.* 1986;7(5):132–134.

4. Roenn JV, et al. *J Clin Oncol.* 1987;5(1):150–159.

5. Bach F, Sachs D. *New Engl J Med.* 1987;317(8):489–492.

6. Flier J, Underhill L. *New Engl J Med.* 1985;312(17):1100–1111.

7. Pardoll D, et al. *Faseb J.* 1987;1:103–109.

8. Reinherz E. *Nature (London).* 1987;325:660–663.

9. Dustin M, et al. *J Exp Med.* 1987;165:677–692.

10. Meuer S, et al. *Cell.* 1984;36:897–906.

11. Hamaoka T, Fujiwara H. *Immunol Today.* 1987;8(9):267–269.

12. Anichini A, et al. *Immunol Today*. 1987;8:385–389.

13. Hersey P, Bolhuis R. *Immunol Today*. 1987;8(7 and 8):233–239.

14. Greene W. *Clin Res*. 1987;439–450.

15. Farrar WL, et al. *Immunol Rev*. 1986;92:49–65.

16. Greene W, et al. *Immunol Rev*. 1986;92:29–48.

17. Phillips J, Lanier L. *J Exp Med*. 1986;164:814–825.

18. Ortaldo JR, et al. *J Exp Med*. 1986;164:1193–1205.

19. Alt F, et al. *Science*. 1987;238:1079–1087.

20. Honjo T. *Annu Rev Immunol*. 1983;1:499–528.

21. Tonegawa S. *Nature (London)*. 1983;302:575–581.

22. Dubois P. *J Immunol*. 1987;139(6):1927–1934.

23. Bernstein I, et al. Monoclonal antibodies: Prospects for cancer treatment. In Mihich E, ed. *Immunological Approaches to Cancer Therapeutics,* 1982:277–297.

24. Henkart P. Mechanism of NK-cell mediated cytotoxicity. In Herberman RB, ed. *Cancer Immunology: Innovative Approaches to Therapy*. 1986:123–150.

25. Schmidt R, et al. *J Clin Invest*. 1987;79:305–308.

26. Gorelik E, Herberman R. Role of natural killer (NK) cells in the control of tumor growth and metastatic spread. In Herberman RB, ed. *Cancer Immunology: Innovative Approaches to Therapy*. 1986:151–176.

27. Stutman O. The immunological surveillance hypothesis. In Herberman RB, ed. *Basic and Clinical Tumor Immunology*. 1983:1–81.

28. Nathan CF, Cohn ZA. Cellular components of inflammation: Monocytes and macrophages. In Kelly E, et al. eds. *Textbook Rheumatology*. 1985:144–169.

29. Somers S, et al. Destruction of tumor cells by macrophages: Mechanisms of recognition and lysis and their regulation. In Herberman RB, ed. *Cancer Immunology: Innovative Approaches to Therapy*. 1986:69–122.

30. Meltzer M, et al. *Fed Proc*. 1982;41(6):2198–2205.

31. Dinarello C, Mier J. *New Engl J Med*. 1987;317(15):940–945.

32. Buckley RH. *JAMA*. 1987;258(20):3841–2850.

33. Cunningham-Rundles C, et al. *J Clin Immunol*. 1987;7(4):294–299.

34. Purtillo D. Immune deficiency, Epstein-Barr virus (EBV) and lymphoproliferative disorders. In Purtillo D, ed. *Immune Deficiency and Cancer*. 1982:vii–ix, 1–10.

35. Levine A. *Seminars Oncol*. 1987;14(2, suppl. 3):34–39.

36. Prehn R, Prehn L. *Cancer Res*. 1987;47(4):927–932.

37. Holm L, et al. *New Engl J Med*. 1985;312(10):601–604.

38. Marrack P, Kappler J. *Science*. 1987;238:1073–1078.

39. Poljak R. *Ann Inst Pasteur/Immunol*. 1987;138:175–180.

40. Marrack P, Kappler J. *Adv Immunol*. 1986;38:1–30.

41. Lamon E. *Transplantation*. 1980;29(1):1–3.

42. Rosenberg S, Lotze M. *Annu Rev Immunol*. 1986;4:681–709.

43. Grimm E, Rosenberg S, et al. *J Exp Med*. 1982;155:1823–1841.

44. Cheever M, et al. Antigen-specific T-cells can mediate tumor therapy and provide long-term immunologic memory in vivo. In *Cellular Immunotherapy of Cancer*. Alan R. Liss Inc; 1987:49–58.

45. Galili U, et al. *Cancer Immunol Immunother.* 1979;6:129–133.

46. Rosenberg S. *Cancer Treat Rep.* 1984;68(1):233–255.

47. Miwa H. *Acta Med Ikayama.* 1984;38(3):215–218.

48. Fliedner V, et al. Colongenic and functional potential of T-lymphocytes infiltrating human solid tumors. In *Cellular Immunotherapy of Cancer.* Alan R. Liss Inc; 1987:223–232.

49. Vose B. *Int J Cancer.* 1982;30:135–142.

50. Itoh K, Balch, C, et al. *Cancer Res.* 1986;46:3011–3017.

51. Vose B, Meure M. *Int J Cancer.* 1979;24:579–585.

52. Vose B, Moore M. *Seminars Hematol.* 1985;22(1):27–40.

53. Kagan J, Fahey J. *JAMA.* 1987;298(20):2988–2992.

54. Nordman E, et al. *Cancer Immunol Immunother.* 1985;20:38–42.

55. Autologous bone-marrow transplantation. *Lancet.* 1987;1(8528):303–304.

56. Humblet, et al. *J Clin Oncol.* 1987;5(12):1864–1873.

57. Cadhan-Raj S, et al. *New Engl J Med.* 1987;317(25):1545–1552.

58. Siegel B. *Int Rev Cytol.* 1985;96:89–120.

59. Smalley R, et al. Biologic response modifiers: Current status and prospects as anti-cancer agents. In Herberman R, ed. *Basic and Clinical Tumor Immunology.* 1983:257–300.

60. Guinan P, et al. *Urology.* 1987;30(6):515–519.

61. Renoux G. *Drugs.* 1980;19:89–99.

62. Klefstrom P. *Cancer.* 1987;60:936–942.

63. Livingston P, et al. Specific active immunotherapy in cancer treatment. In Mihich E, ed. *Immunological Approaches to Cancer Therapeutics.* 1982:363–404.

64. Borden E. *Ann Int Med.* 1979;91:472–479.

65. Goldstein D, Laszlo J. *Cancer Res.* 1986;46:4315–4329.

66. Gutterman J, et al. *Ann Int Med.* 1980;93:399–406.

67. Gutterman J, et al. *Ann Int Med.* 1982;96:549–556.

68. Kohler M, Milstein C. *Nature (London).* 1975;256:494–497.

69. Schlom J. *Cancer Res.* 1986;46:3225–3238.

70. Carter P. *J Biol Response Modifiers.* 1985;4:325–339.

71. Brady L, et al. *Int J Radiat Oncol Biol Phys.* 1987;13:1535–1544.

72. Morgan A, Foon K. Monoclonal antibody therapy of cancer: Preclinical models and investigations in humans. In Herberman RB, ed. *Cancer Immunology: Innovative Approaches to Therapy.* 1986:177–200.

73. Sondel PM, et al. Overview: Cellular Immunotherapy of Cancer. In Truitt RL, Gale RP, Bortin MM, eds. *Cellular Immunotherapy of Cancer.* New York: Alan R. Liss, Inc; 1987:3–14.

74. Kohler PC, et al. *Cancer.* 1985;55:552–560.

75. Taniguchi, et al. *Nature (London).* 1983;302:305–307.

76. Andriole G, Rosenberg S, et al. *J Immunol.* 1985;135(9):2911–2913.

77. Sondel PM, et al. Clinical testing of IL-2: In vivo administration of IL-2 induces IL-2 dependent non-MHC restricted cytotoxicity (NRC). In Truitt RL, Gale RP, Bortin MM, eds. *Cellular Immunotherapy of Cancer.* New York: Alan R. Liss, Inc; 1987:161–172.

78. Rosenberg S. Adoptive immunotherapy of cancer using lymphokine activated killer cells and recombinant interleukin-2. In DeVita V, Hellman S, Rosenberg S, eds. *Important Advances in Oncology.* Philadelphia, PA: J.B. Lippincott; 1986:55–91.

79. Rosenberg S, Lotze M, Mule J. *Ann Int Med.* 1988;108:853–864.

80. Rosenberg S, et al. *New Engl J Med.* 1985;313(23):1485–1492.

81. Sondel P. *J Immunol.* 1986;137(2):502–511.

82. Sosman J, et al. *J Natl Cancer Inst.* 1988;80(1):60–63.

83. Beutler B, Cerami A. *New Engl J Med.* 1988;316(7):379–385.

84. Gray P, et al. *Nature (London).* 1984;312:721–724.

85. Agarwal B, et al. *Nature (London).* 1985;318:665–667.

86. Watanabe N. *Cancer Res.* 1988;48:650–653.

87. Rosenberg S, et al. *Science.* 1986;233:1318–1321.

CLINICAL IMMUNOLOGY

CHAPTER 11

Immunity to Infectious Diseases: The Influence of Phagocytic Cells

Mary Catherine Harris

University of Pennsylvania School of Medicine, The Children's Hospital of Philadelphia, 34th Street and Civic Center Boulevard, Philadelphia, PA 19104 USA

Mervin C. Yoder

Indiana University Medical Center, Indianapolis, IN 46223 USA

Introduction

The host response to infection involves a complex interplay of several aspects of the immune system, among them circulating antibody, cell-mediated components, complement, and phagocytic cells.[1-3] Multiple physical, biochemical, and cellular mechanisms are involved in the successful encounter between the microorganism and the host; this response is further augmented by cooperation between different cell types. Of all the wings of the immune system, phagocytic cells represent the most important acute defense against invading microorganisms.[4] This chapter reviews the structure and function of both polymorphonuclear and mononuclear phagocytes in host defense and highlights several specific immune deficiencies that affect the phagocytic response to infectious challenge.

Before the time of birth, the fetus lives and develops in a sterile, immunologically protected environment provided by the amniotic fluid and the placenta.[2] Shortly after birth, however, the infant becomes colonized on the skin and mucous membranes with microorganisms derived from the maternal vaginal flora. From this time forward, the infant becomes a biological reservoir for bacteria, viruses, fungi, and parasites.[5] The host then ultimately acquires a rich natural microflora on all body surfaces, within all orifices and throughout the gastrointestinal tract. The normal host lives in harmony with this microbial environment. The presence of the physical barriers mentioned above and intact host defense mechanisms maintain potentially pathogenic microorganisms at controllable levels.[6,7] Fortunately, these interactions between the host and surrounding microorganisms only rarely produce symptomatic infection, as well as the need for antimicrobial therapy.

Host responses to infectious pathogens are both local and systemic, nonspecific and specific, and humoral and cellular.[2,7] Nonspecific mechanisms function effectively without prior exposure to a microorganism or its antigens and include physical barriers, chemical barriers (gastric acid, digestive enzymes, bacteriostatic fatty acids of the skin), as well as phagocytic cells and complement. Nonspecific factors generally are more primitive and function early on in the course of bacterial infection. Specific host defenses, such as antibody- and cell-mediated immunity, in contrast, provide a fast and aggressive response to familiar antigens, enabling the host to eliminate organisms efficiently on repeated challenge. Specific factors are more complex and function both early and late in the evolution of the infectious process. In general, however, infectious agents stimulate multiple overlapping host defense mechanisms of both a specific and nonspecific nature.

The Phagocyte System

The phagocytic cells represent the most important acute defense against invading microorganisms.[3,8] They are cells of hematopoietic origin that recognize, ingest, and kill offending bacteria and other microbes. There are two systems of phagocytes: the polymorphonuclear leukocytes and the mononuclear phagocytes. Although both types of specialized phagocytic cells possess many similar antimicrobial properties, these cells differ with respect to lifespan and bone marrow reserve, distribution in the blood stream and tissues, and capability to synthesize immune mediators.[4,8]

Neutrophil Development and Maturation

Neutrophils arise in the bone marrow from undifferentiated hematopoietic pluripotent stem cells, which are capable of producing all classes of human blood cells.[8–10] Both cell division and differentiation of progenitor cells depend on the presence of glycoproteins known as granulocyte/macrophage colony-stimulating factors (CSF). These growth-promoting factors stimulate progenitor cells to develop as discrete macrophage or neutrophil cell lines. Beyond the myeloblast stage of differentiation, the cells become restricted in their potential for terminal differentiation only into neutrophils. This process is further aided by the presence of colony-stimulating factors that stimulate neutrophil development exclusively.[9,11] Microscopically, this commitment of myeloid precursors to differentiate into neutrophils is recognizable at the promyelocyte stage of development, with the formation of cytoplasmic granules. The azurophilic (primary) granules have been shown to be present from the promyelocyte stage of differentiation, while the specific (secondary) granules appear slightly later in development (Figure 11-1).[12,13]

Following this maturation process in the bone marrow, neutrophils are released into the blood stream continually and in large numbers; 3×10^{10} neutrophils are present in circulating adult human blood at any one time.[4] Neutrophils demonstrate a half life of 6½ h from their release from the marrow into the circulation and then exit to the tissues, where they are generally considered terminally differentiated

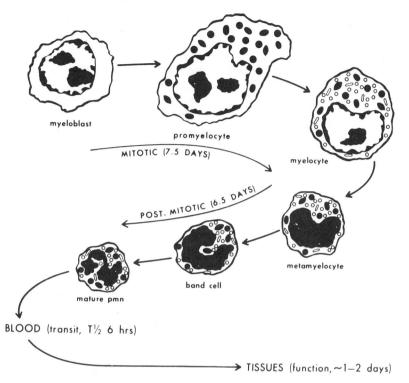

Figure 11-1. The life cycle and stages of neutrophil maturation. (Reproduced from Ref 13 with permission.)

cells.[8] Normally, the bone marrow has a reserve of 3×10^{12} neutrophils to supply fresh circulating cells as those in the blood stream become senescent. Most neutrophil functions (ie, phagocytosis and bacterial killing) are performed at tissue sites after leaving the blood stream in response to chemotactic stimulation and tissue inflammation.

Neutrophil Morphology

The mature neutrophil is an end cell, no longer capable of cell division. It contains a multilobed nucleus, clumps of glycogen particles, cytoskeletal elements including microtubules and microfilaments, and an abundance of cytoplasmic granules. The plasma membrane of the neutrophil is composed of a phospholipid bilayer, which appears as a membrane in excess and actively forms pseudopods and ruffles over portions of the cell surface.[12] The membrane actively transports sugars, adenosine, and ionic substances. In addition, it is rich in receptors for various substrates, among them insulin, lectins, complement components (C3b and C3bi), the Fc portion of immunoglobulin, C5a, and formylated oligopeptides.[8,14,15] A number of enzyme systems have also been detected in the plasma membrane, which function to hydrolyze nucleotides on the exterior of the cell. The cytoskeletal elements of the neutrophil consist of both microtubules and microfilaments. The microtubules are often seen to radiate from the centriole of the cell and consist of the microtubular protein, tubulin, which polymerizes into microtubular structures.[16] Microtubules are involved in neutrophil adherence, orientation, polarity, and motility and are thought to provide a cytoskeleton utilized in the movement of intracellular organelles.

Actin microfilaments are cytoskeletal elements with a critical role in cell adherence, motility, membrane movement, and phagocytosis.[17] The polymerization of actin is thought to generate the force necessary for cell shape change and movement.[16] Actin is a very abundant protein in leukocytes, where it may represent as much as 15–20% of the total cell protein. In the resting state, actin exists in a monomeric or globular form with a molecular weight of 43,000 d, which upon stimulation assembles into long filaments of polymerized or F actin.[17] The formation of actin filaments is a two-step reaction consisting of nucleation and elongation. The nucleation phase is the rate-limiting phase in which two or three actin molecules come together in a specific geometric configuration. Elongation then proceeds rapidly, forming a double-helical filament.[17] Actin polymerization is regulated by several actin-associating and -fragmenting proteins. Filamen is a highly efficient crosslinking protein that promotes actin gelation. Profilin, on the other hand, sequesters actin monomers, while acumentin and gelsolin nucleate the growth of actin polymers by binding to one of the ends of the actin filament. Actin binding protein is responsible for crosslinking fibers into a three-dimensional polymer, while myosin participates in the formation of actin networks to allow an active contraction of the cytoplasmic gel.[8,16,17]

Neutrophils contain two kinds of cytoplasmic granules. The primary or azurophilic granules predominate in the early stages of neutrophil maturation, but in the mature cell, secondary or specific granules contribute two-thirds of the total granule content.[4,18,19] As a response to stimulation, secondary granules present their contents to the external surface of the cell. In contrast, primary granules fuse with phagosomes to form the phagolysosomes which are the primary site of bacterial killing. During the process of inflammation, there is evidence for preferential secretion from secondary granules, particularly following stimulation with chemoattractants, such as IL-1 and PMA.[20,21] Secondary granule secretion may therefore amplify the early inflammatory response. Primary granules, in contrast, are important in the modulation of this response, and secretory products from primary granules such as collagenase and elastase may facilitate neutrophil movement into tissues by degrading extracellular matrix. Later on, primary granule release may provide negative feedback to limit the extent of inflammation.[18]

Neutrophil Function

The neutrophil is qualitatively and quantitatively the most powerful and most significant killing element of host defense. Effective neutrophil function requires several coordinated steps including adherence of the cell to the vascular endothelium, shape change and chemotaxis toward the inflammatory stimulus, attachment and phagocytosis of the offending microorganism, and killing, which requires a metabolic burst on the part of the neutrophil.[12]

The neutrophil response to inflammation is initiated following the interaction or binding of the chemotactic factor to receptors located on the surface of the cell. The biochemical and physiological events subsequent to the chemotactic factor–receptor interaction are termed neutrophil activation and initiate responses such as superoxide anion generation, degranulation, and aggregation.[22] Following stimulation, neutrophils demonstrate rapid changes in cellular calcium permeability and a rise in intracellular calcium. These changes occur prior to the onset of other physiological responses, which amplify the neutrophil inflammatory response.[23,24] For this reason, calcium has been termed a second messenger. In contrast, if the cell is stimulated with phorbol esters, which bypass receptor-mediated events, cell activation may be initiated without a rise in cytosolic calcium. This complex response also involves changes in membrane potential, the breakdown of phosphoinositol into inositol triphosphate and diacylglycerol, the activation of protein kinase C, sodium influx, alkalinization of the cytoplasm, and an increase in cell volume.[25] These events are termed signal transduction and produce a reduction in the negative charge of the neutrophil membrane.

Neutrophil adherence to a substrate is an important prerequisite for migration in vitro and in vivo. This adhesion must be reversible so that the cells can effectively crawl along substrates. The dimeric glycoproteins CR3, LFA-1, and p150,95 comprise a structurally and functionally related family that plays a crucial role in adherence-related functions of neutrophils (Table 11-1).[2,26,27] The glycoproteins are comprised of an identical β subunit that has a molecular weight of approximately 95 kd; however, each glycoprotein has a different α subunit of 150–180 kd.

Following stimulation with chemoattractants, there is an increased surface expression of membrane CR3 receptors from intracellular pools. This translocation of CR3 receptors appears to be essential for cell adherence, as well as the related phenomena of cell-surface spreading, leukoaggregation, and cell movement.[27,28] The LFA-1 glycoprotein present on neutrophils, monocytes, and B cells promotes the adherence of cytotoxic T lymphocytes to target cells and may participate in adherence-related functions as well.[29] The p150,95 glycoprotein has unknown functions and is incompletely categorized to date.[2] The release of lactoferrin from

Table 11-1. Adhesion-Promoting Receptors of Leukocytes

Receptor	Mabs Against a Chain	Cellular Distribution	Function
CR3	OKM1, OKM10, 44a	Monocytes, macrophages PMNs	C3bi receptor LPS receptor
LFA-1	TA-1, TS1/22	Monocytes, macrophages PMNs, T and B cells	NK target binding T-cell target binding MO tumor binding LPS receptor
P150,95	LeuM5, 3.9	Monocytes, macrophages PMNs	? LPS receptor

Source: reproduced from Ref 2 with permission.

neutrophil-specific granules following chemotactic factor stimulation may also enhance the adhesion process.[30]

Aggregation is a premigratory response involving the adhesion of neutrophils to each other, to increase cell density at the site of inflammation.[12] Following stimulation with chemotactic factors, neutrophils normally demonstrate a biphasic aggregation–deaggregation pattern. The temporary aggregation phase functions to amplify the initial inflammatory response, by recruiting additional neutrophils to endothelial surfaces near the inflammatory focus.

Chemotaxis is the directed movement of the cell in response to a concentration gradient of a mediator.[31] During the acute inflammatory response, neutrophils are mobilized from the bone marrow and migrate, deform, and diapedese through the capillary endothelium to the site of tissue injury.[4,12] An important determinant of this neutrophil response is the ability of the cell to change shape and assume a polarized morphology. Cytoskeletal elements, such a microtubules, microfilaments, and intermediate fibers are crucial to this process.

In the resting state the cell has a round, symmetrical shape and configuration of organelles. Upon stimulation, there is a ruffling of the cell membrane, followed by the development of a fusiform configuration of the cell body.[32] The cell orients toward the gradient forming a broad thin veil (lamellipodium) at the advancing front, and a knoblike tail (uropod) and retraction fibers at the rear (Figure 11-2).[33] When viewed microscopically the lamellipodial region of the cell excludes organelles, such as granules and the nucleus. Instead it is a very fluid area of cytoplasm containing microfilaments and other associated contractile proteins, as well as microtubules.[17,34] It is thought that the microtubules provide the directional determinant for the neutrophil, while the microfilament system supplies the mechanical work.

This formation of lamellipodium at the leading front of the cell is then followed by a myosin-based contraction which pulls the remainder of the cell forward, a process similar to muscle contraction.[16,17,32] Both the adherence of the lamellipodia to the substrate and detachment of the rear or uropod region are required for net cell movement. The elongated shape of the cell body during locomotion is the consequence of the tug of war between the anterior, forward-extending lamellipodia

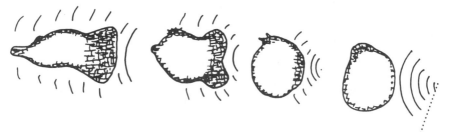

chemotactic factor gradient

Figure 11-2. Schematic drawing of a neutrophil moving toward a chemotactic stimulus. (Reproduced from Ref 17 with permission.)

and the few adherent sites in the posterior portion of the cell. Energy is required for the function of the contractile machinery of the cell, and evidence to date suggests that this is largely supplied through ATP generated by anaerobic glycolysis.[12]

Phagocytosis is the process of engulfment, by which the exterior membrane of the cell forms pseudopods that gradually surround foreign particles, sequestering them into the intracellular phagocytic vacuole.[12,35] Before phagocytosis can take place, there is a preliminary phase whereby neutrophils recognize microorganisms coated with opsonins, such as IgG and C3b. In addition to its adherence-related functions, CR3 is an important opsonic receptor, with high specificity for the C3bi component of complement. Along with the complement receptor type one (CR1), which has affinity primarily for C3b, it mediates binding of complement-coated particles to the neutrophil. The opsonic activity of complement is also synergistic with the effect of immunoglobulin, which binds via its Fc domain to specific receptors (FcR) on the cell surface of the phagocyte. These particle-bound opsonins then bind to specific receptors on the neutrophil surface. Recent evidence suggests that Fc receptors become localized at the leading edge of the cells, where they will come into direct contact with the offending microorganisms.[36] Although phagocytosis is strikingly enhanced by the presence of opsonins, certain particles may be ingested without prior opsonization.[4]

Following contact of the opsonized particle with cell-surface receptors, the plasma membrane infolds and develops pseudopods.[12] This process occurs secondary to the gelation and contraction of actin and myosin filaments, anchored to the microtubules in the cytoplasm. Pseudopods gradually surround the microorganism until engulfment is complete. Initially, the phagocytic vacuole retains its connection to the cell surface by a membranous stalk; however, the phagosome is quickly interiorized. Phagocytosis is dependent upon ATP generation through glycolysis.

Following ingestion of the microorganism, neutrophil granules in close proximity to the phagosome fuse with the vacuole and discharge their contents into the vacuolar space.[4] This converts the phagosome into a phagolysosome. Secondary granules are the first to fuse with the phagolysosome, but both primary and secondary granules participate in the degranulation process.[8,12] This degranulation may result in the complete and irreversible disappearance of granules from the cell cytoplasm as granule formation does not occur beyond the myelocyte stage of neutrophil development.[18] Degranulation may also occur into the extracellular fluid, particularly following incomplete closure of the phagocytic vacuole to the interior of the cell, a process called "regurgitation during feeding."[12] This extracellular degranulation may in fact potentiate inflammation and tissue injury.

Following the pertubation of the plasma membrane during phagocytosis, neutrophils exhibit a metabolic or respiratory burst.[12] Oxygen consumption is greatly increased, as is glucose oxidation via the hexose monophosphate shunt. An NADPH oxidase is activated in the cell membrane, which catalyzes the reduction of oxygen to superoxide (O_2^-), $NADP^+$, and H^+.[4] Two superoxide molecules may then form hydrogen peroxide, H_2O_2, a reaction assisted by superoxide dismutase. The intermediate products, O_2^- and H_2O_2, can then combine to generate highly reactive hydroxyl radicals, $OH^{\cdot}$. The hydrogen peroxide can also undergo halogenation, which is catalyzed by the lysosomal enzyme myeloperoxidase. The product hypophalite (OCL^-) disrupts the cell walls of bacteria and forms singlet oxygen by reaction with H_2O_2.[37] Both oxidized halogen and hydroxyl radicals demonstrate strong bactericidal activities.

The antimicrobial systems of the neutrophil are composed of both oxygen-dependent and oxygen-independent mechanisms.[12] The oxygen-dependent systems are divided into those which require myeloperoxidase and those which function independently of this enzyme. Oxygen-independent mechanisms include acid pH, lysozyme, cationic proteins, and lactoferrin. Acidification of the phagocytic vacuole is optimal for the function of many lysosomal hydrolases and may enhance the reduction of superoxide to hydrogen peroxide.[8] Lactoferrin binds iron and may deprive the microorganism of iron required for growth. Cationic proteins bind to negatively charged gram-negative bacteria and function optimally under alkaline conditions. Lysozyme, in contrast, disrupts the peptidoglycan molecules that form the cell walls of gram-positive bacteria.[25]

Following bacterial killing, there is evidence of microorganism degradation. The bacterial cell wall first appears thickened or fuzzy and loses its integrity. Subsequently, complete dissolution of the cell wall and digestion of all of the cellular components occur.[38] In most instances, organisms are susceptible to more than one antimicrobial system in the vacuolar space. These multiple systems are present so that if one mechanism fails, additional killing mechanisms can compensate. This overkill capacity of the neutrophil provides adequate protection from most microorganisms.

The Mononuclear Phagocyte System

The mononuclear phagocyte system (MPS) is comprised of bone marrow monocyte precursors, circulating monocytes, and macrophages in all tissues including lung, liver, spleen, adrenal glands, intestine, and bone marrow.[39] All mononuclear phagocytes demonstrate certain common functional characteristics. These cells are highly phagocytic and participate in the eradication of invading microorganisms and clearance of damaged or scenescent autologous tissue. They also play an active role in antigen processing and presentation to T lymphocytes to generate the primary immune response. Furthermore, mononuclear phagocytes are capable of secreting numerous biologically active molecules.[40–42] Thus, in concert with circulating and tissue neutrophils, the MPS serves as a fundamental component of host immune defense.

Mononuclear Phagocyte Development-Maturation

The mononuclear phagocyte cell lineage originates in the bone marrow (Figure 11-3) from a committed progenitor cell called the colony-forming unit–granulocyte-macrophage (CFU-GM). At least four of the human colony-stimulating factors (CSF) influence mononuclear phagocyte production. These include interleukin-3, granulocyte-macrophage CSF, granulocyte CSF, and macrophage CSF (CSF-1).[43,44] Of

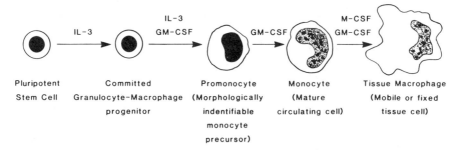

Figure 11-3. Mononuclear phagocyte lineage. (Reproduced from Ref 53 with permission.)

these CSF, CSF-1 predominantly drives the committed progenitor cell toward production of mononuclear phagocytes.[45] Mononuclear phagocyte production in the bone marrow has been estimated at between 7×10^5 and 7×10^6 monocytes per kilogram of body weight per hour with a daily turnover of nearly 4×10^8 cells.[46-48]

The promonocyte is the first immature mononuclear phagocyte readily identifiable in the marrow environment (an earlier cell, the monoblast is usually difficult to identify). The highly replicative promonocytes divide once in the marrow, producing two daughter monocytes. These monocytes are functionally and morphologically indistinguishable from the circulating blood monocyte.[46] After maturing in the marrow for nearly 60 h, monocytes leave the bone marrow compartment, circulate for approximately 72 h, and then proceed to migrate into body tissues, where they replenish the resident tissue macrophage population. The stimulus for the migration of the blood monocyte into the tissues remains undetermined. Once localized in a tissue, the surrounding extracellular milieu probably plays an important role in modulating macrophage differentiation and may explain the morphological and functional heterogeneity observed when comparing tissue macrophages from several different organs, such as the lung, liver, spleen, and central nervous system.[49] Although the ultimate fate of tissue macrophages is not known, experiments have been performed to demonstrate that these cells are long lived and can be observed to be active for several months in human tissue.[50,51]

Mononuclear Phagocyte Morphology

The characteristic features of a peripheral blood monocyte stained (Wright's stain) on a glass slide are the eccentrically placed kidney-shaped nucleus, the pale gray-blue cytoplasm with a variable number of pink and purple granules, and an overall diameter of 10–18 μm.[42,52] When examined by scanning electron microscopy, the most characteristic feature of the monocyte is a flattened spread-out appearance with a very ruffled plasma membrane.[42] At the ultrastructural level, the monocyte cytoplasm consists of well-developed Golgi complex with a small amount of endoplasmic reticulum; there are many mitochondria present, and prominent microvilli are distributed along the outer plasma membrane. Numerous small (<0.2 μm) lysosomal enzyme-laden granules are distributed throughout the cytoplasm.[53] As monocytes develop into tissue macrophages, they increase in cell size and may achieve a diameter of 25–70 μm.[54] On Wright's stained films, the macrophage nucleus is eccentrically placed and the nuclear chromatin has become tightly clumped against the nuclear membrane. The number of granules and clear vacuoles along the peripheral border of the cell has increased with many of these lysosomal granules observed to be fusing with phagosomes (ingested material surrounded by plasma membrane) to form secondary lysosomes. Similar to the neutrophil, the macrophage has a well-developed cytoskeletal apparatus, which is prominently involved in moving the cell and modifying its shape.[55]

There are several cytochemical stains that have proved to be useful in identification and classification of mononuclear phagocytes. While no single cytochemical stain is specific for the MPS, the application of several cytochemical tests is useful in identifying cells at a particular point of differentiation. It is apparent that the mononuclear phagocyte phenotype is a composite of the stage of cellular maturity and the tissue of origin and is subject to changes in the tissue extracellular milieu.[56]

The most reliable cytochemical marker for human mononuclear phagocytes is nonspecific esterase activity demonstrated with α-naphthyl butyrate as the substrate.[57] While the nonspecific esterases are enzymes present in many cell types, distinct isoenzymes are expressed by the mononuclear phagocyte lineage, which are inhibited by sodium fluoride.[56] Therefore, analysis of sodium fluoride inhibition of the nonspecific esterase reaction allows for the discrimination between peripheral blood monocytes and all other circulating formed blood elements. Other useful cytochemical stains include acid phosphatase, peroxidase, and the constitutively synthesized enzyme lysozyme.[58]

All cells of the mononuclear phagocyte lineage express plasma membrane receptors for immunoglobulin G (IgG). At present three distinct IgG receptors have been identified. The first, FcγRI, is expressed by monocytes, macrophages, and activated neutrophils. This receptor binds monomeric IgG through the Fc portion of the molecule.[59] The second IgG receptor, FcγRII, is more widely distributed and is expressed by monocytes, platelets, neutrophils, B and T lymphocytes, and some human endothelium. This receptor binds complexed IgG and may be involved in T-lymphocyte proliferative responses.[60] The third IgG receptor, FcγRIII, also preferentially binds immune complexes of IgG and is expressed by natural killer cells, neutrophils, and tissue macrophages. This receptor appears late in the differentiation of the mononuclear phagocyte and is not present on peripheral blood monocytes.[61]

Mononuclear phagocytes also express several distinct receptors for complement component fragments.[60] Both monocytes and macrophages express complement receptor 1 (CR1), which binds dimeric C3b. Complement receptor 3 (CR3) binds the complement fragment C3bi but does not recognize further cleavage products of C3bi or the complement fragment C3b.[62] As discussed earlier in the section of this chapter on neutrophils, this complement receptor is a heterodimeric glycoprotein comprised of an α chain with a molecular weight of 185 kd and a β subunit of 95 kd. This receptor, along with the leukocyte antigens LFA-1 and p150,95, comprise a family of leukocyte adhesion molecules called the leukocyte integrin subfamily.[28] Recent reviews of the structure and function of the immunoglobulin receptors, complement receptors, and the integrin supergene family of receptors are available.[60,61,63]

Monoclonal antibody techniques have recently provided a more precise description of the mononuclear phagocyte lineage and differentiation sequence. Table 11-2 is a partial listing of some specific antigens that have been identified on the plasma membrane of the mononuclear phagocyte lineage. Most of the cluster of differentiation (CD) antigens identified on mononuclear phagocytes are also expressed by granulocytes, lymphocytes, and even platelets. The CD14 antigen is the most specific antigen for the human MPS.[64] Recent cloning of the gene for this glycoprotein may help in examining its physiology and function.[65] Additionally important antigens include the class-II major histocompatibility antigens that have recently been reviewed.[66]

Because of the diversity in morphological appearance and functional behavior of monocytes, macrophages, and their precursor cells, a consensus statement was published in 1972 to outline those features that best described the mononuclear phagocyte lineage.[67] All members of the mononuclear phagocyte lineage ultimately arise from a single hematopoietic stem cell. Additionally, all of these cells contain a single nucleus, adhere to glass surfaces, express IgG receptors, and phagocytose IgG-coated particles. By these criteria, some members of the reticuloendothelial system are not included in the mononuclear phagocyte system. Those cells include Langerhan's cells in the skin, dendritic cells of lymphoreticular organs, and some phagocytic microglial cells present in the central nervous system.

Table 11-2. Cluster of Differentiation (CD) Antigens[a]

CD Antigen	Monoclonal Examples	Cellular Reactivity	Additional Comments
CD4	Leu3a, OKT4	T cells, monocytes, macrophages	T4 antigen, AIDS virus receptor
CD11a	LFA-1	Leukocytes	LFA-1, α chain
CD11b	Mac-1, OKM-1, Mol, Leu15	Monocytes, granulocytes, NK cells, T cells	C3bi(CR3); Mac-1, α chain
CD11c	3.9, LeuM5	Monocytes, granulocytes (weak)	p150,95, α chain
CD14	MY4, UCHM1, LeuM3, MO2	Monocytes, granulocytes (weak)	
CD16	Leu11	Granulocytes, NK cells, macrophages	FcγR111
CD18	60.3	Leukocytes	β chain of CD11a,b,c
CDw32	IV.3	Monocytes, granulocytes, platelets, B cells	FcγR11
CD33	MY9, L4F3	Myeloid progenitors	
CD34	MY10, B1-3C5	Myeloid/lymphoid progenitors	HPCA-1
CD35	E11,To5	Granulocytes, monocytes	CR1
CD45	2D1	Pan leukocyte	T200
CD45R	2H4, Leu18	B cells, T cells, granulocytes, monocytes	Restricted T200

Source: adapted from Refs 42, 53, and 62.

Mononuclear Phagocyte Function

Like the circulating neutrophil, an effective mononuclear phagocyte response to infection depends upon the ability of these cells to migrate and accumulate at the nidus of the inflammatory focus. Both neutrophils and mononuclear phagocytes are capable of responding to specific chemotactic factors with oriented migration (chemotaxis). These chemoattractants may also activate the phagocytes to greater random migration in the absence of a chemotactic gradient (chemokinesis). The chemotactic substances to which phagocytes respond include products generated through activation of the complement, fibrinolytic, and kinin systems.[68] Additional chemotactic factors are secreted by activated lymphocytes and some are released by bacterial organisms directly. Mononuclear phagocytes appear to utilize the same signal transduction mechanisms that have been well described for the neutrophil.[69] Furthermore, the cytoskeletal alterations that result in cell-shape changes are very similarly regulated in the mononuclear phagocyte and the circulating neutrophil.[55]

To play a central role in wound healing, inflammation, and immune responses, mononuclear phagocytes are required to interact in an adhesive fashion with a variety of cells and tissues. Using time-lapse photography, in vivo experiments have shown that neutrophils and mononuclear phagocytes adhere to vascular endothelium prior to moving into tissues that are inflamed. This leukocyte–endothelial interaction appears to be a temperature-dependent and a magnesium-requiring event and is enhanced by a number of biologically active substances.[70] Interleukin-1 (IL-1), tumor necrosis factor, interferon-γ, (IFN-γ), and lipopolysaccharide (LPS) all increase leukocyte–endothelial adhesion.[71] These agents modify the adhesive nature of the endothelial cell surface membrane for the circulating phagocyte. Other chemotactic factors and phorbol esters appear to stimulate primarily the cell surface of the circulating phagocyte to enhance its interaction with the endothelium.[72] As previously mentioned, the LFA-1 (CD11a), Mac-1 (CD11b), and p150,95 (CD11c) adhesion molecules and their common β subunit (CD18) are functionally important in leukocyte–endothelial adhesion. The physiological relevance of these leukocyte adhesion molecules became apparent when approximately two dozen patients and one dog were described with congenital absence or severe deficiency of the glycoprotein CD18 on the surface of their circulating leukocytes.[73] All of these patients suffer from persistent leukocytosis, recurrent gingivitis, necrotic soft tissue lesions, impaired wound healing, and an apparent inability to accumulate phagocytic cells in the area of inflamed tissues. This disorder has been termed leukocyte adherence deficiency disease (LAD).[74]

Multiple deficiencies in adhesion-dependent neutrophil and mononuclear phagocyte functions have been documented in vitro in patients with LAD. "Blocking" of the CD18 glycoprotein on the leukocyte surface with specific monoclonal antibodies mimics the congenital abnormality in these patients and results in similar in vitro deficiencies in leukocyte adhesion-dependent functions.[75] Use of these specific monoclonal antibodies has helped assess the pathophysiological role of activated neutrophils and mononuclear phagocytes in a wide variety of experimentally induced disorders, such as acute myocardial infarction[76] and acute hemorrhagic shock.[77]

The capacity of mononuclear phagocytes to ingest particulate material is crucial to their immunological function. Endocytosis is important in antimicrobial resistance, removal of scenescent cells, antigen processing, and numerous other mononuclear phagocyte functions. The major forms of endocytosis utilized by the macrophage include pinocytosis and phagocytosis.[50] While these mechanisms are believed to be similar, the distinction between these processes relates to the size and composition of the particulate matter being ingested. Pinocytosis refers to the ingestion of microscopic fluid droplets, while phagocytosis is a better description of the ingestion of large particulate matter. Both endocytic processes involve translocation of the particle into the cell interior through extension of the plasma membrane to surround the particle (phagosome).[78] Once ingested, the phagosome fuses with lysosomal granules to form secondary lysosomes in which mononuclear phagocyte proteolytic enzymes begin the digestion of the particulate matter. As with the neutrophil, phagocytosis is enhanced when particulate matter opsonized with IgG or complement components binds to specific mononuclear phagocyte plasma membrane receptors.[62] The ability of mononuclear phagocytes to recognize and ingest unopsonized particles, as well, may be particularly important to the resolution of inflammation and tissue injury as the macrophages ingest fluids, proteins, and tissue debris, including damaged or scenescent neutrophils.[79]

Interaction of free or fixed tissue mononuclear phagocytes with particulate or soluble stimuli leads to a marked increase in oxygen consumption (respiratory burst) and the elaboration of reactive oxygen intermediates. Similar to the neutrophil, the activation of a transmembrane NADPH oxidase results in the generation of superoxide anion.[80] This molecule, which may be directly toxic to some proteins and membrane constituents, is frequently converted to the more powerful microbicidal agent hydrogen peroxide.[81] Hydrogen peroxide is highly toxic to a number of pathogenic organisms and tumor cells and is a major oxygen-dependent mechanism for killing by mononuclear phagocytes. While peripheral blood monocytes contain myeloperoxidase in cytoplasmic granules, the number of granules is approximately one-third the number quantitated in peripheral blood neutrophils.[82] Mononuclear phagocytes utilize myeloperoxidase and hydrogen peroxide to oxidize halides (iodide, bromide, chloride) to hypohalous acids.[83] These halide oxidation products are powerful oxidants that can attack essential bacterial cell wall constituents and can lead to microbial dissolution.

The in vitro differentiation of monocytes into tissue macrophages is associated with a decrease in oxygen-dependent microbicidal mechanisms.[84] The magnitude of the respiratory burst decreases and the peroxidase-containing granules disappear from the cytoplasm of mature tissue macrophages.[85] While hydrogen peroxide continues to be an important microbicidal agent, the relative lack of myeloperoxidase would suggest that mature tissue macrophages are less capable of amplifying the toxicity of this molecule. However, the highly pinocytic nature of the macrophage results in the ingestion of peroxidase-containing granules released from other degranulating granulocytes, such as neutrophils, eosinophils, or monocytes, during an inflammatory response and these exogenous peroxidases may amplify the hydrogen peroxide formed by the tissue macrophage.[86]

Mononuclear phagocyte oxygen-independent antimicrobial systems include the synthesis and secretion of cationic proteins (defensins, lipid hydrolases, proteases, and nucleases).[87] Activation of the alternative complement pathway also serves to enhance mononuclear phagocyte antimicrobial activity. The extent to which these oxygen-independent mechanisms participate in bactericidal activity in vivo has never been convincingly established. A clinically relevant demonstration of the importance of these mechanisms, however, has been observed in patients with chronic granulomatous disease.[88] These patients suffer from a heritable deficiency in generating reactive oxygen intermediates by both neutrophils and monocytes. In these patients, despite a deficiency in oxygen-dependent antimicrobial activity, mononuclear phagocytes are very capable of killing microbial pathogens.

Mononuclear phagocytes are not only capable of killing invading microorganisms, but under certain pathophysiological conditions, these cells may also destroy normal circulating formed elements of the blood, normal tissue cells, and tumor cells. Mononuclear phagocyte cellular cytotoxicity may occur in the presence of specific antibodies (antibody-dependent cellular toxicity) or may occur in the absence of specific anti-target cell antibody.[89] Antibody-independent cellular cytotoxicity is characterized by a highly efficient killing of a variety of malignant cells without damage to tissue-matched nonmalignant cells. This process is generally nonphagocytic, highly specific for malignant cells, and usually dependent on cell-to-cell contact.[90] Some evidence suggests that plasma membrane receptors on the mononuclear phagocyte exist for these target cells and are involved in this cell-to-cell interaction. Other evidence has been presented for the important role of tumor necrosis factor, reactive oxygen intermediates, and a putative 40-kd serine protease as the major cytotoxic secretory products involved in antibody-independent cellular cytotoxicity.[91]

Antibody-dependent cellular toxicity may be directed toward normal or malignant tissues. In antibody-dependent cellular cytotoxicity, the IgG-bound target interacts with the Fc surface receptor on the mononuclear phagocyte. This binding of the antibody-coated target is necessary but not sufficient for the cellular destruction of the target.[92] Hydrogen peroxide appears to be the major secretory product of the mononuclear phagocyte that is involved in the lysis of the bound target.[93] The roles of tumor necrosis factor and the 40-kd serine protease have not been clearly defined in antibody-dependent cellular cytotoxicity exhibited by mononuclear phagocytes.

The participation of mononuclear phagocytes in acute inflammatory reactions is not limited to the phagocytosis and killing of specific targets. Macrophages secrete nearly 100 biologically active molecules that are important regulatory elements in nearly all aspects of acute and chronic inflammatory reactions. Nathan[94] recently reviewed all published secretory products derived from mononuclear phagocytes and catalogued these products according to certain characteristics. These secretory products included polypeptide hormones, complement components, coagulation factors, other enzymes, inhibitors of enzymes and cytokines, extracellular matrix-like proteins, other binding proteins, bioactive oligopeptides, bioactive lipids, sterol hormones, purine and pyrimidine products, reactive oxygen intermediates, and reactive nitrogen intermediates. Some of these secretory products are produced constitutively, while others are secreted only under specific conditions. Mononuclear phagocytes are highly responsive cells, and as previously mentioned, the final development of the macrophage in the tissue is influenced to a large degree by a number of factors, including the tissue-specific extracellular milieu, prevailing oxygen tension of the tissue, and the presence of inflammatory mediators.

The secretory phenotype of the quiescent tissue macrophage may be dramatically altered during an acute inflammatory response when activated T lymphocytes release numerous biologically active polypeptide hormones. Adams and Hamilton[91] have recently reviewed the effect of the activated T-lymphocyte hormone IFN-γ on mononuclear phagocyte functional and secretory activities. They stressed the important role IFN-γ plays in activating mononuclear phagocytes to a greater competence in destroying microbial pathogens and tumor cells. Once activated, not only are macrophages functionally more competent to destroy these target cells, but there are certain physiological capacities, such as the secretion of reactive oxygen intermediates and proteolytic enzymes, or expression of cell surface receptors, that are also enhanced. These investigators propose a model of macrophage activation in which responsive mononuclear phagocytes are initially primed by IFN-α, IFN-β, or IFN-γ. This enhances the functional and secretory capacity of the macrophages but also makes them further responsive to additional signals, such as lipopolysaccharides (LPS), which then fully activates the cell for its increased competence to kill tumor cells and microbial pathogens.

Once the acute inflammatory reaction is controlled, the mononuclear phagocytes play a regulatory role in the wound healing response.[79] Circulating monocytes are recruited to the inflammatory site, where these cells participate in remodeling the connective tissue matrix that had been damaged during the acute inflammatory reaction. Mononuclear phagocytes release such proteolytic enzymes as elastase, collagenase, and plasminogen activator, which are potent agents in degrading fibronectin, collagen, and elastin, as well as extracellular matrix proteoglycans.[95] Once the tissue matrix is degraded into smaller fragments, resident macrophages can ingest and further degrade the matrix constituents. Additional roles that macrophages play in the remodeling response include the secretion of growth factors for fibroblasts and other mesencyhmal cells,[96] the synthesis and secretion of angiogenic factors for endothelial cells,[97] and secretion of factors that modulate the biosynthesis of extracellular matrix proteins by fibroblasts that are repopulating the wound area.[98] In summary, the mononuclear phagocyte plays an essential role not only in the resolution of the acute inflammatory reaction but in the degradative and reparative phases of wound healing that follow.

In addition to serving as phagocytic scavengers of invading microbial pathogens, the MPS is intimately involved in several other aspects of the establishment of an effective immune response. Mononuclear phagocytes are not the only cell type to serve as antigen-presenting cells (dendritic cells of lymphoreticular organs, B lymphocytes, and endothelial cells in certain circumstances); however, there are several specific interactions with T lymphocytes that mononuclear phagocytes do not share with other antigen-presenting cells.

For most antigenic material, the initial event in immune detection and host response is mononuclear phagocyte ingestion and intracellular processing of that antigen.[99] Although the precise mechanisms involved in antigen processing remain undetermined, a portion of the antigenic molecule appears to be salvaged from extensive proteolysis and becomes accessible to the immune system through display on the mononuclear phagocyte plasma membrane.[100] This processing of antigen appears to occur in the acid environment of the lysosomal granules. Processing of the antigen alone, however, does not insure that the mononuclear phagocyte can express the antigen in a proper fashion to interact with antigen-specific CD4-positive T lymphocytes.[101] Both processed antigen and major histocompatibility (MHC) class-II antigens must be concomitantly expressed on the plasma membrane in order for antigen-specific T cells to recognize the antigen. The density of MHC class-II expression on different populations of mononuclear phagocytes appears to correlate with antigen presentation to CD4-positive T cells.[102] Lymphokines, such as IFN-γ, increase the expression of class-II MHC antigens on mononuclear phagocytes and enhance antigen presentation, whereas prostaglandin E_2, α-fetoprotein, and glucocorticoids inhibit MHC class-II antigen expression and impair antigen presentation.[103]

Interleukin-1 also plays an important role in mononuclear phagocyte antigen presentation to CD4-positive T cells.[99] Mononuclear phagocytes secrete IL-1 after the CD4-positive T cells interact with the MHC class-II antigens presented on the mononuclear phagocyte plasma membrane. The binding of IL-1 to its receptor on the CD4-positive T cell induces T-cell proliferation primarily through induction of T-cell IL-2 receptors and through stimulation of IL-2 synthesis. This T-cell activation results in the generation of a number of additional lymphokines such as IFN-γ and CSF factors, which in turn can activate the microbicidal and tumoricidal behavior of the mononuclear phagocyte. Secretion of other molecules, such as B-cell growth factor and B-cell differentiation factor, by T lymphocytes causes proliferation of B lymphocytes and maturation of these cells to antibody-secreting plasma cells.

In summary, mononuclear phagocytes share many properties with the neutrophil in localizing, ingesting, and killing microorganisms that have invaded the host. In addition, mononuclear phagocytes participate in antigen processing and presentation to antigen-specific T lymphocytes. Once stimulated, the T lymphocytes proceed to elaborate a number of lymphokines that not only enhance their own proliferative state but also enhance the production of antibody-secreting B lymphocytes and further enhance mononuclear phagocyte microbicidal and tumoricidal activity. Once armed with the primary immune response, the host is better capable of warding off future invasion by that particular microbial pathogen.

Disorders of Phagocyte Function

Abnormalities of Phagocyte Function in Newborn Infants

The newborn infant is uniquely susceptible to infection during the first few months of life, primarily because of deficiencies in neonatal host defense mechanisms.[104] In general terms, the neonatal immune system may be described as anatomically competent, yet antigenically inexperienced and functionally deficient.[105] Recent investigations have identified abnormalities in every wing of the newborn immune response, including deficiencies of T and B cells, circulating antibody and complement levels, and mononuclear and polymorphonuclear leukocyte defense mechanisms.[3]

Abnormalities of Neutrophil Function

The neutrophil plays a central role in host defense against infection, and significant abnormalities of granulocyte function contribute to the incidence of severe infections in newborn infants.[24,105] Although many investigations of neutrophil function have been performed in healthy neonates, most studies have reported conflicting results, depending on the specific experimental conditions used. Of all the neutrophil functions investigated (adherence, chemotaxis, phagocytosis, oxidative metabolism, and bactericidal capacity), the most consistently abnormal results have been reported in studies of newborn neutrophil chemotaxis.[106,107]

At the current time, the activation sequence in neutrophils from newborn infants is incompletely understood. Studies of receptors on neonatal neutrophils have demonstrated normal N-formylmethionylleucyl phenylalanine (FMLP) binding at both 4 and 37°C as assessed by receptor number, affinity, and kinetics.[106,108] In a recent study employing the fluorescent probe, Quin 2/AM, Sacchi found defective membrane potential changes and diminished levels of intracellular free calcium following chemotactic factor stimulation.[109] In additional experiments, Strauss noted normal calcium influx from extracellular stores,[110] suggesting that defective calcium mobilization in neonates reflected diminished mobilization from intracellular pools. Hill also measured subsequent events in the activation sequence and demonstrated diminished cAMP generation by neonatal neutrophils.[111] Using cell elastimetry, Miller noted markedly decreased deformability when neonatal neutrophils were compared with adult cells.[112] In studies using colchicine to disrupt microtubules, and concanavalin A, however, neonatal cells failed to show a significant increase in capping over spontaneous levels.

Investigations of neutrophil orientation have shown diminished rate, magnitude, and duration of orientation in neonatal as compared to adult cells.[113] Neonatal neutrophil suspensions showed decreased microtubule number and polymerized tubulin mass product, although cytoplasmic tubulin content was comparable to that of adult cells. We have recently examined some of the morphological correlates of these biochemical events.[114] Following FMLP stimulation, both neonatal and adult neutrophils were able to change shape in suspension. A maximally effective concentration induced comparable numbers of cells with a bipolar configuration, confirming that ligand–receptor interactions were normal. Neutrophils from newborn infants failed to redistribute adhesion sites to the uropod, however, following sequential chemotactic factor stimulation, a defect that was more pronounced in sick or stressed rather than healthy neonates. Thus, newborn neutrophils failed to demonstrate complete morphological changes and uropod formation, as occurred when normal adult neutrophils were exposed to chemoattractants. In additional experiments, we have examined actin polymerization by neonatal neutrophils, as a mechanism underlying abnormalities of newborn neutrophil polarity and chemotaxis.[115] Despite similar basal levels of F-actin, neutrophils from newborn infants had significantly diminished actin polymerization when compared to adults.

Studies of the adherence response of neutrophils from newborn infants have revealed similar unstimulated adherence values.[107] However, sequential chemotactic factor stimulation was required to enhance the adherence of neonatal neutrophils as normally observed after a single exposure of adult cells. Our laboratory has recently investigated neutrophil adherence in healthy term neonates, and those stressed with a variety of acute respiratory illnesses.[116] Neutrophils from healthy infants demonstrated significantly diminished adherence values when compared to stressed neonates, which was attributed to diminished amounts of neutrophil membrane fibronectin. Although the mechanisms responsible for the adherence defects are incompletely understood, there is strong evidence that they are functionally linked to abnormalities in the plasma membrane expression of CR3.[117] Neutrophils from term infants stimulated with FMLP expressed significantly less CR3 than neutrophils from adults, and this impairment was directly correlated with the degree of impairment in stimulated adherence.[117,118] Using monoclonal antibodies and flow cytometry, we have recently demonstrated significantly diminished CR3 expression, when neutrophils from fetuses, preterm, and term infants were compared to adults.[119] Moreover, neutrophils from newborn infants demonstrated irreversible aggregation in response to C5a, rather than the usual biphasic aggregation–deaggregation pattern seen in the adult.[120]

Several investigations have demonstrated deficient motility by neutrophils from healthy infants following stimulation with chemotactic factors generated from *Escherichia coli, Staphylococcus aureus,* antigen–antibody complexes, or zymosan-activated serum.[107,108] Since cord blood contains a higher percentage of band forms than adult blood, investigations have examined the chemotactic response of granulocytes from cord blood as a function of cellular maturation.[121] Band forms from cord blood had a mean migrating distance less than multilobed forms, suggesting that the stage of neutrophil development contributed to chemotactic responsiveness. Krause used the monoclonal antibody 31D8 which binds heterogeneously to adult neutrophils, to determine the effect of subpopulations on neutrophil chemotaxis in newborn infants.[122] The larger proportion of immature, poorly motile neonatal neutrophils also expressed less surface antigen as identified by the monoclonal antibody.

Previous studies have reported normal phagocytic activity of neonatal neutrophils in the presence of concentrations of adult serum in excess of 10%, but decreased activity at lower serum concentrations.[123,124] Studies from our laboratory have demonstrated increased phagocytosis of group B *Streptococcus* when neutrophils from stressed or healthy newborn infants were compared to adults.[125] In assessing the function of neutrophil opsonic receptors, the expression of CR1 by stimulated neutrophils from term infants was comparable to adults.[117,118] Our recent studies have also demonstrated diminished expression of CR1 on neutrophils from preterm infants; CR3 on neutrophils from fetal, preterm, and term infants; and FcR on neutrophils from preterm and term infants.[119] Pross has also reported normal numbers of Fc receptors on neutrophils from term infants using rosetting techniques.[126] Deficiencies in the expression of FcR and CR3, along with a possible deficiency of CR1 in preterm infants, may contribute to the phagocytic defects observed in neonatal neutrophils tested with low concentrations of opsonins.

Studies concerning the bactericidal capacity of neonatal granulocytes have produced controversial results. Forman and McCracken[127,128] found normal bactericidal functions in neutrophils from newborn infants. However, Quie demonstrated depressed bactericidal activity when newborn neutrophils were challenged with *E. coli* at large bacteria to neutrophil ratios.[129] Wright noted decreased bactericidal capacity in neutrophils from newborn infants with a variety of clinical abnormalities, including sepsis, respiratory distress syndrome, meconium aspiration, hyperbilirubinemia, or prolonged rupture of membranes.[130] Studies from our laboratory have demonstrated diminished killing of group B *Streptococcus* by neutrophils from newborn infants; however, this capacity was not further compromised by severe stress.[131]

Shigeoka found an impaired chemiluminescence response to zymosan in stressed neonatal neutrophils, despite elevated superoxide generation.[132] In contrast, the chemiluminescence response to phorbol myristate acetate in stressed neonates was significantly elevated. The authors proposed either a defect in the reaction of superoxide anion to form the later high-energy oxygen products, a defect in hexose monophosphate shunt activity, or a stimulus-specific abnormality in respiratory burst activity. Ambruso further demonstrated that neutrophils from newborn infants produced relatively less hydroxyl radical than superoxide following stimulation with zymosan or phorbol esters.[133] The lactoferrin content of neonatal-specific granules was also decreased when compared to adults.[134] These data, therefore, may perhaps provide an explanation for the normal activity of the respiratory burst despite decreased bactericidal capacity of neonatal cells.

In summary, several abnormalities of neutrophil function have been described in newborn infants that contribute to their increased susceptibility to bacterial infection. Deficiencies of granulocyte function are probably further exaggerated by stress, such as that induced by severe illness or infection. Future investigations may suggest insights toward the therapeutic enhancement of neonatal neutrophil function, and toward the control and prevention of neonatal morbidity and mortality.

Abnormalities of Mononuclear Phagocyte Function

Like the neutrophil, a number of functional abnormalities have been reported for mononuclear phagocytes isolated from the blood of newborn infants. Mononuclear phagocytes isolated from newborn infants demonstrate impaired migration to an area of inflammation in response to a chemotactic agent.[135] Yegin[136] reported that prior to 6 years of age, monocyte chemotaxis was significantly lower than that of cells isolated from adult patients. He and other investigators[137] reported that monocytes isolated from cord blood in many instances were able to move toward a chemotactic stimulus in a fashion equivalent to monocytes isolated from the peripheral blood of adult patients. However, when monocytes were isolated from peripheral blood of newborn infants at 2–6 days of age, a dramatic decrease in monocyte migration toward the chemotactic stimulus was documented. Random migration in response to the chemotactic agent appeared to be similar to the migration of adult blood monocytes. One technical problem encountered by the investigators performing the above studies was that the method utilized to obtain the mononuclear phagocytes resulted in a mixed population of immature granulocytes, lymphocytes, and mononuclear phagocytes. This poses a particular problem because large immature lymphocytes, myelocytes, and some metamyelocytes belonging to the neutrophil series, and the monocytes isolated from cord blood and the blood of newborn infants share many morphological similarities. Unless special cytochemical, monoclonal antibody phenotyping, or ultrastructural analyses are performed, these cells may not be readily classified. Considering these study limitations, the most convincing evidence suggests that monocyte chemotactic activity is decreased during the neonatal period but gradually improves during the first 6 years of life.

The adhesive properties of monocytes isolated from fetal blood and from the blood of newborn infants has only been examined in a preliminary fashion. Boner et al.[138] have reported that mononuclear phagocytes isolated from cord blood or adult blood demonstrate equivalent capacity to attach to glass coverslips in vitro. Similarly, Speer et al.[139] demonstrated that 85% of nonspecific esterase-positive mononuclear phagocytes in cord and adult blood samples adhere to nylon wool packed columns. When analyzed in another fashion, monocytes isolated from the blood of fetuses as early as 14 weeks gestation, express the CR3 (CD11b) receptor.[140] The expression of this leukocyte-adhesion molecule is increased following stimulation with a chemotactic stimulus (formyl peptide). Recently increased expression of this leukocyte-adhesion molecule was reported on monocytes isolated from the cord blood of term gestation newborn infants.[141] Whether increased expression of the CR3 receptor on monocytes isolated from cord blood is associated with increased adhesion-related functions by these cells remains to be examined.

Monocytes isolated from the cord blood of infants at birth appear to be less efficient in the endocytosis of nonopsonized particles compared with monocytes isolated from adult peripheral blood.[142] Furthermore, cord blood monocyte phagocytosis of group B streptococci and *Staphylococcus aureus* has been reported by some investigators.[143] Jacobs et al.[144] recently reported that the adhesive glycoprotein fibronectin was highly effective in enhancing cord blood monocyte phagocytosis of group B streptococci. While fibronectin alone was not sufficient to increase the phagocytosis of the microbial pathogen, fibronectin when combined with intravenous IgG in vitro resulted in significant mononuclear uptake of ingested organisms. Furthermore, the fibronectin enhancement of group B streptococcal opsonophagocytosis was associated with greater monocyte microbicidal activity.

Speer[145] and co-workers have reported that following a 10-d culture period, cord blood monocyte-derived macrophages ingest complement opsonized *Staphylococcus aureus* to a degree equivalent to that demonstrated by macrophages derived from adult peripheral blood monocytes. These results are consistent with those reported by other investigators, who found that paraffin oil particles, latex particles, *Staphylococcus aureus, Toxoplasma gondii,* type II herpes simplex virus, and *Escherichia coli* are phagocytized by cord blood mononuclear phagocytes to the same extent as mononuclear phagocytes isolated from adult peripheral blood.[146] In summary, mononuclear phagocytes appear to have an appropriately developed endocytic capacity (during the neonatal period) for most microbial pathogens encountered.

Mononuclear phagocyte activation may be impaired during the perinatal period. This generalization is drawn from a composite of reports published on the function of mononuclear phagocytes isolated from newborn infants since no comprehensive analysis of the activation process has been examined for mononuclear phagocytes in this age group. Wilson and Westfall[147] reported that both newborn and adult mononuclear phagocytes are deficient in their ability to kill the organism *Toxoplasma gondii.* Furthermore, as the mononuclear phagocytes differentiate in vitro they became more permissive for the replication of this organism. When mononuclear phagocytes from adult and newborn infant's blood are exposed to IFN-γ, however, the mononuclear phagocytes demonstrate a greater competence to kill or inhibit the replication of the organism. When they examined T-lymphocyte production of IFN-γ during the incubation of lymphocytes and mononuclear phagocytes with *Toxoplasma gondii,* they noted a significant decrease in the amount of IFN-γ produced by cord blood T lymphocytes. Furthermore, the cord blood T lymphocyte IFN-γ failed to activate mononuclear phagocytes from cord blood to the level demonstrated by mononuclear phagocytes isolated from adult volunteers. They concluded that subtle defects in the activation of mononuclear phagocytes may occur in newborn subjects and this may contribute to the enhanced susceptibility on newborn infants to infection with such intracellular pathogens as *Toxoplasma gondii.*

Treatment of both adult and cord blood monocyte-derived macrophages with LPS or muramyl dipeptide serves to prime these cells for enhanced production of superoxide anion following a soluble stimulus. When monocytes isolated from cord blood or from the peripheral blood of adult volunteers are cultured in vitro for more than 3 d, the release of superoxide anion by the cord blood monocyte-derived macrophages has been demonstrated to be significantly less than that by monocyte-derived macrophages isolated from adults.[148] Both cord blood and adult monocyte-derived macrophages release less superoxide anion after in vitro culture than when monocytes are freshly isolated from the blood samples. However, as recently reported by Speer et al.,[148] when both adult and cord monocyte-derived macrophages are cultured in the presence of LPS or muramyl dipeptide, the ability to release superoxide anion in response to soluble or particulate stimuli is primed so that superoxide anion generating capacity is nearly equivalent to that of freshly isolated blood monocytes. In these same experiments, cord blood monocyte-derived macrophages failed to respond to the LPS or muramyl dipeptide to the same degree as the adult monocyte-derived macrophages, and therefore, following 3 d of in vitro culture, significantly less superoxide anion was released by the primed cord blood monocyte-derived macrophages. These authors proposed that these results may indicate a diminished capacity of mononuclear phagocytes from newborn infants to undergo maturation into activated macrophages.

Lipopolysaccharide has been shown to increase the synthesis of the third component of complement (C3) and factor B of the alternative complement pathway in mononuclear phagocytes isolated from human adult volunteers.[149] The lipid-A portion of the LPS molecule appears to be the active moiety that induces increased biosynthesis of C3 and factor-B components as well as enhancing superoxide anion, hydrolytic enzyme, and prostaglandin E_2 biosynthesis in mononuclear phagocytes. When biosynthesis of C3 and factor B was examined in cord blood mononuclear phagocytes stimulated by lipid A, no increase in biosynthesis of these molecules was observed. This was significantly different from the response of adult mononuclear phagocytes, which in the presence of lipid A increased C3 synthesis by greater than 11-fold and factor B synthesis by greater than threefold. When cord blood mononuclear phagocytes were co-incubated with adult mononuclear phagocytes in the presence of LPS, a significant enhancement of C3 and factor B synthesis in cord blood mononuclear phagocytes was observed. In this same study, the biosynthesis of superoxide anion and phagocytosis of complement opsonized sheep erythrocytes was enhanced in both cord blood and adult mononuclear phagocyte cultures when these cells were exposed to LPS. These authors concluded that since both cord blood and adult mononuclear phagocytes responded with enhanced reactive oxygen intermediate production and phagocytosis following LPS exposure that qualitative differences in the cell populations did not appear to account for the apparent inability of cord blood monocytes to augment complement biosynthesis in the presence of LPS or lipid A. These studies support a specific difference between cord blood and adult mononuclear phagocytes in the recognition or response to LPS.

Many areas of mononuclear phagocyte immunobiology remain to be examined in the fetal period and the early neonatal period. Further development of techniques to isolate purified populations of mononuclear phagocytes with a detailed examination of the morphological, cytochemical, and plasma membrane antigenic phenotype will enhance our ability to study specific mononuclear phagocyte functions in this age group. Preliminary evidence suggests that mononuclear phagocytes isolated from newborn infants are impaired in their ability to respond to certain activation agents. A more detailed analysis of mononuclear phagocyte activation in newborn infants should elucidate the mechanisms for this impaired response and may provide clues to therapeutic immunomodulation.

Congenital Phagocyte Dysfunction Syndromes

In addition to the leukocyte-adhesion deficiency syndrome described earlier in this chapter, there are several other congenital phagocyte dysfunction syndromes, including chronic granulomatous disease, Chediak-Higashi syndrome, and hyperimmunoglobulin E recurrent infection (Job's) syndrome. These disorders affect both neutrophils and members of the MPS.

Chronic granulomatous disease (CGD) is comprised of a group of phagocyte oxidative metabolic disorders that share a common phenotype. These disorders are inherited as X-linked, autosomal recessive or autosomal dominant patterns.[150] The major clinical features of this disease include recurrent life-threatening infections and the formation of granulomas due to an excessive inflammatory response. The central underlying defect in this disease appears to be abnormalities in the structure, function, or activation of the NADPH oxidase and the associated membrane-bound electron transport system.[151] Impairment in any one of these enzymatic steps in the generation of reactive oxygen intermediates associated with impaired activity of the hexose monophosphate shunt can account for the clinical features of this disease. Affected patients usually present in the first year of life with skin and soft tissue infections, suppurative lymphadenitis, pneumonia with lung abscesses, and occasionally osteomyelitis. Most of these serious infections are caused by *Staphylococcus aureus* and some gram-negative bacteria. Although granulocytes from patients appear to ingest these microorganisms normally, intracellular killing is deficient because of the failure to generate reactive oxygen intermediates. When granulocytes from patients with CGD are studied in vitro, IFN-γ exposure significantly increases superoxide anion production and bactericidal capacity.[152] Recently human recombinant IFN-γ was administered subcutaneously to several patients with CGD.[153] After a 4- to 6-d treatment, neutrophils and monocytes isolated from these patients exhibited five- to tenfold increases in superoxide anion production and significant improvement in phagocyte bactericidal activity against *Staphylococcus aureus*. These preliminary studies are encouraging and suggest that in some patients with CGD, IFN-γ administration may provide some amelioration of phagocyte dysfunction and potentially improve their clinical course.

The Chediak-Higashi syndrome is an autosomal recessive inherited disorder resulting in an increased susceptibility to infection because of a depressed inflammatory response.[154] The major cellular defects that have been identified include impaired neutrophil and mononuclear phagocyte migration and degranulation.[155] In many of these phagocytes, giant lysosomal granules are readily observed by light microscopy. Numerous biochemical defects including abnormal cyclic nucleotide metabolism, disorders of cytoskeletal assembly, and exaggerated oxygen consumption and hydrogen peroxide production are observed in the phagocytes of many of these patients.[156] Currently it is not clear how any of these cellular defects relate to the pathogenesis of this disease. Ascorbate has been utilized in some patients with this disorder. An improvement in neutrophil function in vitro in response to the drug has been observed.[157] A similar disease has been described in beige mice, albino whales, partial albino cattle, and Aleutian mink.[151] Determination of therapeutic agents that correct the neutrophil and mononuclear phagocyte dysfunction in these animals may help identify clinically useful agents for human patients.

Job's syndrome is an eponym that describes a clinical disorder in which patients present with recurrent furunculosis, cellulitis, sinusitis, otitis, and staphylococcal pneumonia.[158] Characteristic laboratory abnormalities include elevated serum IgE concentration with a decreased or absent secretory IgA concentration, a slight elevation of IgM concentration, and a persistent low-grade eosinophilia. Impaired neutrophil and mononuclear phagocyte chemotaxis has been documented in vitro.[159] In some patients with this disorder, mitogen-induced and antigen-induced lymphocyte transformation is also impaired, especially when challenged with *Candida* antigen.[160] This may account for the increased susceptibility of these patients to mucocutaneous candidiasis. Despite enumeration of abnormalities in the in vitro function of lymphocytes and phagocytes from these patients, no specific biochemical defect has been defined.

Conclusions

Phagocytic cells constitute critical elements in the host defense against invading microorganisms. Neutrophils are quantitatively the most important of the phagocytic cells and the first to provide an acute inflammatory response. Mononuclear cells function in the blood in a fashion similar to neutrophils; however, they also migrate into tissues where they differentiate into long-lived tissue macrophages. In this general fashion, the function of neutrophils and monocytes are complimentary and provide a most effective and sustained response to an inflammatory focus. We present only a few selected disorders of phagocytic cell function; many other disorders have been described for which excellent reviews are available.

References

1. Hirsch JG. Host resistance to infectious diseases. In Gallin JI, Fauci AS, eds. *Advances in Host Defense Mechanisms,* Vol. 1, *Phagocytic Cells.* New York: Raven Press; 1982:1–12.
2. Gallin JI, Goldstein IM, Snyderman R. *Inflammation Basic Principles and Clinical Correlates.* New York: Raven Press; 1988.
3. Fulginiti VA, Sieber OF. Immune mechanisms in infectious diseases. In Stiehm ER, Fulginiti VA, eds. *Immunologic Disorders in Infants and Children.* Philadelphia: W.B. Saunders Co; 1973:551–564.
4. Mims CA. The encounter of the microbe with the phagocytic cell. In Mims CA, ed. *The Pathogenesis of Infectious Diseases.* New York: Academic Press, Inc; 1987:63–91.
5. Harris, MC, Polin RA. *Clin Lab Med.* 1985;5:545.
6. Polin RA. *Eur J Clin Microbiol.* 1984;3:387.
7. Drutz DJ. Immunity and infection. In Fudenberg HH, Sites DP, Caldwell JL, Wells JV, eds. *Basic and Clinical Immunology.* Los Altos, California: Lange Medical Publications; 1976:182–194.
8. Stossel TP. The phagocyte system: Structure and Function, In Nathan DG, Oski FA, eds. *Hematology of Infancy and Childhood.* Philadelphia: W.B. Saunders Co; 1987:779–796.
9. Metcalf D. *Blood.* 1986;67:257.
10. Lipton JM, Nathan DG. The anatomy and physiology of hematopoiesis. In Nathan DG, Oski FA, eds. *Hematology of Infancy and Childhood.* Philadelphia: W.B. Saunders Co; 1987:128–158.
11. Curnutte JT, Boxer LA. Disorders of granulopoiesis and granulocyte function. In Nathan DG, Oski FA, eds. *Hematology of Infancy and Childhood.* Philadelphia: W.B. Saunders Co; 1987:797–847.
12. Klebanoff SJ, Clark RA. *The Neutrophil: Function and Clinical Disorders.* New York: North-Holland Publishing Co; 1978:5–72.
13. Bainton DF, Ullyot JL, Farquhar MG. *J Exp Med.* 1971;134:907.
14. Chenoweth DE, Erickson BW, Hugli TE. *Biochem Biophys Res Commun.* 1979;86:227.
15. Arnaout MA, Todd RF, Dana N, Melamed J, Schlossman SF, Colten HR. *J Clin Invest.* 1983;72:171.

16. Alberts B, Bray D, Lewis J, Raff M, Roberts K, Watson JD. *Molecular Biology of the Cell.* New York: Garland Publishing Inc; 1983:549–609.

17. Southwick FS, Stossel TP. *Seminars Hematol.* 1983;20:305.

18. Gallin JI. *Clin Res.* 1984;32:320.

19. Wright DG. The neutrophil as a secretory organ of host defense. In Gallin JI, Fauci AS, eds. *Advances in Host Defense Mechanisms,* Vol. 1, *Phagocytic Cells;* New York: Raven Press; 1981:75–110.

20. Wright DG, Bralove DA, Gallin JI. *Am J Pathol.* 1977;87:273.

21. Gallin JI, Wright DG. *J Clin Invest.* 1978;62:1364.

22. Korchak HM, Rutherford LE, Weissman G. *J Biol Chem.* 1984;259:4070.

23. Korchak HM, Vienne K, Rutherford LE, Wilkenfeld C, Finkelstein MC, and Weissman G. *J Biol Chem.* 1984;259:4076.

24. Skylar LA, Oades AG. *J Biol Chem.* 1985;600:11,468.

25. Hill HR. *Pediatr Res.* 1987;22:375.

26. Malech HL, Gallin JI. *New Engl J Med.* 1987;317:687.

27. Gallin JI. *J Infect Dis.* 1985;152:661.

28. Dana N, Styrt B, Griffin JD, Todd RF III, Klempner MS, Arnaout MA. *J Immunol.* 1986;137:3259.

29. Krensky AM, Robbins E, Springer TA, Burakoff SJ. *J Immunol.* 1984;132:2180.

30. Oseas R, Yang HH, Baehner RL, Boxer LA. *Blood.* 1981;57:939.

31. Snyderman R, and Goetzl EJ. *Science.* 1981;213:830.

32. Stossel TP. The mechanism of leukocyte locomotion. In Gallin JI, Quie PG, eds. *Leukocyte Chemotaxis: Methods, Physiology, and Clinical Implications.* New York: Raven Press; 1978:143–160.

33. Zigmond SH, Hirsch JG. *J Exp Med.* 1973;137:387.

34. Stossel TP. *New Engl J Med.* 1974;290:717.

35. Weissman G, Smolen JE, Korchak HM. *New Engl J Med.* 1980;303:27.

36. Walter RJ, Berlin RD, Oliver AM. Asymmetric Fc receptor distribution on human PMN oriented in a chemotactic gradient. *Nature (London).* 1980;286:724.

37. Babior BM. *J Clin Invest.* 1984;73:599.

38. Elsbach P. *Rev Inf Dis.* 1980;2:106.

39. Nathan CF, Cohn ZA. In Kelley WN, Harris Jr, ED, Ruddy S, Sledge CB, eds. *Textbook of Rheumatology,* Vol. 1, 2nd ed. Philadelphia: W. B. Saunders Co; 1985:144.

40. vanFurth R. Cells of the mononuclear phagocyte system: nomenclature in terms of sites and conditions. In vanFurth R, ed. *Mononuclear Phagocytes—Functional Aspects.* Martinus Nijhoff: Dordrecht; 1980:1.

41. Johnston Jr, RB. *New Engl J Med.* 1988;318:747.

42. Johnston Jr, RB, Zucker-Franklin D. Monocytes and macrophages. In Zucker-Franklin D, Greaves MF, Grossi CE, Marmont AM, eds. *Atlas of Blood Cells: Function and Pathology.* Philadelphia: Lea and Febiger; 1988:323.

43. Broxmeyer HE. *Int J Cell Cloning.* 1986;4:378.

44. Sieff CA. *J Clin Invest.* 1987;79:1549.

45. Bartocci A, Mastrogiannis DS, Migliorati G, Stockert RJ, Wolkoff AN, Stanley ER. *Proc Natl Acad Sci (USA).* 1987;84:6179.

46. vanFurth R, Raeburn JA, vanZwet TL. *Blood.* 1979;54:485.

47. Meuret G, Batara E, Furst HO. *Acta Haematol.* 1975;54:261.

48. Whitelaw DM. *Cell Tissue Kinet.* 1972;5:311.

49. Morahan PS, Volkman A, Melnicoff M, Dempsey WL. Macrophage heterogeneity. In Heppner GH, Fulton AM, eds. *Macrophages and Cancer.* Boca Raton, FL: CRC Press; 1988:1.

50. Douglas SD, Hassan NI, Blaese RM. The mononuclear phagocytic system. In Steihm ER, ed. *Immunologic Disorders in Infants and Children.* New York: W.B. Saunders Co; 1989:81.

51. Cohn ZA. *Harvey Lect.* 1983;77:63.

52. Johnson WD, Mei B, Cohn ZA. *J Exp Med.* 1977;146:1613.

53. Yoder MC, Hassan NI, Douglas SD. Mononuclear phagocyte system. In Polin RA, Fox WW, eds. *Neonatal and Fetal Medicine.* Philadelphia: W.B. Saunders Co; (in press).

54. Zuckerman SH, Ackerman SK, Douglas SD. *Immunology.* 1979;38:401.

55. Hartwig JH. Actin filament architecture and movements in macrophage cytoplasm. In *Biochemistry of macrophages* (Ciba Foundation Symposium 118, April 16–18, 1985). New York: John Wiley & Sons; 1986:42.

56. vanFurth R, Diesselhoff-den Dulk MMC, Sluiter W, vanDissel JT. New perspectives on the kinetics of mononuclear phagocytes. In vanFurth R, ed. *Mononuclear phagocytes: characteristics, physiology and function.* Martinus Nijhoff: Dordrecht; 1985:201.

57. Hayhoe FGJ, Quaglino D, eds. Esterases. In *Haematological Cytochemistry.* New York: Churchill Livingstone; 1980:146.

58. Radzun HJ, Parwaresch MR, Wittke JW. *Cell Immunol.* 1981;63:400.

59. Huber H, Fudenberg HH. *Seminars Haematol.* 1970;3:160.

60. Unkeless JK, Wright SD. Phagocytic cells: Fc, and complement receptors. In Gallin JI, Goldstein IM, Snyderman R, eds. *Inflammation.* New York: Raven Press; 1988:343.

61. Hogg N. *Immunol Today.* 1988;9:185.

62. Wright SD, Griffin Jr, FM. *J Leuk Biol.* 1985;38:327.

63. Hynes RO. *Cell.* 1987;48:549.

64. Todd RF III Schlossman SF. *Blood.* 1982;59:775.

65. Ashmun RA, Peiper SC, Rebentisch MB, Look AT. *Blood.* 1987;69(3):886.

66. Lechler RI. *Immunol Today.* 1988;9:76.

67. vanFurth R, Cohn ZA, Hirsch JG, Humphrey JH, Spector WG, Langevdort HL. *WHO Bull.* 1972;46:845.

68. Kozin F, Cochrane CG. The contact activation system of plasma: biochemistry and pathophysiology. In Gallin JI, Goldstein IM, Snyderman R, eds. *Inflammation.* New York: Raven Press; 1988:101.

69. Snyderman R, Uhing RJ. Phagocytic cells: Stimulus-response coupling mechanisms. In Gallin JI, Goldstein IM, Snyderman R, eds. *Inflammation.* New York: Raven Press; 1988:309.

70. Pawlowski NA, Abraham EL, Pontier S, Scott WA, Cohn ZA. *Proc Natl Acad Sci (USA).* 1985;82:8208.

71. Pohlman TH, Stanness KA, Beatty PG, Ochs HD, Harlan JM. *J Immunol.* 1986;136:4548.

72. Wallis WJ, Beatty PG, Ochs HD, Harlan JM. *J Immunol.* 1985;135:2323.

73. Todd RF III, Freyer DR. *Hematol Oncol Clin North Am.* 1988;2:13.

74. Anderson DC, Springer TA. *Annu Rev Med.* 1987;38:175.

75. Arfors KE, Lundberg CL, Lindbom L, Lundberg K, Beatty PG, Harlan JM. *Blood.* 1987;69:338.

76. Simpson PJ, Todd RF III, Fantone JC, Mickelson JK, Griffin JD, Lucchesi BR. *J Clin Invest.* 1988;81:624.

77. Vedder NB, Winn RK, Rice CL, Chi EY, Arfors KE, Harlan JM. *J Clin Invest.* 1988;81:939.

78. Griffin FM Jr, Griffin JA, Leider JE, Silverstein SC. *J Exp Med*. 1975;142:1263.

79. Riches DWH. The multiple roles of macrophages in wound healing. In Clark RAF, Henson PM, eds. *The Molecular and Cellular Biology of Wound Repair*. New York: Plenum Press; 1988:213.

80. Chaudhry AN, Santinga, JT, Gabig TG. *Blood*. 1982;60:979.

81. Box A, Wever R, Roos D. *Biochim Biophys Acta*. 1979;525:37.

82. Baehner RL, Johnston Jr, RB. *Blood*. 1972;40:31.

83. Klein SM, Cohen G, Cederbaum AI. *FEBS Lett*. 1980;116:220.

84. Musson RA, McPhail LC, Shafran H, Johnston Jr, RB. *J Reticuloendothel Soc*. 1982;31:261.

85. Nakagawara A, DeSantis NM, Nogueira N, Nathan CF. *J Clin Invest*. 1981;68:1243.

86. Locksley RM, Wilson CB, Klebanoff SJ. *J Clin Invest*. 1982;69:1099.

87. Elsbach P, Weiss J. Phagocytic cells: Oxygen-independent antimicrobial systems. In Gallin JI, Goldstein IM, Snyderman R, eds. *Inflammation*. New York: Raven Press; 1988:334.

88. Elsbach P, Weiss J. *Rev Infect Dis*. 1983;5:843.

89. Adams DO, Hamilton TA. *Annu Rev Immunol*. 1984;2:283.

90. Adams DO, Johnson WJ, Marino PA. *Fed Proc*. 1982;41:134.

91. Adams DO, Hamilton TA. Phagocytic cells: cytotoxic activities of macrophages. In Gallin JI, Goldstein IM, Snyderman R, eds. *Inflammation*. New York: Raven Press; 1988:471.

92. Adams DO, Cohen MS, Koren HS. Activation of mononuclear phagocytes for cytolysis: Parallels and contrasts between activation for tumor cytotoxicity and for ADCC. In Koren HS, ed. *Macrophage Mediated Antibody-Dependent Cellular Cytoxicity*. New York: Marcel Dekker; 1983:43.

93. Somers SD, Johnson WJ, Adams DO. Destruction of tumor cells by macrophages: Mechanisms of recognition and lysis and their regulation. In Herberman R, ed. *Basic and Clinical Tumor Immunology*. New York: Marcel Dekker; 1986:69.

94. Nathan CF. *J Clin Invest*. 1987;79:319.

95. Jones PA, Werb Z. *J Exp Med*. 1980;152:1527.

96. Martin BM, Gimbrone MA, Unanue ER, Cotran RS. *J Immunol*. 1981;126:1510.

97. Polverini PJ, Cotran RS, Gimbrone MA, Unanue ER. *Nature (London)*. 1977;269:804.

98. Ross R, Benditt EP. *J Biochem Cytol*. 1961;11:677.

99. Unanue ER, Allen PM. *Science*. 1987;246:551.

100. Ziegler HK, Unanue ER. *J Immunol*. 1981;127:1869.

101. Ashwell JD, Schwartz RH. *Nature (London)*. 1986;320:176.

102. Unanue ER. *Annu Rev Immunol*. 1984;2:395.

103. Snyder DS, Beller DI, Unanue ER. *Nature (London)*. 1982;299:163.

104. Harris MC, Polin RA. *Pediatr Clin N Am*. 1983;30:243.

105. Miller ME. In Oliver TK, ed. *Host Defenses in the Human Neonate*. New York: Grune and Stratton; 1978:59.

106. Anderson DC, Hughes BJ, Smith CW. *J Clin Invest*. 1981;68:863.

107. Miller ME. *Pediatr Res*. 1971;5:487.

108. Strauss RG, Snyder EL. *Pediatr Res*. 1984;18:63.

109. Sacchi F, Hill HR. *J Exp Med*. 1984;160:1247.

110. Strauss RG, Nyder ELS. *J Leuk Biol*. 1985;37:423.

111. Hill HR, Augustine NH, Newton JA, Shigeoka AO, Morris E, Sacchi F. *Am J Pathol*. 1987;128:307.

112. Miller ME. *Clin Immunol Immunopathol*. 1979;14:503.

113. Anderson DC, Hughes BJ, Wibel LJ, Perry GJ, Smith CW, Brinkley BR. *J Leuk Biol.* 1984;36:1.

114. Harris MC, Douglas SD. *Pediatr Res.* 1986;20:386a.

115. Harris MC, Shalit M, Southwick FS. *Pediatr Res.* 1987;21:408a.

116. Harris MC, Levitt J, Douglas SD, Gerdes JS, Polin RA. *J Clin Microbiol.* 1985;21:243.

117. Anderson DC, Freeman KB, Heerdt B, Hughes BJ, Jack RM, Smith CW. *Blood.* 1987;70:740.

118. Bruce MC, Baley JE, Medvik KA, Berger M. *Pediatr Res.* 1987;21:306.

119. Smith JB, Campbell DE, Douglas SD, Garty BZ, Ludomirsky A, Polin RA, Harris MC. *Pediatr Res.* 1988;22:468a.

120. Mease AD, Burgess DP, Thomas PJ. *Am J Pathol.* 1981;104:98.

121. Boner A, Zeligs BJ, Bellanti JA. *Infect Immun.* 1982;35:921.

122. Krause PJ, Malech HL, Kristie J, Kosciol CM, Herson VC, Eisenfeld L, Pastuszak WT, Kraus A, Seligman B. *Blood.* 1986;68:200.

123. Dossett JH, Williams RC, Quie PG. *Pediatrics.* 1969;44:49.

124. Miller ME. *J Pediatr.* 1969;74:255.

125. Harris MC, Stroobant J, Cody CS, Douglas SD, Polin RA. *Pediatr Res.* 1983;17:358.

126. Pross SH, Hallock JA, Armstrong R, Fishel CW. *Pediatr Res.* 1977;11:135.

127. McCracken GH Jr, Eichenwald HF. *Am J Dis Child.* 1971;121:120.

128. Forman ML, Stiehm ER. *New Engl J Med.* 1969;281:926.

129. Quie PG, Mills EL. *Peds Supp.* 1979;64:719.

130. Wright WC, Ank BJ, Herbert J, Stiehm ER. *Pediatrics.* 1975;56:579.

131. Stroobant JS, Harris MC, Cody CS, Polin RA, Douglas SD. *Pediatr Res.* 1984;18:634.

132. Shigeoka AO, Charette RP, Wyman ML, Hill HR. *J Pediatr.* 1981;98:392.

133. Ambruso DR, Altenburger KM, Johnston RB Jr. *Pediatrics.* 1979;64:722.

134. Ambruso DR, Bentwood B, Henson PM, Johnston RB Jr. *Pediatr Res.* 1984;18:1148.

135. Bullock JD, Robertson AF, Bodenbender JG, Kontras SB, Miller CE. *Pediatrics.* 1969;44:58.

136. Yegin O. *Pediatr Res.* 1983;17:183.

137. Raghunathan R, Miller ME, Everett S, Leake RD. *J Clin Immunol.* 1982;2:242.

138. Boner A, Zeligs BJ, Bellanti JA. *Infect Immun.* 1982;35:921.

139. Speer ChP, Wieland M, Ulbrich R, Gahr M. *Eur J Pediatr.* 1986;145:418.

140. Bhoopat L, Taylor CR, Hofman FM. *Clin Immunol Immunopathol.* 1986;41:184.

141. Adinolfi M, Cheetham M, Lee T, Rodin A. *Eur J Immunol.* 1988;18:565.

142. Schuit KE, Powell DA. *Pediatrics.* 1980;65:501.

143. Marodi L, Leijh PCJ, vanFurth R. *Pediatr Res.* 1984;18:1127.

144. Jacobs RF, Kiel DP, Sanders ML, Steele RW. *J Infect Dis.* 1985;152:695.

145. Speer CP, Gahr M, Wieland M, Eber S. *Pediatr Res.* 1988;24:213.

146. Speer CP, Johnston Jr, RB. Phagocyte function. In Ogra PL, ed. *Neonatal Infections.* Orlando, FL: Grune & Stratton; 1984:21.

147. Wilson CB, Westall J. *Infect Immun.* 1985;49:351.

148. Speer CP, Ambruso DR, Grimsley J, Johnston Jr, RB. *Infect Immun.* 1985;50:919.

149. St. John Sutton MB, Strunk RC, Cole CF. *J Immunol.* 1986;136:1366.

150. Gallin JL, Buescher ES, Seligmann BE, Nath J, Gaither TE, Katz P. *Ann Int Med.* 1983;99:657.

151. Gallin JI. Phagocytic cells: disorders of function. In Gallin JI, Goldstein IM, Snyderman R, eds. *Inflammation*. New York: Raven Press; 1988:493.

152. Ezekowitz RAB, Phil D, Dinauer MC, Jaffe HS, Orkin SH, Newburger PE. *New Engl J Med*. 1988;319:146.

153. Sechler JMG, Malech HL, White CJ, Gallin JI. *Proc Natl Acad Sci (USA)*. 1988;85:4874.

154. Wolff SM, Dale DC, Clark RA, Root RK, Kimball HR. *Ann Int Med*. 1972;76:293.

155. Clark RA, Kimball HR. *J Clin Invest*. 1971;50:2645.

156. Nath J, Flavin M, Gallin JL. *J Cell Biol*. 1982;95:519.

157. Boxer LA, Watanabe AM, Rister M, Besch Jr, HR, Allen J, Bachner RL. *New Engl J Med*. 1976;295:1041.

158. Donabedian H, Gallin JL. *Medicine*. 1983;62:195.

159. Donabedian H, Gallin JI. *Infect Immun*. 1983;40:1030.

160. Gallin JL, Wright DG, Malech HL, Davis JM, Klempner MS, Kirkpatrick CH. *Ann Int Med*. 1980;95:520.

CHAPTER 12

Immunodeficiency Diseases

Naynesh R. Kamani

Division of Allergy-Immunology, Children's Hospital of Philadelphia, 34th Street and Civic Center Boulevard, University of Pennsylvania School of Medicine, Philadelphia, PA 19104 USA

Introduction

The normal host immune response involves a complex series of interactions between the four major arms of the immune system: the cellular immune system, the humoral immune system, phagocytic cells, and the complement system. A brief overview of the immune response follows.

The Normal Immune Response

The primary function of the immune system is to discriminate "self" from "nonself." In order to do this, a complex but well-orchestrated series of interactions must take place between different components of the afferent and efferent limbs of the immune response following an encounter with a nonself antigen.[1,2] The afferent limb of the immune response involves the processing and presentation of the antigen by "antigen-presenting cells" to immunocytes that can specifically recognize antigen. Monocytes and macrophages are the principal antigen-presenting cells, although B cells, vascular endothelial cells, and dendritic cells can also serve in this capacity. When first encountered by macrophages, antigen may be ingested and processed by unfacilitated phagocytosis. Upon subsequent exposure, however, the presence of antibody (opsonin) and complement greatly facilitate phagocytosis via the macrophage Fc and C3b receptors. Once ingested, antigen is partially degraded into smaller fragments, which can then be reexpressed on the macrophage cell surface in the context of major histocompatibility complex (MHC) molecules for specific recognition by T and B cells. During the process of antigen presentation, monocytes and macrophages release many cytokines, including interleukin-1 (IL-1) and α-interferon, which serve to activate T cells and enhance their ability to recognize antigen. These activated T cells, in turn, aid in the afferent arm of the immune response by releasing other cytokines that facilitate the antigen-processing and -presenting function of macrophages; these include γ-interferon and macrophage inhibitory factor (MIF).

Once antigen has been presented to T and B cells, the effector arm of the immune response is set in motion. Specific recognition of antigen occurs via the T-cell antigen receptor (T3–Ti complex) on T lymphocytes and via surface immunoglobulin on B cells. Helper–inducer T cells bearing CD4 play a central role in the effector response. They elaborate interleukin-2, which promotes entry of resting T lymphocytes into S phase and their subsequent proliferation. Interleukin-2 induces helper cells to produce other lymphokines and enhances the function of other lymphocyte subsets, such as CD8-bearing suppressor T cells or cytotoxic T cells. Activated helper T cells also release several B-cell lymphokines, including B-cell growth factor (BCGF), B-cell differentiation factor (BCDF), and IL-4, that induce the differentiation of antigen-driven B cells into antibody-secreting plasma cells.[3] Cytotoxic T cells recognize antigen on the surface of only those target cells that express the same class-I molecules as the effector T cells (ie, in the context of self-MHC class-I molecules) and cause direct target cell death. Suppressor T cells elaborate suppressor factors that can regulate the function of T and B cells. γ-Interferon released by activated T lymphocytes can promote the activity of natural killer cells (NKC) that have the ability to kill target cells, such as tumor cells, in the absence of antibody. The complement system, which consists of over 20 immunologically and chemically distinct plasma proteins, is an integral component of the effector arm of the immune response. The activation of the complement cascade by antigen–antibody complexes or aggregated immunoglobulins via the classic pathway leads to the generation of mediators of inflammation and of the terminal attack complex, which can cause direct cell damage of opsonized targets.[4]

Immunodeficiencies

Immunodeficiency diseases can be broadly classified into primary immunodeficiencies, ie, those that arise from primary defects of the immune system, and secondary immunodeficiencies, ie, those that occur secondary to other underlying causes.[5] Primary immunodeficiencies can be divided into several major categories based on the arm of the immune system that is affected. These are listed in Table 12-1 along with examples of immunodeficiencies in each category. There are numerous causes of secondary immunodeficiencies (see Table 12-2). Acquired immune deficiency syndrome (AIDS) secondary to infection with the human immunodeficiency virus (HIV) is a classic example of a secondary immunodeficiency.

Primary immunodeficiencies can result from abnormalities of any component of the host immune system. Defects such as those resulting from the absolute deficiency or impairment of function of cellular components, immunoglobulins, complement components, cytokines, or as yet undefined factors can render the host defenseless against endogenous or exogenous microorganisms and result in increased susceptibility to infection. If left untreated, these defects can result in the eventual death of the host.

The cardinal manifestation of primary immune deficiency is an increased susceptibility to infections. Although recurrent infections are the hallmark of primary immune deficiencies in children and adults, it is important to note that the majority of children with recurrent infections do not have primary immune defects. Since

Table 12-1. Classification of Primary Immunodeficiencies

1. Defects of humoral (B-cell) immunity
   X-Linked agammaglobulinemia (hypogammaglobulinemia)
   X-Linked immunodeficiency with hyper-IgM
   Selective IgA deficiency
   Transient hypogammaglobulinemia of infancy
2. (a) Defects of cellular (T-cell) immunity
      DiGeorge syndrome
      Chronic mucocutaneous candidiasis
   (b) Combined B-cell and T-cell immunodeficiencies
      Severe combined immunodeficiency (X-linked or autosomal recessive)
      Wiskott-Aldrich symdrome
      Ataxia–telangiectasia
      Adenosine deaminase deficiency
3. Phagocytic dysfunction syndromes
   Chronic granulomatous disease
   Chediak-Higashi syndrome
   Leukocyte-adhesion (LFA-1) deficiency
4. Complement deficiencies
   C1q, C1r, and C1s deficiency
   C2 deficiency
   C8 deficiency

Table 12-2. Causes of Secondary Immunodeficiencies

Infections
   Congenital infections: HIV, cytomegalovirus, rubella virus
   Acquired immunodeficiency syndrome, secondary to HIV infection
   Systemic viral, bacterial, or fungal infections
Malnutrition
   Protein–calorie
   Iron; zinc
Stress
Malignancies
Protein-losing states
   Protein-losing enteropathy
   Nephrotic syndrome
Immunosuppressive therapy
   Radiation
   Drugs: corticosteroids, cyclosporine, cyclophosphamide
Prematurity
Pregnancy
Aging
Other disorders
   Down's syndrome
   Diabetes mellitus, sarcoidosis
   Uremia, burns,
   Splenectomy

normal, immunocompetent children can have frequent and recurrent infections, the differentiation of the normal child from a truly immunodeficient one is important. There are several other causes for recurrent infections in childhood and these need to be excluded before a diagnosis of immunodeficiency is made. Some of these causes are listed in Table 12-3.

The majority of immune deficiencies manifest themselves in infancy or early childhood. Most immunodeficiency disorders are congenital; many are inherited either as sex-linked or autosomal recessive traits. Primary immunodeficiencies are significantly more common in males, especially in children under age 15. Common variable hypogammaglobulinemia, which generally manifests itself in the second or third decade of life, occurs more frequently in females.

Most primary immunodeficiencies occur infrequently and a few are extremely rare. It has been estimated that the overall incidence of primary immunodeficiency disorders is about $1:50,000$ general population. This does not take into account selective IgA deficiency, which is believed to occur at a frequency of $1:600$ population. Many cases of selective IgA deficiency, however, go undiagnosed or unreported because most patients with this immunodeficiency have few, if any, clinically significant infections secondary to the IgA deficiency.

A thorough history and physical examination should lead to the recognition of the immunodeficient individual in the majority of cases. Since different immunodeficiencies have different modes of presentation, the delineation of the underlying immune defect can often be made on the basis of a careful history, physical examination, and an immunodeficiency screening laboratory workup.

The history should look into the frequency, severity, and types of infections; the age of onset of infections; the effects of therapy on the course of the infections; and the presence of accompanying symptoms, such as chronic diarrhea and growth failure. Individuals with immunodeficiencies have an increased frequency of severe and protracted infections, often with complications and unusual manifestations. Opportunistic infections, ie, infections with organisms of low pathogenicity, are

Table 12-3. Causes of Recurrent Infections in Immunocompetent Children

Unusual exposure
   eg, attendance at daycare centers; siblings attending school
Integumental defects
   eg, eczema; immotile cilia syndrome
Congenital anomalies
   eg, Tracheoesophageal fistula; congenital cardiac defects
Inherited disorders
   eg, cystic fibrosis; α-1-antitrypsin deficiency; sickle cell
   disease
Atopic disorders
   eg, bronchial asthma; allergic rhinitis
Foreign bodies
   eg, inhaled foreign bodies; central venous catheter
Secondary immunodeficiency states

quite common in immunodeficient hosts. In general, children with humoral immunodeficiencies do not manifest infections until about 5–6 months of age because they are protected up to that age by passively acquired maternal antibody. Children with T-cell immunodeficiencies, on the other hand, present with infections very early in infancy. An analysis of the types of infections often aids in determining the nature of the underlying immunodeficiency; eg, recurrent bacterial infections are common in hypogammaglobulinemia, whereas infections with fungi and intracellular microbes such as viruses and protozoa are more frequently seen in children with cellular immunodeficiencies. Individuals with neutrophil dysfunction syndromes often have superficial and deep-seated staphylococcal and fungal infections. Recurrent infections with neisserial organisms are a hallmark of deficiencies of the later complement components (Table 12-4).

Because many immunodeficiencies are inherited, a detailed family history with the construction of a pedigree is vital. The family history on the maternal side has obvious relevance in sex-linked disorders. A history of early deaths or recurrent infections or autoimmune disorders in siblings or other relatives can be an important clue. Special scrutiny of the skin, lymphoid tissues, lungs, and reticuloendothelial organs, along with an evaluation of the physical growth of the patient is essential as part of a thorough physical examination. There are a number of specific findings that are associated with specific immunodeficiency disorders eg, partial albinism in Chediak-Higashi syndrome, tetany in DiGeorge syndrome.

An immunological workup that screens for defects of each component of the immune system should be performed in all patients in whom an underlying immunodeficiency is suspected. Such a workup can be performed in most hospital laboratories and can lead to a diagnosis in over 75% of cases of immunodeficiencies. The remainder can generally be identified after specialized and more sophisticated tests of immune function are performed. A screening workup should include a complete blood count with a differential count; measurement of serum IgG, IgA, IgM, and IgE; delayed hypersensitivity skin testing; evaluation of antibody responses to spe-

Table 12-4. Infectious agents in Primary Immunodeficiencies

Humoral
   Bacterial: *Pneumococcus, Hemophilus, Pseudomonas*
   Viral: ECHO virus, poliovirus
   Protozoal: *Giardia, Pneumocystis carinii*
   Other: *Mycoplasma, Ureaplasma*
Cellular
   Bacterial: Mycobacteria, *Salmonella*
   Fungal: *Candida albicans, Cryptococcus*
   Protozoa: *P. carinii, Toxoplasma, Cryptosporidium*
   Viral: CMV, HSV, EBV, RSV, adenovirus, rotavirus
Phagocytic
   Bacterial: *Staphylococcus, Klebsiella, Escherichia coli*
   Fungal: *C. albicans, Aspergillus*
Complement
   Bacterial: *Pneumococcus, Neisseria, Klebsiella, Hemophilus*

cific antigens, such as tetanus toxoid; isohemagglutinin titers to evaluate for the presence of functional IgM antibody; nitroblue tetrazolium dye reduction to evaluate neutrophil oxidative metabolism; and hemolytic complement (CH50) to assess functional activity of complement components.

Immunodeficiency diseases can be classified into four major categories based on the specific component of the immune system that is affected: (1) B-cell or humoral immunodeficiencies, (2) T-cell or cellular immunodeficiencies, (3) phagocytic dysfunction disorders, and (4) complement deficiencies. An additional category may include those disorders in which there is a combined humoral and cellular defect(s).[6,7] A detailed discussion of all the immunodeficiencies is beyond the scope of this chapter. In the discussion that follows, the major manifestations of prototypic immunodeficiencies from each major category are described, and the pathogenesis and therapy of immunodeficiency disorders are reviewed.

B-Cell Immunodeficiencies

Humoral immunodeficiency disorders constitute just over half of all immunodeficiencies encountered in clinical practice. These deficiencies are predominantly of B-cell function but because of the interaction between T and B cells during the immune response, abnormalities of the T-cell system may coexist in some of these disorders. Antibody immunodeficiency disorders may range from a disorder with a marked paucity of all immunoglobulin isotypes, eg, X-linked hypogammaglobulinemia, to one where only a single immunoglobulin class or subclass may be absent, eg, selective IgA deficiency or IgG2 subclass deficiency.

The characteristic manifestations of defects of humoral immunity are recurrent bacterial infections, often involving the respiratory and gastrointestinal tracts. Symptomatology is generally milder in those deficiencies where only a single class of antibody is deficient. Infections generally do not manifest until after 6 months of age, when passively acquired maternal IgG has been completely eliminated from the infant's circulation. Normal serum levels of IgG, IgA, IgM, and IgE and the presence of functional antibodies as assessed by titers of isohemagglutinins (IgM) and antibodies to specific antigens such as diphtheria or tetanus (IgG) will for the most part rule out an underlying B-cell defect. A more thorough evaluation of B-cell immunity should include a measurement of circulating B cells, lymphocyte proliferative responses to T-cell-independent B-cell mitogens (staphylococcal protein A- Cowan I strain), in vitro immunoglobulin synthesis, and specific antibody responses following in vivo immunization.[8]

X-Linked Hypogammaglobulinemia

This X-linked humoral immunodeficiency disorder is characterized by the onset of recurrent pyogenic infections of the respiratory tract after 6 months of age.[9] Chronic pulmonary disease is seen as a long-term sequela in a significant number of patients. Sepsis, meningitis, and osteomyelitis can also occur. Most of the infections in these patients are caused by encapsulated bacteria, streptoccocci and *Pseudomonas aeruginosa.* A marked paucity or even absence of lymphoid tissues is the cardinal physical finding. Lymphoid tissues from these patients show no plasma cells, lymphoid follicles, or germinal centers. B cells cannot be demonstrated in the peripheral circulation by routine immunofluorescent techniques. There is a marked deficiency or absence of all immunoglobulin isotypes in the serum. Although most patients have no problem in dealing with viral infections, some develop indolent, progressive, and often fatal chronic ECHO virus infections. Vaccine-associated poliomyelitis after inadvertent immunization has been seen in a number of patients. Prompt institution of parenteral gammaglobulin therapy replacement can lead to normal physical growth and delay in the onset of or even prevention of chronic pulmonary disease.

T-Cell Immunodeficiencies

Cellular immunodeficiency disorders and combined B- and T-cell immunodeficiencies account for over a third of all immunodeficiency disorders. Frequent and recurrent viral, fungal, and other opportunistic infections starting in early infancy associated with growth failure are common presenting features. The degree of immunodeficiency varies from disorder to disorder and is most severe in the syndrome of severe combined immunodeficiency (SCID) characterized by thymic dysplasia, absent cellular immunity, and low to absent serum immunoglobulins.

Many of the T-cell immunodeficiencies are characterized by relative or absolute lymphopenia, although its absence does not rule out the presence of an underlying cellular immune defect. Investigations of T-cell immunity should include delayed hypersensitivity skin testing to recall antigens; quantitation of circulating T cells and their subsets; evaluation of lymphocyte proliferative responses to mitogens, antigens, and allogeneic cells, and when appropriate, the determination of levels of enzymes of the purine metabolic pathway.

DiGeorge Syndrome

This is a cellular immunodeficiency arising from abnormal embryologic development of the pharyngeal pouches. It is characterized by a congenital absence or hypoplasia of the thymus, hypocalcemic tetany secondary to hypoparathyroidism, congenital heart disease, and an unusual facies. A wide spectrum of thymic deficiency with differing clinical presentations and courses has been observed. Patients with an early onset of recurrent viral infections, persistent oral candidiasis, or opportunistic infections and other features of this syndrome should be worked up for DiGeorge syndrome. Recalcitrant hypocalcemia, especially during the neonatal period, is a common finding. A number of congenital heart defects, including interrupted aortic arch and persistent truncus arteriosus, have been reported.[10] Some children with milder forms of this syndrome have shown progressive improvement in cellular function over time. Others will require interventional therapy with either bone marrow transplantation or fetal thymic transplantation.

Severe Combined Immunodeficiency

This is a group of congenital diseases of diverse etiology that result in deficiencies of both the T- and B-cell immune systems and death, in the absence of treatment, within the first 2 years of life in the majority of patients.[11] Most patients demonstrate marked lymphopenia, hypogammaglobulinemia, and recurrent viral, bacterial, fungal, and protozoal infections. Both X-linked and autosomal recessive forms of SCID have been described. Approximately half of all autosomal recessive cases (20% of all cases) are caused by adenosine deaminase (ADA) deficiency.[12] Deficiency of ADA, an enzyme that catalyzes the conversion of adenosine and deoxyadenosine to inosine and deoxyinosine during normal purine catabolism, results in the accumulation of metabolites that inhibit lymphocyte function and are toxic to lymphocytes. The treatment of choice for SCID is bone marrow transplantation from a histoidentical sibling donor. In the absence of such a donor, a T-cell depleted haploidentical bone marrow transplant from one of the parents can result in normal immunoreconstitution in over 70% of cases.[13]

Phagocyte Dysfunction Syndromes

Primary defects of phagocyte function occur infrequently and are responsible for less than 10% of all primary immunodeficiencies. Secondary defects are much more common and are seen in association with diseases such as diabetes, systemic lupus erythematosus (SLE), and rheumatoid arthritis, in malnutrition, and following immunosuppressive or cancer chemotherapy. Patients with phagocytic defects have a propensity for developing bacterial (especially staphylococcal) and fungal infections of the skin, lungs, liver, and bone. Periodontal infections are not uncommon in many patients with these defects. Most patients with phagocytic defects have intact cellular and humoral immunity. Workups for phagocyte dysfunction should include a complete blood count and differential count, evaluation of polymorphonuclear neutrophil (PMN) granule morphology, myeloperoxidase content, in vitro chemotaxis, and in vivo Rebuck skin window. Polymorphonuclear neutrophil oxidative metabolism can be assessed by a number of assays, including chemiluminescence, superoxide generation, and microbicidal assays. Nitroblue tetrazolium dye (NBT) reduction by neutrophils is a simple test for PMN oxidative metabolic function. Leukocyte cell-surface expression of plasma membrane glycoproteins involved with granulocyte adherence (C3bi receptor) can be determined with the help of monoclonal antibodies. When indicated, levels of leukocyte enzymes, such as glucose-6-phosphate dehydrogenase (G6PD) and glutathione peroxidase, should be measured.

Chronic Granulomatous Disease (CGD)

This inherited disorder of phagocyte function is characterized by an inability of patient PMNs to produce superoxide anion upon ingestion of catalase-positive microorganisms. It is due to a defect in the membrane-associated NADPH oxidase enzyme system.[14] The majority of patients have the X-linked form of the disease. Patients with CGD have an early onset of recurrent purulent infections of the skin, reticuloendothelial organs, and lungs caused by catalase-positive bacteria and fungi, such as staphylococci and *Candida*. Therapy for most patients consists of life-long antibiotic prophylactic therapy and aggressive treatment of infections. Bone marrow transplantation may be considered if a matched sibling donor is available and offers the only potential for long-term cure of this disorder.[15] γ-Interferon has recently been shown to increase in vitro and in vivo bactericidal activity of PMNs from some patients with CGD and may hold some promise.[16]

Complement Deficiencies

Primary defects of complement components have now been described for the majority of serum complement glycoproteins. Patients with these defects have a propensity for developing autoimmune disorders and recurrent bacterial infections. Deficiencies of complement components occur as secondary phenomena in a number of collagen–vascular diseases. All primary complement deficiencies, with the possible exception of properdin deficiency, are inherited in an autosomal fashion. These defects are extremely rare and account for less than 5% of all primary immunodeficiencies.[17] Workups of patients suspected of having complement deficiencies should start with determination of total hemolytic complement (CH50) which is a good screen for the functional integrity of the complement cascade and C3 and C4 levels. These can be readily determined in most hospital laboratories. When indicated, individual complement components can be immunochemically and functionally assayed in specialized laboratories.

Autoimmune diseases, especially systemic lupus erythematosus, and recurrent pneumococcal infections are characteristically seen in patients with deficiencies of the earlier complement components such as C1, C4, and C2. Patients with terminal complement component defects typically have recurrent systemic neisserial infections. Despite the fact that these deficiencies are inherited, neisserial infections in these patients often manifest for the first time during the second decade of life. There is no optimal therapy for complement deficiencies. Early detection and aggressive treatment of bacterial infections are the mainstay of therapy. Vaccination with pneumococcal and meningococcal vaccines appears not to offer additional protection against infection since these patients have intact natural humoral immunity. Because of the short in vivo half life of complement proteins, transfusions of fresh frozen plasma may be clinically useful only during acute infectious episodes.

Pathogenesis of Immunodeficiencies

Deficiencies of the immune system can result from a number of underlying aberrations. Examples of different etiologic mechanisms include (1) embryologic maldevelopment, such as that seen in the DiGeorge syndrome; (2) a failure of differentiation of lymphoid stem cells into T and B cells, such as that postulated in X-linked

SCID; (3) a purine metabolic pathway enzyme deficiency (ADA or PNP) that leads to accumulation of metabolites that may be toxic to or inhibit the function of lymphocytes; (4) genetically mediated absence of synthesis of complement components, eg, C4 deficiency; (5) gene defects resulting in the absence or defective synthesis of cell-surface glycoproteins (eg, LFA-1) or cellular enzyme components (eg, phagocyte NADPH oxidase) that are vital to the normal functioning of cells involved in host defence.[2,5]

Although significant progress has been made in recent years in delineating the pathogenetic mechanisms of many primary immunodeficiencies at the cellular and molecular levels, most of the underlying defects remain undefined. Primary immunodeficiencies, for the most part, are inherited either as sex-linked recessive or autosomal traits. By definition, the genetic defects in the X-linked immunodeficiencies, such as X-linked hypogammaglobulinemia (XLA), X-linked SCID, and X-linked CGD, must be located on the X chromosome. In several of the immunodeficiencies the genes affected have been identified using DNA linkage analysis and reverse genetics. In CGD, for example, the specific protein defect has not been definitively identified but monocytes from CGD patients have been shown to lack the mRNA transcript of the putative CGD gene believed to be confined to the Xp21.1 locus on the X chromosome. Since most CGD patients do not have gene deletions or rearrangements, it is believed that the genetic defect in most patients results from limited mutations involving a few or perhaps single nucleotides.[18] Gene defects have been localized in the Xq21.3.q22 locus in patients with XLA and to the Xq12.q13 locus in patients with X-SCID.[19]

Leukocyte-adhesion deficiency is an autosomal recessively inherited immunodeficiency disorder characterized by recurrent, purulent infections of the oral, gastrointestinal, respiratory, and genital mucous membranes. The gene defect consists of a mutation in the gene that codes for the β-subunit shared by the heterodimers LFA-1, MAC-1, and p150,95 expressed on leukocyte surfaces. The absence or deficient expression of this adhesive glycoprotein results in an inability of patient phagocytes to adhere to endothelial surfaces and migrate to sites of infection.[20] In patients with the Wiskott-Aldrich syndrome, there is absence or dysfunction of a 115,000 mol wt surface sialoglycoprotein, sialophorin, normally present on the surfaces of lymphocytes and the absence of a glycoprotein 1b on platelets.[21]

Therapy

Over the past several years, the outlook for the majority of patients with primary immunodeficiencies has become brighter than ever before. Reasons for this include the advances that have made haploidentical bone marrow transplantation feasible and the availability of safe and efficacious intravenous gammaglobulin preparations. With the delineation of the precise gene defects responsible for many of the immunodeficiencies and the much anticipated advent of gene therapy, it is hoped that most patients with immunodeficiencies will be able to undergo beneficial therapy in the near future.

The early detection of infection and prompt institution of antimicrobial therapy during infections is of paramount importance in all immunodeficiencies. Measures to prevent the acquisition of nosocomial infections should be strictly followed in patients with cellular immunodeficiencies. Continuous antibiotic prophylaxis is still the most rational therapy for patients with CGD or the hyper-IgE syndrome and in patients with agammaglobulinemia who continue to have recurrent infections despite replacement gammaglobulin therapy. In patients with neutrophil dysfunction syndromes such as CGD, granulocyte transfusions should only be used as an adjunct to therapy in overwhelming bacterial or fungal infections when there is a failure to respond to appropriate antimicrobial therapy.

Periodic intravenous (IV) or intramuscular (IM) gammaglobulin is the mainstay of therapy for most patients with humoral immunodeficiency disorders and has virtually replaced fresh frozen plasma as a therapeutic modality for this purpose. Despite their cost, IV gammaglobulin preparations are generally more desirable than the im product because they are as safe, are less painful, and allow for the achievement of normal or close to normal circulating immunoglobulin levels. It is also quite likely that institution of periodic IV gammaglobulin therapy during infancy or early childhood will help prevent the sequelae of chronic sinopulmonary infection.

Transfer factor (TF), which is a dialyzable extract of immune leukocytes, has been used as therapy for a number of disorders of cellular immunity, including chronic mucocutaneous candidiasis and the Wiskott-Aldrich syndrome. Since well-controlled clinical trials demonstrating its efficacy are lacking and because of inconsistencies in the potency of different TF extracts, its use has always been controversial. Other cytokines such as interferon-γ (in CGD) and interleukin-2 (in certain cellular immunodeficiencies) are being evaluated for their therapeutic potential. Enzyme replacement therapy is an option for patients with ADA deficiency. Promising results have recently been reported by Hershfield and co-workers using weekly injections of polyethyleneglycol-modified bovine ADA in several patients with ADA deficiency.[22]

Bone marrow transplantation (BMT) from histocompatible donors is considered to be the therapy of choice for patients with SCID syndromes and other fatal primary T-cell immunodeficiencies. In the past several years, many patients with SCID have been successfully immunoreconstituted following T-cell-depleted haploidentical bone marrow transplantation. A number of other primary immunodeficiencies, including the Wiskott-Aldrich syndrome, CGD, leukocyte-adhesion LFA-1 deficiency, and the Chediak-Higashi syndrome, can also be corrected with allogeneic BMT. Fetal liver and thymus transplants and cultured thymic epithelial transplants have all been utilized in T-cell immunodeficiencies and SCID with limited and often transient improvement. Somatic gene therapy appears to be on the horizon, especially for disorders such as ADA deficiency where the manifestations of the gene defect are most severely expressed in bone marrow-derived cells, where BMT is curative, and where there are no other somatic manifestations of any significance.[23]

Efforts aimed at preventing immunodeficiencies can be expected to be of use only in disorders like Immunodeficiency with hyper-IgM which has been seen in association with congenital rubella. Similarly, the immunodeficient state that follows congenital or acquired human immunodeficiency virus infection can be prevented. Genetic counselling and, where feasible, prenatal diagnosis are clearly very important in all inherited disorders. Because of the higher incidence of dysgammaglobulinemia in relatives of patients with humoral immunodeficiency disorders, determination of immunoglobulin and complement levels on family members and other relatives may aid in the diagnosis of asymptomatic but immunodeficient individuals.

In summary, primary immunodeficiency diseases are a diverse but generally uncommon group of diseases that all result in an increased susceptibility to infection. The types and severity of infections encountered vary depending on the underlying immune defect. When left untreated, significant morbidity and mortality is the rule rather than the exception. Specific curative or supplementation therapy is now available for a number of these disorders. This, along with early and aggressive antimicrobial therapy for infectious complications and good supportive care, has resulted in an improved prognosis for most of these patients.

The Acquired Immunodeficiency Syndrome (AIDS)

The acquired immunodeficiency syndrome (AIDS) was described in young homosexual men with opportunistic infections and Kaposi's sarcoma in 1981. It was declared an epidemic a year later. The immunodeficiency seen in AIDS is secondary to infection with the human retrovirus, human immunodeficiency virus (HIV). AIDS represents the most severe manifestation of the clinical spectrum of HIV infection. As of December 1988, between 5 and 10 million people are estimated to be HIV infected and over 125,000 cases of AIDS have been reported worldwide. HIV is transmitted in a fashion similar to the hepatitis B virus, ie, by means of homosexual or heterosexual contact, or by parenteral transmission via blood products (eg, hemophiliacs or blood transfusion recipients) or contaminated needles (eg, IV drug users). Thus, in the United States, intravenous drug abusers and homosexuals constitute the major high-risk groups for HIV infection. In Africa, almost 80% of HIV infection is acquired heterosexually.[24,25] Pediatric HIV infection can be acquired perinatally by in utero transmission, at the time of or immediately following delivery, or postnatally via breast milk. Children can also become infected after receiving contaminated blood or blood products.[26,27]

Following infection with HIV, some patients develop an acute infectious mononucleosis-like illness with nonspecific symptoms, such as fever, fatigue, arthralgias, pharyngitis, skin rash, and lymphadenopathy. Most patients then remain asymptomatic for varying periods of time before developing signs and symptoms of what has been referred to as the AIDS-related complex (ARC).[28] Symptoms include fevers, diarrhea, weight loss, persistent generalized lymphadenopathy, and oral candidiasis. Progression to full-blown AIDS can then occur within a period of months to years, with a mean time of progression from ARC to AIDS estimated to be about 3.5 years in adult male homosexuals. The incubation period for AIDS, ie, the duration of time from the point of infection to the development of symptoms of disease, is long and variable. Estimations of the incubation period in cases of transfusion-associated AIDS suggest that approximately half of the transfused recipients will develop AIDS 5–9 years after infection. Perinatally infected infants may have shorter incubation periods, with a significant number of infected infants developing AIDS in the first year of life. Seroconversion generally occurs within 6–10 weeks following infection. The anti-HIV IgG antibody response is sustained for several years. Titers of antibodies to the HIV core protein antigen, p24, appear to wane with the onset of full-blown AIDS. There is a brief period of antigenemia soon after infection, followed by disappearance of HIV p24 antigen from the serum for long periods of time. Reappearance of antigenemia often occurs concurrently with clinical progression to AIDS.

Infections with opportunistic microorganisms, such as *Pneumocystis carinii,* cytomegalovirus, cryptosporidium, and *Toxoplasma gondii,* is the cardinal manifestation of AIDS. A list of the opportunistic infections seen in patients with AIDS is shown in Table 12-5. Recurrent bacterial infections are common in children with HIV infection.[27] A significant proportion of infected children develop lymphoid interstitial pneumonitis (LIP), a chronic and indolent interstitial lung disorder characterized by varying degrees of respiratory compromise and characteristic bilateral, diffuse nodular densities on chest x-ray. Histological examination reveals a florid, lymphoid and plasmacytoid cell hyperplasia in the interstitial and peribronchial areas. Lymphoid interstitial pneumonitis has been described in a small number of adults with HIV infection. Although its precise etiology is unknown, studies suggest that LIP may represent hyperplasia of pulmonary lymphoid tissue secondary to an Epstein-Barr virus (EBV)-associated polyclonal lymphoproliferation. Whether HIV has a primary role in the pathogenesis of LIP is presently unclear.[24]

Malignancies, especially non-Hodgkins lymphoma and Kaposi's sarcoma, are frequently seen in patients with AIDS. Direct HIV infection of the central and peripheral nervous system results in a wide spectrum of neurologic abnormalities.

Table 12-5. Opportunisitic Infections in AIDS Patients

Bacterial
Mycobacterium avium intracellulare
Salmonella spp.
Fungal
Candida spp.
Cryptococcus neoformans
Coccidioides immitis
Histoplasma capsulatum
Viral
Cytomegalovirus
Herpes simplex virus
Varicella zoster virus
Adenovirus
Protozoal
Pneumocystis carinii
Toxoplasma gondii
Cryptosporidium
Isospora belli

The AIDS–dementia complex is the most common clinical syndrome seen. It is a progressive disorder of subcortical dementia consisting of slowing of mental processes, disorders of concentration and attention, slowing of motor control, and parallel behavioral changes. The end stage consists of a nearly vegetative state with paraparesis or paraplegia and rudimentary intellectual function. Central nervous system infections and neoplasms are frequent complications. Clinical and pathologic manifestations attributable to virtually every organ system have now been described in patients with AIDS and HIV infection.

Immunodeficiency in AIDS is a cellular immunodeficiency caused by infection of CD4-bearing helper T lymphocytes. The most severe immunologic abnormalities are seen in patients with AIDS. Early on, there is an elevation in suppressor–cytotoxic CD8+ T cells, to be followed over time by a decline in helper-inducer CD4+ T cells. This results in a marked lymphopenia and a reversal of the helper to suppressor T cell (CD4/CD8) ratio. The absolute CD4 count in most adult patients with AIDS is less than 400 mm^{-3}. Evaluation of lymphocyte function reveals reduced to absent proliferative responses to mitogens and antigens. Polyclonal hypergammaglobulinemia is another hallmark of HIV infection. Despite this, patients often fail to mount specific antibody responses to immunizations. Other abnormalities include the presence of circulating immune complexes, reduced natural killer cell activity, and reduced lymphokine production by T cells. Complement levels and polymorphonuclear oxidative metabolic functions are generally normal.

Mononuclear phagocytes serve as one of the principal targets for human immunodeficiency virus infection. The effect of HIV infection on T cells is typically cytopathic. Monocytes, however, are quite resistant to the cytopathic effects of the virus, suggesting that they may play a role in viral latency and subsequent dissemination of the virus. The CD4 molecule, which is the major receptor for HIV on CD4+ helper-inducer T cells, also serves as the HIV receptor on monocytes and macrophages. Alternative mechanisms of viral entry, eg, via the Fc receptor, may be operative in HIV infection of mononuclear phagocytes. Defects of monocyte function can be demonstrated in HIV-infected individuals, including decreased chemotaxis, decreased IL-1 production or production of an inhibitor of IL-1, and decreased microbicidal activity. Since mononuclear phagocytes are antigen-presenting and -processing cells in the immune response, HIV infection of these cells may contribute to the immunological dysfunction seen early on in the course of HIV infection.[29]

Curative therapy for AIDS would be one that is able to inhibit the replication of the retrovirus and reverse the immunological abnormalities resulting from HIV infection. Such therapy is presently unavailable. In the last several years, the advent of the antiretroviral agent, zidovudine (3'-azido-3'-deoxythymidine or AZT), has offered some hope for affected patients. Treatment with AZT has resulted in some improvement in clinical and immunological parameters and a decrease in mortality rate. In children treated with AZT, significant amelioration of HIV-induced encephalopathy has been observed in phase I–II trials. Toxicity is related to dose and duration of AZT therapy and consists predominantly of myelosuppression with resultant anemia and neutropenia. Other side effects include headaches, nausea, myalgia, insomnia, and possible neurotoxicity. Since disease progression would occur when therapy is discontinued, AZT has to be given indefinitely if tolerated. A number of immunostimulatory agents and thymic factors have been tried in patients with AIDS but have generally been unsuccessful. Along with antiretroviral therapy, patients with AIDS need multidisciplinary supportive care. As with primary immunodeficiencies, early diagnosis and aggressive treatment for infectious complications is of paramount importance. Effective therapies exist for most of the opportunistic infections encountered in these patients. Despite all these efforts, the prognosis for patients with the full-blown syndrome of AIDS remains grim. As of December 1988, over 55% of the AIDS patients reported to the CDC have died.

Serological screening of blood donors has now greatly reduced the spread of HIV infection via blood transfusions, at least in the developed countries. Similarly, the use of donor-screened, heat-treated factor VIII concentrates has been implemented and will protect uninfected hemophiliacs. The sexual transmission of HIV infection to uninfected adolescents and adults can only be prevented through education and modification of unsafe and high-risk sexual behavior. Intensive efforts are underway for the development of an effective vaccine for HIV infection. However, there are several formidable obstacles that need to be overcome before a safe and effective vaccine can become a reality. In the meantime, global control of HIV infection can only be approached through public education campaigns.

References

1. Nossal GJV. *New Engl J Med.* 1987;316:1320.

2. Rosen FS, Cooper MD, Wedgwood RJ. *New Engl J Med.* 1984;311:235, 300.

3. Lanzavecchia A. *Nature (London).* 1985;314:537.

4. Brown EJ, Joiner KA, Frank MM. *Springer Seminars Immunopathol.* 1983;6:349.

5. Stiehm ER. Immunodeficiency disorders—General considerations. In Stiehm ER, ed. *Immunologic Disorders in Infants and Children,* 3rd ed. Philadelphia, PA: W.B. Saunders Co; 1989:157–195.

6. Rosen FS, Wedgwood RJ, Eibl M, et al. *Clin Immunol Immunopathol.* 1986;40:166.

7. Ammann A. Immunodeficiency diseases. In Stites DP, Stobo JD, Wells JV, eds. *Basic & Clinical Immunology,* 6th edition. Norwalk, CT: Appleton & Lange; 1986:317–355.

8. Buckley RH. *Clin Immunol Immunopathol.* 1986;40:13–24.

9. Lederman HM, Winkelstein JA. *Medicine.* 1985;64:145–156.

10. Conley ME, Beckwith JB, Mancer JFK, Tenckhoff MD. *J Pediatr.* 1979;94:883–890.

11. Gelfand EW, Dosch H. Diagnosis and classification of severe combined immunodeficiency disease. In Wedgwood RJ, Rosen FS, Paul NW, eds. *Primary Immunodeficiency Diseases,* Vol. 19. March of Dimes Birth Defects Foundation, Birth Defects, Original Article Series. New York: A.R. Liss, Inc; 1983:65–72.

12. Hirschhorn R. *Clin Immunol Immunopathol.* 1986;40:157–165.

13. Buckley RH, Schiff SE, Sampson HA, et al. *J Immunol.* 1986;136:2398–2407.

14. Curnutte JT, Babior BM. *Adv Hum Genetics.* 1987;16:229–297.

15. Kamani N, August CS, Campbell DE, Hassan NF, Douglas SD. *J Pediatr.* 1988;113:697–700.

16. Ezekowitz RAB, Dinauer MC, Jaffe HS, Orkin SH, Newburger PE. *New Engl J Med.* 1988;319:146–151.

17. Ross SC, Densen P. *Medicine*. 1984;63:243–273.

18. Dinauer MC, Orkin SH. *Immunodef Rev*. 1988;1:55–69.

19. Kwan SP, Kunkel L, Bruns G, Wedgwood RJ, Latt S, Rosen FS. *J Clin Invest*. 1986;77:649–652.

20. Anderson DC, Springer TA. *Annu Rev Med*. 1987;38:175–194.

21. Remold-O'Donnell E, Kenney DM, Parkman R, Cairns L, Savage B, Rosen FS. *J Exp Med*. 1984;159:1705–1723.

22. Hershfield MS, Buckley RH, Greenberg ML, et al. *New Engl J Med*. 1987;316:589–596.

23. Williams DA, Orkin SH. *J Clin Invest*. 1986;77:1053–1056.

24. Broder S, ed. *AIDS: Modern Concepts and Therapeutic Challenges*. New York: Marcel Dekker Inc; 1987:245–262.

25. Adler MW, Gold JWM, Weber JN, eds. *AIDS 1988*. AIDS Vol 2, Suppl. 1. London: Gower Academic Journals; 1988.

26. Kamani N, Krilov L. *Pediatr Rev Commun*. 1987;1:101–121.

27. Falloon J, Eddy J, Wiener L, Pizzo PA. *J Pediatr*. 1989;114:1–30.

28. Kamani N, Lightman H, Leiderman I, Krilov LR. *Pediatr Infect Dis*. 1988;7:383–388.

29. Fauci AS. *Science*. 1988;239:617–622.

CHAPTER 13

Autoimmune Diseases

Sharad D. Deodhar

Department of Immunopathology, Cleveland Clinic Foundation, Cleveland, OH 44195-5131 USA

Introduction

The past two decades have seen rapid progress in the field of immunology, not only in its basic, theoretical aspects, but also in its clinical laboratory applications. There is no area of immunology that involves the clinical laboratory more than that of autoimmune diseases. Most of the laboratory tests performed at present in a typical clinical immunology laboratory are directed toward the diagnosis and/or management of one or more of the diseases of autoimmunity. Technological developments in the area of immunologic testing have been equally significant and rapid during the same period, and it is important for both the practitioners of laboratory medicine as well as the bioscientists representing the industry to become aware of these developments in immunobiology and laboratory testing as related to diseases of autoimmunity.

The primary purpose of this chapter is to provide a brief review of autoimmune diseases with focus on current understanding of the mechanisms involved, emphasizing present and future developments from the clinical laboratory perspective. This review is intended not as a comprehensive treatment of the subject but as an attempt to provide a perspective into certain selected autoimmune diseases with respect to laboratory methodology, clinical relevance, and general concepts concerning mechanisms involved. Those interested in greater detail about these diseases may refer to some excellent monographs and review articles that have appeared recently on this subject.[1-4]

Mechanisms of Autoimmunity

Immune mechanisms are not always protective or beneficial to the host. Under certain conditions they produce tissue injury and clinical disease. Normally, immunological attack is directed against agents that are foreign or nonself. However, under certain conditions, an individual's own tissue components become participants in immunological reactions and injury, resulting in clinical disease. Thus, autoimmune diseases are those which result from immunological reactions, humoral and/or cellular, directed against the individual's own tissue components. In recent years, many clinical diseases have been assigned an autoimmune origin, but the evidence is not equally convincing for all.

Factors Involved in Autoimmunity

Forbidden Clone Theory

The mechanisms by which the immune system differentiates between self and nonself are not clear. One hypothesis postulates that those clones of cells capable of responding to autologous (self) tissue components are suppressed or forbidden during embryonic development by contact with the respective autoantigens.[5] These clones, under certain conditions, become activated and immune responses against self tissue components occur, resulting in tissue injury and clinical disease. The effectors in the production of tissue injury, in addition to the relevant immune complexes, include the complement system; the coagulation system; such cellular elements as cytotoxic lymphocytes, natural killer cells, macrophages, neutrophils, basophils, eosinophils, and various lymphokines; and the vasoactive and inhibitory molecules resulting from interactions of these systems. Initiation of autoimmunity is thought to be the result of disturbance in immune regulation and various factors have been implicated in the process.

Genetic Factors

It is well known that autoimmune diseases in general show a highly significant familial predisposition.[6] Relatives of a patient with a given autoimmune disease are known to be at a high risk for developing the same disease, and also the relevant autoantibodies are known to occur in a much higher frequency among patients' relatives than in the general population. Also, multiple autoimmune diseases are known to occur in the same patient. These findings suggest involvement of genetic factors that in recent years have been linked to the human lymphocyte antigen (HLA) system. The HLA system of antigens, particularly the HLA-DR system, identified serologically and, in some cases, by cellular techniques, has shown important associations with numerous autoimmune diseases, including systemic lupus erythematosus and related immune complex diseases (connective tissue diseases); autoimmune renal, skin, and gastrointestinal diseases; insulin-dependent diabetes (type I); autoimmune endocrine diseases; multiple sclerosis; myasthenia gravis; and many others.[7] The current hypothesis implicates an autosomal dominant primary autoimmune gene acting in collaboration with secondary HLA-linked genes controlling the expression of autoimmunity. The technology involved in studying these HLA–disease associations is currently in a state of flux and it is anticipated that as DNA technology becomes more widely used, the techniques of choice in these studies will be the restriction fragment length polymorphisms (RFLP) and oligonucleotide probes for the HLA genes.

Defect in Immune Regulation

The immune response is controlled mainly by the regulatory influence of the two lymphocyte subsets, T cells and B cells. These cells operate in close cooperation and they are subject to an intricate network of feedback control mechanisms. The two important elements in this control system are the T-helper (T_H) and T-suppressor (T_S) cells and the initiation and duration of a given immune response are the result of the balance of activities of these two T-cell subsets. In normal individuals, the ratio of T_H to T_S cells in peripheral blood is approximately 2:1, whereas in almost all of the autoimmune diseases studied so far, particularly in the active phase, this ratio tends to be considerably greater, often approaching 10 or 15:1. Thus, in autoimmune diseases, the T_H activity is relatively increased and this has been attributed, in most cases, to a decrease in T_S cell activity. For example, in systemic lupus erythematosus, the prototype of autoimmune diseases, there is a significant decrease in T_S cells during the active phase of the disease; during clinical remission this suppressor activity is restored, causing the T helper–suppressor ratio to return to a normal value.[8] There is great interest at the present time in exploring the possibility that soluble factor (S) produced by T_S cells may be helpful in correcting the T_S cell defect noted in autoimmune diseases. Such factors are under intense investigation at present. Other examples of relationship between disturbed immune regulation and autoimmune disease include (1) the association between aging and development of autoantibodies, (2) association between various congenital and familial immune deficiency syndromes and autoimmune phenomena, and finally (3) the more recently described autoimmune phenomena in patients with acquired immune deficiency syndrome (AIDS).[9] In all of these situations, it appears that defects in immune regulation trigger autoimmune reactivity and eventually cause autoimmune disease.

Hormonal Factors

It is well known that autoimmune diseases occur far more commonly in females than they do in males, with the ratio of female to male involvement often reaching 10:1 or 12:1 in certain diseases. The mechanisms involved are completely unclear; however, sex hormones only provide a partial answer. In the animal model for systemic lupus erythematosus, the NZB-NZW mouse, the disease occurs far earlier and in a more severe form in the females than it does in the males. It was reported that treatment of female mice with androgens, male sex hormones, delayed the onset of the disease and decreased severity of the disease, whereas treatment of male mice with estrogens, female sex hormones, accelerated the onset of the disease and caused it to appear in a more severe form.[10] However, in neither situation could the disease be completely prevented. The mechanisms by which sex hormones alter the disease process are not understood at present.

Defect in the Idiotype–Anti-Idiotype Network

Another possible mechanism for initiation of autoimmune phenomena and formation of autoantibodies may lie in the idiotype–anti-idiotype network. Idiotypes are the unique structural moieties in the variable portions of the heavy and light chains of an antibody molecule that are capable of serving as immunogens in a given individual. Thus, an immune response to such idiotypes results in formation of anti-idiotypic antibodies. The anti-idiotypic antibody can then bind with the respective structures (idiotypes) in the variable region of a given antibody. There is increasing evidence being reported at present demonstrating that abnormalities of the idiotype–anti-idiotype network can lead to autoreactive immune responses.[11] The development of anti-idiotypic antibodies to autoantibodies has been shown in several human autoimmune diseases, such as systemic lupus erythematosus, rheumatoid arthritis, myasthenia gravis, and certain possible autoimmune central nervous system diseases.[12] Of great interest in these studies has been the demonstration of an inverse relationship between serum levels of anti-idiotypic antibodies and those of the corresponding autoantibodies. Furthermore, it appeared that the serum levels of these anti-idiotypic antibodies had a significant bearing on the patient's clinical course with respect to a given autoimmune disease. For instance, in patients with systemic lupus erythematosus, it was noted that in those patients undergoing spontaneous remission, there was concomitant increase in serum levels of anti-idiotypic antibodies to the anti-DNA autoantibodies. Similar correlations were also observed in patients with myasthenia gravis.[12] These exciting studies show great promise for future therapeutic modalities for various human autoimmune diseases. Thus, it may be possible to manipulate the idiotype–anti-idiotype network in such a way as to provide a highly specific form of immunotherapy in a given autoimmune disease.

General Characteristics of Autoimmune Diseases

Autoimmune disorders as a group demonstrate some common clinical and laboratory features; however, it should be emphasized that the diagnosis of a specific autoimmune disease often rests in the demonstration of the specific autoantibody or autoantibodies associated with that disease.

Elevation of Serum Immunoglobulin Levels

Serum levels of immunoglobulins, especially IgG and IgA, are usually increased in autoimmune diseases. These elevations are usually of a polyclonal nature and can be detected by serum electrophoresis and/or immunoelectrophoresis. In rare cases, such as primary biliary cirrhosis, the IgM level is significantly increased and this can be utilized as a diagnostic criterion in the clinical laboratory.

Presence of Immunoglobulins and/or Lymphocytes in Tissue Biopsies

In most autoimmune diseases, the diseased tissues often show the presence of one or more of the immunoglobulin classes by immunohistochemical techniques and the presence of lymphocytes and its subsets by conventional histochemical techniques. The presence of these components is often used as evidence for the participation of immune mechanisms in a given tissue injury process. These immunohistochemical techniques have become very necessary for complete evaluation of many of the autoimmune diseases.

Decrease in Serum Complement Level

Additional evidence for the role of immune mechanisms in many of these diseases comes from the finding that complement levels, particularly the C3 and C4 components, are often diminished during the acute phase of the disease process. In, for example, systemic lupus erythematosus the complement component levels can be very helpful in monitoring disease activity and evaluating response to appropriate therapy.

Role of Cell-Mediated Immune Reactions

In recent years, a number of autoimmune diseases have been demonstrated to involve cell-mediated immunological injury rather than the conventional, humoral antibody-mediated injury known for many years. In such diseases as polymyositis, primary cardiomyopathy, type I diabetes mellitus, multiple sclerosis, inflammatory bowel diseases, and autoimmune liver diseases, the immunological injury appears primarily mediated by cytotoxic T cells and their products.

Beneficial Effects of Immunosuppressive Agents

Since the pathogenesis of all autoimmune diseases involves immunological injury, immunosuppressive therapy would be expected to provide a beneficial effect. Indeed, most autoimmune diseases respond well clinically, to such agents as corticosteroids and cytotoxic agents such as azathioprine or imuran, cyclophosphamide or cytoxan, methotrexate, and others. These agents are currently the preferred therapeutic modalities for almost all of these diseases. The current success noted with the use of cyclosporin, a powerful anti-T-cell agent, in clinical transplantation has stimulated interest in the use of this agent in the treatment of various autoimmune diseases. Many clinical trials are currently in progress with this agent, and final results are anxiously awaited.

Association with Cancer

According to the immune surveillance theory, one of the important functions of the immune system is to recognize abnormal, potentially malignant cells and to destroy them by appropriate mechanisms. Any disturbance in the immune system would therefore be expected to result in an increased incidence of neoplastic disease. This, indeed, has been demonstrated to be true in naturally occurring immune deficiency diseases as well as in clinically induced states of immune suppression.[13] Since autoimmune diseases are characterized by disturbance in the immune system, here also one would expect a concomitant, higher incidence of malignant disease or cancer. This has been well documented in many instances and examples of this are the high incidence of gastric cancer in pernicious anemia, gastrointestinal cancer in ulcerative colitis, lymphomas in Sjogren's syndrome, thymoma in myasthenia gravis, and a generally higher incidence of cancer in dermatomyositis, nephrotic syndrome, and systemic lupus erythematosus. On the other side of the coin, autoimmune phenomena have been reported to be more common in patients with lymphoid malignancies than they are in the general population.[14] Most of these involve hematological elements in the form of autoantibodies to red cells, platelets, lymphocytes, etc. The precise mechanisms involved in these phenomena are not understood at present.

Laboratory Techniques for Diagnosis of Autoimmune Diseases

Techniques demonstrating specific autoantibodies include immunofluorescence, red cell or latex agglutination, complement fixation, agar diffusion, immunoelectrophoresis, radioimmunoassays, enzyme-linked immunosorbant assays (ELISA), and nephelometric procedures. If the autoimmune mechanisms involve cellular immunity, the techniques for demonstrating sensitized T cells usually include lymphocyte cytotoxicity, blast transformation of lymphocytes with the appropriate antigen, and in some cases, production of migration inhibitory factor or other lymphokines. The study of cellular immunity on a laboratory level is assuming increasingly greater significance in the diagnosis of autoimmune diseases. The details of the procedures involved in diagnosis of the various autoantibodies as they relate to respective autoimmune diseases are available from appropriate sources.[15,16] In Table 13-1,

Table 13-1. Autoimmune Diseases and the Respective Autoantibodies

Disease	Autoantibodies Directed Against:
Lupus Related	
Systemic lupus erythematosus	Nuclear antigens, DNA, Sm
Scleroderma	Nuclear antigen, Scl 1
Sjogren's syndrome	Nuclear antigens SS-A, SS-B
Mixed connective tissue disease	Extractable nuclear antigen (RNP)
Rheumatoid arthritis	Fc portion of IgG (rheumatoid factor)
Other	
Autoimmune thyroiditis	Thyroglobulin, microsomal Ag
Addison's disease	Adrenal cortical cell Ag
Pernicious anemia	Intrinsic factor, parietal cell Ag
Inflammatory bowel disease	Colonic mucosal Ag
Chronic active hepatitis	Smooth muscle Ag
Primary biliary cirrhosis	Mitochondrial Ag
Myasthenia gravis	Acetylcholine receptor
Goodpasture's syndrome	Glomerular basement membrane
Pemphigus vulgaris	Epidermal intercellular substance
Bullous pemphigoid	Skin basement membrane
Autoimmune hemolytic anemia	Red cell membrane Ags
Multiple sclerosis and related demyelinating diseases	Myelin basic protein Ag
Diabetes type 1	Islet cell Ag

some of the more commonly studied autoimmune diseases and their respective autoantibodies are listed. These are among the popular laboratory tests currently performed in clinical laboratories.

Current Trends in the Study of Autoimmune Diseases

Some of the highlights with respect to current developments in the field of autoimmune diseases are presented in this section. Some of the items, such as suppressor factors and their potential for therapy, use of cyclosporin as a powerful agent for suppressing cell-mediated immune responses, and the potential use of anti-idiotypic antibodies to autoantibodies for therapy, have already been discussed briefly. Some of the exciting recent developments have been in the diseases that follow.

1. Autoimmune phenomena associated with AIDS. The human immunodeficiency virus (HIV) causes not only a profound deficient immune response but also a highly disregulated one. One expected outcome of this disregulation would be initiation of autoimmune phenomena. These are being described with increasing frequency in patients with AIDS and AIDS-related complex (ARC).[9] The autoimmune phenomena observed have included circulating immune complexes; autoantibodies, such as antinuclear antibody, rheumatoid factor anti-cardiolipin antibody, anti-platelet, red cell, and lymphocyte antibodies; and others. These observations are important, not only for better understanding of HIV infection but also with respect to strategies for successful management of these patients.

2. Schizophrenia: The central nervous system (CNS)–immune system relationship. Immune studies in the pathogenesis of schizophrenia have demonstrated cellular immune reactions that may participate in producing alterations of the central nervous system.[17] Furthermore, both clinical and animal experimental studies have suggested that activation of the central nervous system by stressful stimuli may be capable of altering immunological function. These highly provocative studies implicate the CNS–immune system–endocrine system axis in the pathogenesis of certain CNS diseases previously thought to have an immunological basis.

3. Inflammatory bowel diseases. Several lines of evidence have suggested that inflammatory bowel diseases such as chronic ulcerative colitis and transmural colitis (Crohn's disease) may involve immunological injury. The histopathology of these diseases and immunological studies involving humoral and cellular events support this hypothesis. Autoantibodies to mucosal components have been demonstrated in these patients; however, recent studies favor a cell-mediated immunological injury in the pathogenesis of these diseases.[18]

4. Autoimmune otologic diseases. Clinical otologic diseases can occur in association with a wide variety of systemic autoimmune diseases. Also, evidence of direct immunological injury have been found in certain cases of hearing loss accompanied by vestibular dysfunction. Present studies support a cell-mediated immunological injury in these phenomena.[19] These highly exciting studies, for the first time, link immune mechanisms to some of the otologic diseases.

5. Systemic lupus erythematosus and related diseases. Most of the laboratory testing in a typical clinical immunology laboratory is related to study of patients with these diseases. Testing for antinuclear antibodies; circulating immune complexes; testing for anti-DNA, the specific marker for systemic lupus erythematosus; measurement of serum levels of complement components for monitoring disease activity, etc., still continue to be the most commonly utilized laboratory procedures for study of patients with these diseases. Another autoantibody, namely, the anti-cardiolipin antibody, has generated considerable interest at present with respect to certain manifestations of systemic lupus erythematosus involving the CNS and coagulation systems.[20] Anti-cardiolipin antibody has also been linked to the spontaneous abortions frequently reported in pregnant females with SLE. Procedures for measuring anti-cardiolipin antibodies are now well established and additional studies are needed to shed further light on the role of anti-cardiolipin antibodies.

These are but a few examples of some of the current exciting developments with respect to studies in autoimmune diseases. These studies are anticipated to lead to more and better diagnostic procedures as well as better and more specific therapeutic approaches.

References

1. Deodhar SD. *Clinics in Laboratory Medicine,* Vol. 8. Philadelphia, PA: W.B. Saunders Co; 1988.

2. Schwartz RS, Rose NR. *Ann NY Acad Sci.* 1986;475.

3. Moller G. *Immunol Rev.* 1986;94.

4. Condemi JJ. *JAMA.* 1987;258:2920.

5. Burnett FM. *The Clonal Selection Theory of Acquired Immunity.* New York: Cambridge University Press; 1959.

6. Shoenfeld Y, Schwartz RS. *New Engl J Med.* 1984;311:1019.

7. Braun WE, Zachary A. In Deodhar SD, ed. *Autoimmune Diseases,* Vol 8. Philadelphia, PA: W.B. Saunders Co; 1988:351–371.

8. Clough JD, Frank S, Calabrese L. *Arthr Rheum.* 1980;23:24.

9. Calabrese LH. In Deodhar SD, ed. *Autoimmune Diseases,* Vol 8. Philadelphia, PA: W.B. Saunders Co; 1988:269–280.

10. Ahmed A, Penhole W, Talal N. *Am J Pathol.* 1985;121:531.

11. Roitt IM, Male DK, Cooke A, Lydyard PM. *Springer Seminars Immunopathol.* 1983;6:51.

12. Abdou NJ. *J Clin Immunol.* 1985;5:365.

13. Harris JE. In Sinkovics JS, ed. *Immunology of Malignant Diseases,* 2nd ed. St. Louis: CW Mosby; 1976:283–339.

14. Chandor SB. In Deodhar SD, ed. *Autoimmune Diseases,* Vol 8. Philadelphia, PA: W.B. Saunders Co; 1988:373–384.

15. Rose N, Friedman H. *Manual of Clinical Immunology,* 2nd ed. Washington DC: American Society for Microbiology; 1982.

16. Nakamura RM, Deodhar SD. *Laboratory Tests in the Diagnosis of Autoimmune Diseases.* Chicago, IL: American Society of Clinical Pathologists Press; 1975.

17. Gangoli R, Rabin BS, Kelly RH, et al. *Ann NY Acad Sci.* 1987;496:676.

18. Keren DF. In Deodhar SD, ed. *Autoimmune Diseases,* Vol 8. Philadelphia, PA: W.B. Saunders Co; 1988:325–336.

19. Barna B, Hughes GB. In Deodhar SD, ed. *Autoimmune Diseases,* Vol 8. Philadelphia, PA: W.B. Saunders Co; 1988:385–398.

20. Triplett D, Brandt J, Musgrave K, Orr C. *JAMA.* 1988;259

DRUGS OF IMMUNE ORIGIN

Therapeutic Aspects of Interleukin-1, Interleukin-2, and Interleukin-1 Antagonists

Robert W. Wilmott and Joseph Kaplan

Department of Pediatrics, Wayne State University School of Medicine and Children's Hospital of Michigan, 3901 Beaubien Boulevard, Detroit, MI 48201 USA

There is a wealth of new information concerning the role of cytokines, such as interleukin-1 (IL-1) and interleukin-2 (IL-2), in modulating the host's response to infection, inflammation, and malignancy. Both of these proteins are now available as recombinant human molecules, their receptors have been cloned, and there is considerable detailed information concerning ligand–receptor interactions.

This chapter reviews this new information in the light of potential therapeutic applications. It is hoped that this perspective will be valuable to clinicians, immunologists, and pharmacologists.

Interleukin-1

IL-1 Review

Interleukin-1 (IL-1) is a protein that is synthesized by stimulated monocytes and macrophages and that has many diverse biological effects. The systemic effects of IL-1 include fever, sleep, anorexia, increased synthesis of hepatic acute-phase proteins, and hypotension.[1]

Interleukin-1 also has many immunologic effects. It augments T-lymphocyte proliferative responses to mitogens, induces B- and T-cell differentiation, activates natural killer (NK) cells, and induces neutrophil release from the bone marrow.

At the cellular level, IL-1 increases the production of several cytokines (IL-2, IL-3, IL-4, and IL-6), as well as interferons and colony-stimulating factors. The increase in acute-phase reactants is mediated by increasing gene expression.[2]

There are many cellular sources for IL-1. The activated mononuclear phagocyte is a very efficient specialized producer of IL-1 and a high proportion of the mRNA in such cells codes for it. Other sources include dendritic cells, Langerhans cells, keratinocytes, epithelial cells, melanocyte cell lines, B lymphocytes, NK cells, astrocytes, gliomas, microglia, mesangial cells, fibroblasts, synovial cells, neutrophils, and endothelial cells.

The cloning of a cDNA for human IL-1 has revealed the existence of at least two mRNA species, coding for two distinct human IL-1 moieties: IL-1α, with a pI of 5.0 and M_r 17 kd, and IL-1β, with a pI of 7.0 and M_r 17 kd.[3] Both forms of IL-1 are translated primarily as 31-kd peptides and cleaved to biologically active 17-kd molecules.[4] So far IL-1α and IL-1β are not reported to exhibit any biological differences[5] and they bind to the same receptor.[6] The specific activity of both forms of IL-1 is $1-6 \times 10^7$ U mg^{-1} in the thymocyte comitogenic assay, which suggests the existence of high-affinity receptors specific for IL-1 on various types of responder cells.

There are many stimuli for IL-1 production and these include microbial products, such as lipopolysaccharide and zymosan; particles, such as silica and latex beads; and membrane-active agents, such as phorbol esters.

The Role of IL-1 in Treatment of Malignancy

The observation that IL-1 stimulates macrophages to exhibit an enhanced tumoricidal state[7] led to further experiments, which revealed that IL-1 alone was directly cytotoxic to certain sensitive tumor cell lines, such as the human melanoma cell line A375.[8] Interleukin-1 therefore may have an antitumor effect in several different ways: (1) by directly inhibiting tumor cells; (2) by enhancing the effect of NK cells[9] and cytotoxic T lymphocytes (CTL),[10] (3) by augmenting the production of other lymphokines, such as IL-2 and interferon, and (4) synergistically acting with IL-2 and interferon in promoting CTL and NK cell activities.[11]

Interleukin-1 is likely to be used as a therapy in the treatment of cancer. In addition to the above data there is some evidence that some patients with extensive tumor burdens produce reduced amounts of IL-1 and that NK cell tumor killing is reduced and responds to exogenous IL-1.[12] The increase in availability of recombinant IL-1 with the cloning of the human IL-1 genes creates the opportunity to study administration of IL-1 either for its antitumor effects or as an immunostimulant.[13]

IL-1 Agonists

Although there are no synthetic agonists for IL-1, apart from recombinant materials, several agents have been shown to increase IL-1 release by mononuclear blood cells. In one study it was shown that patients with pemphigus vulgaris had a deficiency of production of IL-1 and IL-2 by peripheral mononuclear blood cells, as well as decreased expression of the IL-2 receptor on the cells. It was found that these defects resolved following therapy with gold sodium thiomalate. Whether this was a direct or an indirect effect related to remission of the disease was unclear.[14]

However, other studies of rats with adjuvant-induced arthritis have shown increased IL-1 production by adherent splenic cells and normalization of this response after therapy with gold thiomalate.[15]

Glucan, a polyglucose, was shown to enhance the production of IL-1 and IL-2 by splenic cells, and this led to increases in plasma levels of the lymphokines. The increases in lymphokine production could be detected for up to 12 days after glucan administration.[16]

IL-1 Receptor

The IL-1 receptor is a cell-surface protein with a molecular ratio of approximately 80 kd. Scatchard analysis of the binding of radiolabeled IL-1 reveals the existence of 100 receptors on a human T-cell line, 4900 on human gingival fibroblasts, 185 on EL-4 T-lymphoma cells (murine), and 550 on LBRM-33-1A5 murine T-lymphoma cells.[17] The human peripheral blood mononuclear cell appears to have approximately 27 receptors, and human polymorphonucleocytes (PMN) have been shown to have approximately 400 receptors for IL-1 (P. Kilian, Hoffmann Roche Research Center, data in press for *J. Immunol.*).

Studies of the effects of corticosteroids on expression of the IL-1 receptor by peripheral blood mononuclear cells revealed a marked increase in expression following incubation with glucocorticoids. Fractionation of the cells and study of the subpopulations revealed that glucocorticoids predominantly affected B lymphocytes.[18] This result was the opposite of predicted effects in view of the antiinflammatory actions of corticosteroids.

Role of IL-1 in Radiation Sickness

Interleukin-1 has a promising role for the therapy of people exposed to ioinizing radiation. There is no effective treatment for the bone marrow suppression or the secondary infections that develop. Bone marrow transplantation may be useful for small numbers of patients but it would be impractical on a larger scale.

Interleukin-1 and tumor necrosis factor are effective in protecting mice against lethal irradiation when given prior to exposure, whereas IL-2, interferon-γ and GM-CSF are not effective.[19,20] Interleukin-1 does not protect against lethal irradiation when given after exposure,[21] although it does hasten recovery in sublethally irradiated (700 cGy) mice. In a more recent study, the same group has shown that a single injection of IL-1 can protect mice in a dose-dependent manner from a radiation dose that results in death of 95% of control animals within 30 days.[22] It appears that IL-1, as well as tumor necrosis factor (TNF) and interferon-γ may alter the kinetics of repair and recovery during a degenerative phase after radiation exposure.

Role of IL-1 in Other Bone Marrow Suppressive Conditions

Interleukin-1 may also have a role in the therapy of other myelosuppressive conditions. In a mouse system, daily injections of human recombinant IL-1 led to an accelerated recovery of stem cells, progenitor cells, and blood neutrophils following treatment with 5-fluorouracil. It was shown that this protective effect was synergistic with the effects of G-CSF.[23]

Antagonists

Biological Antagonists

There are naturally occurring substances that oppose the activity of IL-1 by binding the molecule,[24] inhibiting the activity of the molecule, or inhibiting the activity of the IL-1 receptor.[25] Therefore, high-titer monoclonal antibodies to IL-1 are likely to have a role as neutralizing antibodies. An alternative strategy might be to block the IL-1 receptor with anti-receptor antibodies.

Pharmacologic Agents

Applications. Because there appears to be altered IL-1 activity that is important in some pathological processes it is feasible to attempt to modulate these processes by pharmacologic intervention. For example, IL-1 may contribute to the pathology of arthritis. In vitro studies of IL-1 (catabolin) have demonstrated loss of proteoglycans and collagen when it is added to cultures of cartilage.[26] Interleukin-1 also inhibits the synthesis of new proteoglycans.[27]

In vivo studies have revealed that intraarticular injection of IL-1 in rabbits leads to cartilage erosion, loss of proteoglycan, and the induction of an inflammatory effusion.[28] It has been shown that human synovial tissue has the capacity to synthesize IL-1.[29] The presence of IL-1 in synovial fluid has also been reported,[30] and IL-1 has been demonstrated in the serum and correlated with disease activity.[31]

Agents. Steroids are very potent downregulators of IL-1 production and appear to inhibit transcription of the IL-1 gene.[32] This may account for some of the anti-inflammatory actions of these agents. Inhibitors of IL-1 production therefore are likely to have a role in the therapy of rheumatoid arthritis.

One such agent is gold thiomalate, which has been recognized as a therapeutic agent in rheumatoid arthritis for many years. In vitro studies show that it inhibits both the production of IL-1 activity by monocytes and the response to IL-1 by C3H/HeJ thymocytes.[33]

New Agents

Lobenzarit. Lobenzarit disodium (disodium-4-chloro-2,2'-iminodibenzoate) is a novel antiinflammatory drug developed in Japan.[34] Lobenzarit, also known as CCA, was shown to inhibit the mixed-lymphocyte reaction, immunoglobulin secretion, and IL-1 generation by lipopolysaccharide (LPS)-stimulated human monocytes. It was shown that addition of IL-1 or IL-2 could restore the autologous MLC reaction and overcome the inhibition by CCA.

Two hundred and thirty patients were studied in a double-blind controlled study of CCA (80 mg tid) with indomethacin versus indomethacin alone. The CCA-treated group had significantly less joint swelling and a significantly improved clinical score compared to the control group. However, both groups complained of gastric irritation, which may have been related to the other drugs being administered concurrently.[35]

Antimalarial Drugs. There has been interest recently in the possible application of antimalarial drugs to the treatment of arthritis. This led to studies of the effects of several antimalarial compounds on IL-1-induced cartilage degradation in vivo. Aminoquinoline and aminoacridine compounds having side chains with a tertiary amino group similar to that of chloroquine were effective in inhibiting degradation of bovine nasal cartilage in response to porcine IL-1α.[36] The most active compound against porcine IL-1α was mefloquine but it was relatively ineffective against human IL-1α. It was suggested that there might be subtle receptor specificity for these drugs and IL-1 in bovine cartilage. The mechanism of action of the drugs is unclear but they may inhibit IL-1-induced transcription of enzymes responsible for destruction of cartilage proteoglycan and collagen.

PAF Antagonists. Another class of agents that may have a role in the treatment of inflammation is the inhibitors of platelet activating factor (PAF). As well as a chemoattractant for neutrophils PAF is a very active inducer of vascular permeability. The observation that IL-1 promoted PAF synthesis by endothelial cells led to the theory that PAF contributed to IL-1-induced inflammation.[37] A study was performed in which interleukin-1 was used to induce inflammatory changes in the anterior chamber of the eye in an animal model; it was shown that a PAF antagonist (SRI 63-441) was effective in preventing these changes. The action of this antagonist was synergistic with a prostaglandin inhibitor, flurbiprofen, and the corticosteroid prednisolone.

Pentyoxifylline. Pentoxyifylline, a methyl xanthine derivative, has been shown to inhibit the inflammatory actions of IL-1 (and tumor necrosis factor-α) on neutrophil function. Specifically, pentoxifylline decreased neutrophil adherence to nylon fibers, reversed the inhibition of directed migration to f-MLP induced by these agents, and decreased neutrophil priming for superoxide production.[38]

Probucol. There is preliminary evidence that probucol, a substituted bis-phenol that is used as an antilipemic agent, also inhibits the release of IL-1 by murine peritoneal macrophages stimulated by LPS. However, this effect could be demonstrated by pretreatment of animals with probucol in vivo but it could not be reproduced in vitro at concentrations from 10^{-9} to 10^{-4} mol L^{-1}. It was proposed that probucol inhibited the modification and uptake of low-density lipoproteins and the subsequent induction of IL-1 release.[39]

Use of IL-1 Antagonists in Other Diseases. There are very few data concerning therapeutic approaches to other diseases using modulators of IL-1 activity. Our laboratory has been active in investigating the role of IL-1 production by the activated alveolar macrophage in causing pulmonary inflammation in children with pulmonary infection such as cystic fibrosis patients. High levels of IL-1β were demonstrated in the bronchoalveolar lavage fluid from cystic fibrosis patients with infection, and the levels correlated with the presence of significant numbers of bacteria and with the presence of neutrophils.[40] These data are in accord with the theory that some lung disease in cystic fibrosis is the result of a secondary immune process complicating recurrent pulmonary infections. It is possible that IL-1 antagonists have a therapeutic role in this disease, which appears to respond favorably to corticosteroids.[41]

In Vivo Administration of Interleukin-2

Interleukin-2 (IL-2) is a lymphokine that stimulates the proliferation and differentiation of T cells,[42–44] natural killer (NK) cells,[45] and B cells.[46,47] It has been used both in vitro and in vivo to generate two distinct types of cytotoxic cells of potential clinical utility in adoptive and active immunotherapy—cytotoxic T lymphocytes (CTL), and lymphokine-activated killer (LAK) cells. Both CTL and LAK cells are capable of killing tumor cells and virus-infected cells, but they differ markedly in their mode of stimulation and target cell recognition. Whereas CTL exhibit immunological memory and major histocompatibility complex (MHC) restriction, LAK cells do not. Thus, tumor-specific or virus-specific CTL are only generated following specific stimulation with tumor-specific or virus-encoded cell-surface membrane antigens seen in the context of self-MHC antigens. By contrast, LAK cells that kill tumor cells or virus-infected cells can be generated by exposure to IL-2 in the absence of prior antigenic stimulation and kill, not only autologous targets, but also allogeneic and even xenogeneic targets. The ability of IL-2 to generate potent killers of tumor cells and virally infected cells in vitro, and the abundant supply of IL-2 made possible by the development of recombinant human IL-2,[48] have led to an accelerating number of investigations of the use of IL-2 in the treatment of tumors and microbial infections.

Interleukin-2 has been used either alone or in combination with other agents, including LAK cells, CTL-like tumor infiltrating lymphocytes, cytotoxic drugs, antibodies, and other cytokines. The following discussion reviews the current status of these in vivo studies with emphasis on therapeutic efficacy, toxicity, and mechanisms of action.

IL-2 Alone

Repeated administration of high-dose recombinant IL-2 has been shown to induce regression of primary and metastatic tumors in experimental animals and in humans.[47,49–54] For example, Rosenberg et al.[55] reported that repeated ip injection of high-dose recombinant IL-2 reduced the numbers of lesions in the lungs of mice bearing established pulmonary metastases from both immunogenic and nonimmunogenic tumors,[50] and Thompson et al.[51] showed that high-dose IL-2 treatment cured 50% of mice previously injected with a lethal dose of viral-induced leukemic cells. In an initial phase-I clinical trial in 39 subjects with advanced cancer treated with IL-2 alone, no tumor regressions occurred. However, after additional subjects were studied, this same group reported response rates of 13%.[56] In a separate study of 40 cancer patients, West et al. reported a 32% response rate using continuous infusion high-dose IL-2.[57]

Several investigations have examined the effectiveness of IL-2 administration in the treatment or prevention of infections. In one study,[58] 5 subjects with chronic HBV hepatitis were given 250–500 U day^{-1} of human recombinant IL-2. All 5 showed decreased HBV replication as measured by serum DNA polymerase activity, and serum hepatitis B early antigen disappeared in 2 of the 5 subjects. This suggests that IL-2 treatment may be useful in certain chronic viral infections. However, the results of another study comparing the efficacy of treatment of AIDS patients with IL-2 or γ-interferon[59] raise the possibility that IL-2 treatment increases the susceptibility to bacterial infections. In that study, 17 of 52 AIDS patients treated with continuous iv IL-2 developed nonopportunistic bacterial infections, whereas no such infections occurred in 22 patients treated with continuous iv γ-interferon. There has been no problem with bacterial infections in cancer patients treated with IL-2, but such patients often receive prophylactic antibiotics.

In most studies in which IL-2 has been given alone, dose-limiting toxicity has occurred at IL-2 doses close to those required to induce tumor regression. In mice, doses of roughly 2 million units kg^{-1} day^{-1} are required for the antitumor effect,[50,55] and doses as low as 4 million units kg^{-1} day^{-1} have been lethal.[49] In one phase-I trial in humans,[60] dose-limiting toxicity occurred at 1 million U kg^{-1} as a bolus dose and at 3000 U kg^{-1} hour^{-1} by continuous iv infusions. The maximum tolerated cumulative dose of IL-2 administered as a daily infusion was 1.5 million units kg^{-1}. In a similar study[61] the maximum tolerated cumulative dose of IL-2 given as a 6-hour iv infusion daily for 2 weeks was 2 million units m^{-2}. Most human subjects given high-dose IL-2 develop flulike symptoms of fever, chills, malaise, arthralgias, myalgias, nausea, vomiting, and diarrhea,[60] and many develop a pruritic, "burning" erythematous macular rash.[62] These symptoms may be mediated by IL-2-induced in vivo production of γ-interferon.[60] However, the major dose-limiting toxic effect of IL-2 treatment is a widespread increase in vascular permeability, manifested by weight gain, fluid retention, ascites, pleural effusions, and hypotension. Although these toxic effects are reversible upon discontinuation of IL-2 treatment, some subjects have required intensive measures, including intravascular expanders, vasoconstrictors, and respiratory support. The capillary leak syndrome may be the result of damage to endothelial cells mediated by IL-2-activated NK cells, which have been shown to adhere to and lyse normal vascular endothelial cells.[63,64] Mice that have been depleted of NK cells by treatment with antibodies to asialo-GM1 or NK1[65] are resistant to the IL-2-induced capillary leak syndrome.

The mechanisms underlying the antitumor effects of IL-2 have not been established with certainty, but they almost certainly involve IL-2-induced proliferation and augmentation of the cytolytic activity of LAK cells and tumor-specific CTL. Continuous or repeated administration of IL-2 causes a rapid but transient depletion in circulating lymphocytes and LAK precursors. This is followed by a marked lymphocytosis and an accompanying increase in both the number and cytolytic activity of circulating LAK cells and CTL.[60,65–72] Therapeutic responses clearly require cell proliferation since IL-2 given alone fails to induce tumor regressions in mice first subjected to sublethal (5 Gy) irradiation.[55] Moreover, as discussed below, the antitumor effects of IL-2 increase when IL-2 is given together with adoptively transferred LAK cells[45,50] or tumor-specific immune T cells.[51,72] Of interest is the observation that coadministration of LAK cells with IL-2 enhances the antitumor effectiveness of the latter even when the recipient mice are first given 5 Gy irradiation.[73] This is in contrast to the lack of IL-2 responsiveness in tumor-bearing mice given a similar dose of prior irradiation and supports the notion that IL-2-mediates anti-tumor activity by increasing both the number and the functional activity of cytolytic cells.

In addition to expanding the number of antitumor cytolytic effector cells in vivo and enhancing the direct cell-mediated killing of tumor cells by these cells, the antitumor effects of IL-2 may also involve stimulation of these and other cells to release other cytokines, including interferons[60,61,74] and tumor necrosis factor.[75] These IL-2-induced cytokines could, in turn, either directly mediate antitumor effects, or indirectly activate antitumor cytolytic activity of lymphocytes and macrophages.

IL-2 and LAK Cells

The in vivo antitumor effects of high-dose IL-2 treatment alone, and the ability of IL-2 to stimulate the in vitro production and activation of LAK cells, led to studies in mice of the efficacy of combined adoptive immunotherapy of tumors with IL-2 and LAK cells. In these studies the combination of IL-2 and LAK cells caused a greater reduction in metastatic foci than treatment of tumor-bearing animals with IL-2 or LAK cells alone.[73,76–78] Based on these results a number of clinical trials of combined IL-2 and LAK cell adoptive immunotherapy have been initiated. The overall approach has been to prime subjects with high-dose IL-2 for 5 days and, following 2 days of rest, obtain circulating lymphocytes by daily leukapheresis for 5 days. These cells are cultured in recombinant IL-2 for 3–4 days and then readministered to the subjects together with another course of high-dose IL-2. The overall response rate in trials conducted at the NIH has been 22%, only a small improvement over the results of treatment by this same group with IL-2 alone.[79] Preliminary results of confirmatory studies carried out by The National Cancer Institute Extramural IL-2/LAK Working Group indicate that significant tumor reductions have occurred in 14 of 83, or 17%, of subjects given both IL-2 and LAK cells.[80] As with treatment with IL-2 alone, combined treatment with high-dose IL-2 and LAK cells has been associated with significant toxicity. In the NCI extramural working group study, 56 of 83 evaluable subjects experienced major toxicity, much of it associated with capillary leak syndrome. In this study no relationship could be established between either response to therapy or toxicity and the numbers or cytotoxic activity of LAK cells infused. More recently reported results of another clinical trial suggest that more prolonged use of lower doses of IL-2 in conjunction with LAK cells results in considerably reduced incidence of serious toxic reactions and at least comparable tumor responses.[81]

The demonstrated antitumor effects of combined use of IL-2 and adoptively transferred LAK cells may not be primarily due to direct tumor cell killing by transferred LAK cells. As shown in a representative study in mice,[82] following intravenous injection most radiolabeled LAK cells distribute in the lung 1 hour after transfer, and during the next 24–72 hours they move gradually into the liver and spleen. Only a minor proportion (4–5%) of injected cells enter tumor tissue outside these organs, and there is no evidence that LAK cells preferentially localize in tumors. Based on these figures, and considering the likelihood that a single LAK cell can only kill a single tumor cell by direct cell-mediated cytolysis, one can make the rough calculation that in order to successfully eliminate by direct LAK cell-mediated killing even the smallest detectable solid tumor eg, a tumor consisting of 10^9 cells, at least 2×10^{11} LAK cells must be injected systemically, a number of cells roughly three times the average dose of LAK cells administered by iv injection in clinical trials to date.

In some instances it may be possible to overcome the problem of inaccessibility of tumor cells to systemically administered LAK cells by injecting IL-2 and LAK cells directly into tumor sites. This approach has been used with some success by Yoshida et al.[83] They treated 23 patients with recurrent malignant glioma by injecting LAK cells and IL-2 directly into the brain tumors via Ommaya reservoirs. Tumor regression occurred in six patients, continuous remission of more than 6 months occurred in three patients, and there was minimal toxicity associated with this treatment.

Taken together, currently available data fail to provide convincing evidence that administration of ex vivo generated LAK cells, a process that is technically demanding and highly labor intensive, yields additional benefit compared to IL-2 alone in the treatment of patients with advanced cancer.

IL-2 and Tumor-Infiltrating Lymphocytes

Rosenberg et al. reported[84] that adoptive transfer of IL-2-expanded tumor-infiltrating lymphocytes (TIL) was 50–100 times more potent than that of LAK cells in mediating regression of established tumors in mice. Successful therapy with TIL depended on pretreatment with high-dose cyclophosphamide or total body irradiation and simultaneous administration of IL-2. This same group recently presented[85] preliminary results of similar treatment of a group of patients with metastatic melanoma. Treatment of a group of 13 patients with cyclophosphamide and IL-2 resulted in 2 partial responses. Addition of TIL to the combination of cyclophosphamide and IL-2 resulted in responses in 9 of 15 patients not previously given IL-2 and in 2 of 5 patients who had previously failed treatment with IL-2 alone. The median dose of TIL infused was 20.5×10^{10} cells; however, the only complete response seen in this trial was in a patient given 3×10^{10} TIL. Toxicity in this regimen was lower than in others using similar doses of IL-2 because the duration of treatment was shorter. The higher response rates seen in this trial compared to previous trials of IL-2 alone and IL-2 + LAK may be because, in contrast to LAK cells, most TIL are MHC-restricted tumor-specific T cells[86] and may preferentially home to tumor sites.[87] However, for any given tumor one or both cell types could play a role, with the relative importance of each perhaps dependent on whether the tumor is immunogenic or nonimmunogenic. One might expect MHC-restricted T cells to play a more important role with immunogenic tumors and LAK cells to be more important with nonimmunogenic tumors.

IL-2 and Chemotherapy

Several studies have demonstrated synergistic antitumor effects with combined therapy of mice bearing immunogenic or nonimmunogenic tumors with cyclophosphamide and IL-2.[52,53,82] The capacity of cyclophosphamide to enhance the antitumor effect of IL-2 could be due to a diminished tumor burden, lowering of IL-2-mediated toxicity,[53] or enhanced penetration of IL-2 stimulated host LAK cells.[82]

Michell et al.[88] recently reported results of a clinical trial of low-dose cyclophosphamide (350 mg m^{-2}) and low-dose intravenous IL-2 (3.6×10^6 U m^{-2} iv qd $\times$ 5 days) in the outpatient treatment of 27 patients with disseminated melanoma. This regimen resulted in 25% response rate, and only two patients required hospitalization during treatment. Therefore it was as effective as regimens involving administration of ex vivo activated LAK cells and resulted in considerably lower toxicity.

IL-2 and Other Cytokines

Synergistic antitumor effects have been observed with combined usage of recombinant tumor necrosis factor α (TNF) and IL-2 in mice bearing immunogenic tumors, but not in mice bearing nonimmunogenic tumors.[89,90] This form of therapy appears to be more effective when treatment with IL-2 precedes treatment with TNF.[89] Phase-I clinical trials of IL-2 combined with TNF and interferons are currently in progress.

IL-2 and Tumor-Specific Monoclonal Antibodies

Based on evidence that LAK cells mediate antibody-dependent cell-mediated cytotoxicity (ADCC), attempts have been made to augment the antitumor efficacy of tumor-specific monoclonal antibodies using IL-2 or IL-2+ LAK cells. Bernstein and Levy[91] showed that treatment of a murine B-cell lymphoma with IL-2 and monoclonal tumor-specific anti-idiotypic antibodies increased the survival of tumor bearing mice. Eisenthal et al.[92] showed an enhanced antitumor effect of combined therapy with LAK cells, IL-2, and tumor-specific monoclonal antibody compared to mice treated with LAK cells alone or treated with combined IL-2 and monoclonal antibody without coadministered LAK cells. These findings suggest that adoptive immunotherapy of human cancer patients with combined LAK cells, IL-2, and monoclonal antibodies warrants study.

Conclusions

This chapter has reviewed the current status of IL-1 and IL-2 in respect to their relationship to human diseases and possible therapeutic applications of human recombinant proteins as well as new agonists and antagonists of IL-1.

References

1. Dinarello CA. *Dig Dis Sci.* 1988;33:25S.

2. Dinarello CA. *Faseb J.* 1988;2:108.

3. Lomedico PT, Kilian PL, Gubler U, Stern AS, Chizzonite R. *Cold Spring Harb Symp Quant Biol.* 1986;51:631.

4. Auron PE, Warner SJ, Webb AC, Cannon JG, Bernheim HA, McAdam KJ, Rosenwasser LJ, LoPreste G, Mucci SF, Dinarello CA. *J Immunol.* 1987;138:1447.

5. Wood DD, Bayne EK, Goldring MB, Gowen M, Hamerman D, Humes JL, Ihrie EJ, Lipsky PE, Staruch MJ. *J Immunol.* 1985;134:895.

6. Kilian PL, Kaffka KL, Stern AS, Woehle D, Benjamin WR, Dechiara TM, Gubler U, Farrar JJ, Mizel SB, Lomedico PT. *J Immunol.* 1986;136:4509.

7. Onozaki K, Matsushim K, Kleinerman ES, Saito T, Oppenheim JJ. *J Immunol.* 1985;135:314.

8. Onozaki K, Matsushima K, Aggarwal BB, Oppenheim JJ. *J Immunol.* 1985;135:3962.

9. Migliorati G, Cannarile L, DAdamio L, Herberman RB, Riccardi C. *Nat Immun Cell Growth Reg.* 1987;6:306.

10. Farrar JJ, Benjamin WR, Hilfiker ML, Howard M, Farrar WL, and Fuller-Farrar J. *Immunol Rev.* 1982;63:129.

11. Oppenheim JJ, Kovacs EJ, Matsushima K, Durum SK. *Immunol Today.* 1986;7:45.

12. Herman J, Kew MC, Rabson AR. *Cancer Immunol Immunother.* 1984;16:182.

13. Dinarello CA. *J Clin Immunol.* 1985;5:287.

14. Blitstein Willinger E. *Clin Exp Immunol.* 1985;62:705.

15. Lee JC, Dimartino MJ, Votta BJ, Hanna N. *J Immunol.* 1987;139:3268.

16. Sherwood ER, Williams DL, McNamee RB, Jones EL, Browder IW. *Int J Immunopharmacol.* 1987;9:261.

17. Dower SK. *Immunol Ser.* 1987;35:159.

18. Oppenheim JJ, Lew W, Akahoshi T, Matsushima K, Neta R. *Arzneimittelforschung.* 1988;38:461.

19. Neta R, Sztein MB, Oppenheim JJ, Gillis S, Douches SD. *J Immunol.* 1987;139:1861.

20. Neta R, Oppenheim JJ, Douches SD. *J Immunol.* 1988;140:108.

21. Neta R, Vogel SN, Oppenheim JJ, Douches SD. *Lymphokine Res.* 1986;5(Suppl. 1):S105.

22. Neta R, Oppenheim JJ. *Blood.* 1988;72:1093, 108.

23. Moore MA, Warren DJ. *Proc Natl Acad Sci (USA).* 1987;84:7134.

24. Brown KM, Muchmore AV, Rosenstreich DL. *Proc Natl Acad Sci (USA).* 83:9119.

25. Balavoine JF, de Rochemonteix B, Williamson K, Seckinger P, Cruchaud A, Dayer JM. *J Clin Invest.* 1986;78:1120.

26. Saklatvala J, Pilsworth LM, Sarsfield SJ, Gavrilovic J, Heath JK. *Biochem J.* 1984;224:461.

27. Benton HP, Tyler JA. *Biochem Biophys Res Commun.* 1988;154:421.

28. Pettipher ER, Higgs GA, Henderson B. *Proc Natl Acad Sci (USA).* 1986;83:8749.

29. Elford PR, Meats JE, Sharrard RM, Russell RG. *FEBS Lett.* 1985;179:247.

30. Wood DD, Ihrie EJ, Dinarello CA. Cohen PL. *Arthr Rheum.* 1983;26:975.

31. Eastgate JA, Symons JA, Wood NC, Grinlinton FM. *Lancet.* 1988;2:706.

32. Lew W, Oppenheim JJ, Matsushima K. *J Immunol.* 1988;140:1895.

33. Drakes ML, Harth M, Galsworthy SB, McCain GA. *J Rheumatol.* 1987;14:1123.

34. Fujimoto M, Sugawara I, Kimoto M, Ishizaka S, Tsujii T. *Int J Immunopharmacol.* 1986;8:323.

35. Shiokawa Y, Horiuchi Y, Mizushima Y, Kageyama T, Shichikawa K, Ofuji T, Honma M, Yoshizawa H, Abe C, Ogawa N. *J Rheumatol.* 1984;11:615.

36. Rainsford KD. *J Pharm Pharmacol.* 1986;38:829.

37. Rubin RM, Rosenbaum JT. *Biochem Biophys Res Commun.* 1988;154:429.

38. Sullivan GW, Carper HT, Novick WJ Jr, Mandell GL. *Infect Immun.* 1988;56:1722.

39. Ku G, Doherty NS, Wolos JA, Jackson RL. *Am J Cardiol.* 1988;62:77B.

40. Wilmott RW, Kassab JT, Kilian PL, Benjamin WR, Douglas SD, Wood RE. *Lymphokine Res.* 1988;7:334.

41. Auerbach HS, Williams M, Kirkpatrick JA, Colton HR. *Lancet* 1985;2:686

42. Morgan DA, Ruscetti FW, Gallo R. *Science.* 1976;193:1007.

43. Gillis S, Baker PE, Union NA, Smith KA. *J Exp Med.* 1979;149:1460.

44. Smith KA, Baker PE, Gillis PE, Ruscetti FW. *Mol Immunol.* 1980;17:579.

45. Bolhuis RLH, Van De Griend RJ, Ronteltap CPM. *Nat Immun Cell Growth Reg.* 1983;3:61.

46. Lantz O, Grillot-Courvalin C, Schmitt C, et al. *J Exp Med.* 1985;161:1225.

47. Zubler RH, Lowenthal JW, Erard F, et al. *J Exp Med.* 1984;160:1170.

48. Taniguchi T, Matsui H, Fujita T, Takaoka C, Kashina N, Yoshimoto R, Hamuro J. *Nature (London)* 1983;302:305.

49. Cheever MA, Peace DJ. *Abst Soc Biol Ther.* 1988;12.

50. LaFreniere R, Rosenberg SA. *J Immunol.* 1985;135:4273.

51. Thompson JA, Peace DJ, Klarnet JP, Kern DE, Greenberg PD, Cheever MA. *J Immunol.* 1986;137:3675.

52. Silagi S, Schaefer AE. *J Biol Resp Mod.* 1986;5:411.

53. Papa MZ, Yang JC, Vetto JT, Shiloni E, Eisenthal A, Rosenberg SA. *Cancer Res.* 1988;48:122.

54. Zimmerman RJ, Aukerman SL, Landre P, Gauny S, Bell D, Young J, Katre N. *Abst Soc Biol Resp Mod.* 1988;18.

55. Rosenberg SA, Mule JJ, Spiess PJ, Reichert CM, Schwartz SL. *J Exp Med.* 1985;161:1169.

56. Lotze M, Chang AE, Seipp CA, et al. *JAMA.* 1986;256:3117.

57. West WH, Tauer KW, Yannelli JR, et al. *N Engl J Med.* 1985;316:1485.

58. Nishioka M, Kagawa H, Shirai M, Terada S, Watanabe S. *Am J Gastro.* 1987;82:438.

59. Murphy PM, Lane HC, Gallin JI, Fauci AS. *Ann Int Med.* 1988;108:36.

60. Lotze MT, Matory YL. Ettinghausen SE, Rayner AA, Sharrow SO, Seipp CAY, Custer MC, Rosenberg SA. *J Immunol.* 1985;135:2865.

61. Kolitz JE, Welte K, Wong GY, Holloway K, Merluzzi VJ, Engert A, Bradley EC, Konrad M, Polivka A, Gabrilove JL, Sykora KW, Miller GA, Fiedler W, Krown S, Oettgen HF, Mertelsmann R. *J Biol Resp Mod.* 1987;6:412.

62. Gaspari AA, Lotze MT, Rosenberg SA, Stern JB, Katz SI. *JAMA*. 1987;258:1624.

63. Aronson FD, Libby PM, Brandon EP, Janicka MW, Mier JW. *J Immunol*. 1988;141:158.

64. Damle N, Doyle LV, Bender JR, Bradley EX. *J Immunol*. 1987;138:1779.

65. Hefeneider SH, Conlon PJ, Henney CS, Gillis S. *J Immunol*. 1983;130:222.

66. Cheever MA, Greenberg PD, Irle C, Thompson JA, Urdal DL, Mochizuki DY, Henney CS, Gillis S. *J Immunol*. 1984;132:2259.

67. Phillips JH, Gemlo BT, Myers WW, Rayner AA, Lanier LL. *J Clin Oncol*. 1987;5:1933–1941.

68. McMannis JD, Fisher RI, Creekmore SP, Braun DP, Harris JE, Ellis TM. *J Immunol*. 1988; 140:1335.

69. Rosenthal NS, Hank JA, Kohler PC, Minkoff DZ, Moore KH, Bechofer R, Hong R, Storer B, Sondel PM. *J Biol Resp Mod*. 1988;7:123.

70. Cheever MA, Thompson JA, Kern DE, Greenberg PD. *J Immunol*. 1985;134:3895.

71. Ellis TM, Creekmore SP, McMannis JD, Braun DP, Harris JA, Fisher RI. *Cancer Res*. 1988; 48:6597.

72. Donohue JH, Rosenstein M, Chang AE, Lotze MT, Robb RJ, Rosenberg SA. *J Immunol*. 1984; 132:2123.

73. Mule JJ, Shu S, Rosenberg SA. *J Immunol*. 1985;135:646.

74. Kasahara T, Hooks JJ, Dougherty SF, Oppenheim JJ. *J Immunol*. 1983;130:1784.

75. Nedwin GE, Sverdersky LP, Bringman TS, Palladino MA, Goiddel DV. *J Immunol*. 1985; 135:2492.

76. Eggermont AMM, Steller EP, Ottow RT, Matthews Jr W, Sugarbaker PH. *J Natl Cancer Inst*. 1987;79:983.

77. Mule JJ, Shu S, Schwarz L, Rosenberg SA. *Science*. 1984;225:1487.

78. LaFreniere R, Rosenberg SA. *Cancer Res*. 1985;45:3735.

79. Rosenberg SA, Lotze MT, Muul LM, et al. *New Engl J Med*. 1987;316:889.

80. Boldt DH, Mills BJ, Gemlo BT, Holden H, Mier J, Paietta E, McMannis JD, Escobedo LV, Sniecinski I, Rayner AA, Hawkins MJ, Atkins MB, Ciobanu N, Ellis TM. *Cancer Res*. 1988; 48:4409.

81. Schoof DD, Gramolini BA, Davidson DL, Massaro AF, Wilson RE, Eberlein TJ. *Cancer Res*. 1988;48:5007.

82. Hosokawa M, Sawamura Y, Morikage T, Okada F, Xu Z-Y, Morikawa K, Itoh K, Kobayashi H. *Cancer Immunol Immunother*. 1988;250.

83. Yoshida S, Tanaka R, Takai N, Ono K. *Cancer Res*. 1988;48:5011.

84. Rosenberg SA, Spiess P, Lafreniere R. *Science*. 1986;233:1318.

85. Rosenberg SA, et al. *New Engl J Med*. 1988;319:1676.

86. Belldegrun A, Muul LM, Rosenberg SA. *Cancer Res*. 1988;48:206.

87. Fisher B, Packard BS, Read EJ, et al. *J Clin Oncol*. (in press).

88. Mitchell MS, Kempf RA, Harel W, Shau H, Boswell WD, Lind S, Bradley EC. *J Clin Oncol*. 1988;6:409.

89. Agah R, Malloy B, Sherrod A, Bean P, Girgis E, Mazumder A. *J Biol Resp Mod*. 1988;7:140.

90. McIntosh JK, Mule JJ, Merino MJ, Rosenberg SA. *Cancer Res*. 1988;48:4011.

91. Berinstein N, Levy R. *J Immunol*. 1987;139:971.

92. Eisenthal A, Cameron RB, Uppenkamp I, Rosenberg SA. *Cancer Res*. 1988;48:7140.

CHAPTER 15

Current Approaches to Immunomodulatory Drug Development: Clinical Development of Interleukin-2 and Identification of Interleukin-2 Antagonists

William Benjamin, Patricia Kilian,
Richard Chizzonite, Maurice Gately,
Bradford Graves, John Hakimi, Grace Ju,
Daniel Levitt, Gary Truitt, Wen-Hui Tsien,
and L. Patrick Gage

Roche Research Center, Hoffmann-LaRoche Inc., Nutley, NJ 07110 USA

Introduction

Cells of the immune system communicate through the elaboration of specific proteins, termed cytokines, which are induced and released following activation. One series of these cytokines has been termed the interleukins because they are produced by immune cells and provide stimulatory signals to other receptive cells of the immune system. Interleukins are typically 15–30 kd glycoproteins that stimulate cells through interaction with specific cell-surface receptors. The key role that many of the interleukins play in immune responses suggests that this family of cytokines contains candidates for pharmaceutical development both as pharmacological agents and as targets for the identification of structures that modulate their function. This chapter illustrates several approaches that are being taken to develop one of these interleukins, interleukin-2 (IL-2), as a pharmaceutical agent for treating cancer patients and to identify and evaluate organic compounds that block IL-2 activity by inhibiting IL-2 binding to its receptor.

Two approaches have been pursued to develop an IL-2 receptor antagonist. One avenue of research focuses on rational drug design. This involves defining the binding sites participating in the IL-2–IL-2 receptor interaction. This, in part, requires the identification of the binding sites within the primary amino acid sequence of the proteins; the solution of the three-dimensional structures of IL-2, the IL-2 receptor, and the IL-2–IL-2 receptor complex; and the design of antagonists by computer-assisted molecular modeling efforts. The second and concurrent approach consists of screening diversified organic structures and natural products from various sources in a highly specific receptor binding assay. Samples identified in the primary drug screen, along with structural analogs, can be further evaluated in specific in vitro bioassays and in various in vivo efficacy models.

Interleukin-2 plays a central role in the induction of immune responses. The clonal expansion of activated T cells, both helper and cytotoxic-suppressor types, is governed by IL-2 produced by activated helper T (T_H) cells and IL-2 receptors expressed on the target cell. In addition, the presence of IL-2 receptors on activated B cells and lymphokine-activated killer (LAK) cells suggests that IL-2 may play a role in antibody production and cell-mediated immune responses by these cells. The central role of IL-2 in immune regulation suggests that it has a powerful use as an immunoenhancer. It is for this reason that IL-2 is currently being evaluated as a therapeutic adjunct in cancer therapy. We also envisage utility for an IL-2 antagonist as an immunosuppressive agent blocking the response of T cells to foreign or self-antigens and thus having potential as a therapeutic in tissue transplants or autoimmune diseases.

The key role that IL-2 plays in immune responses and the evidence that inhibiting its activity may be useful to control diseases characterized by an overactive immune system provide the rationale both for evaluating the clinical utility of recombinant IL-2 (rIL-2) and for setting up a mechanism to identify agents that inhibit the interaction of IL-2 with its receptor.

Preclinical Therapeutic Evaluation of IL-2 for Antitumor Activity

We first evaluated the ability of rIL-2 to inhibit solid tumor growth in mice. In general, rIL-2 was administered shortly after tumor transplant for a duration of 3 weeks before quantitation of tumor growth. The inhibition of primary subcutaneous Lewis lung tumors and the spontaneous pulmonary metastases that resulted from this tumor are shown in Table 15-1. Although daily doses of up to 300,000 units only marginally inhibited the growth of the primary tumor (maximum inhibition of tumor growth of only 28%), there was a significant dose-related inhibition of the number of spontaneous metastases. As reported by others,[1] the antimetastatic effect of rIL-2 was quite marked. This is demonstrated at treatment levels of 10,000 and 30,000 units, which were completely inactive against the primary tumor. The ability of rIL-2 to inhibit the growth of a primary tumor in vivo was demonstrated in experiments with the colon 38 adenocarcinoma model as summarized in Table 15-2. In this model both 50,000 and 100,000 units per treatment of rIL-2 were effective.

Table 15-1. Efficacy of IL-2 Against the Primary Tumor and Spontaneous Pulmonary Metastases in Mice Bearing Lewis Lung Carcinomas[a]

Treatment[b]	Tumor Weight (g) Mean ± SEM (% Inhibition)		Spontaneous Pulmonary Metastases (% Inhibition)	
Untreated	6.51 ± 0.40	—	—	—
Vehicle	6.78 ± 0.68	(0)	15.4 ± 1.7	(0)
10,000 units	6.53 ± 0.91	(4)	8.6 ± 0.9	(44)
30,000 units	6.51 ± 0.63	(4)	8.0 ± 2.1	(48)
100,000 units	5.08 ± 0.46	(25)	3.2 ± 0.7	(79)
300,000 units	4.87 ± 0.55	(28)	1.3 ± 0.3	(92)

[a]Three-tenths mL of a 30% tumor suspension (from in vivo passage) was inoculated sc into BDF$_1$ mice and IL-2 was administered ip once daily, 5 days a week for 3 weeks beginning on the day of tumor transplant. Tumors were excised and weighed and lungs were evaluated for metastases on the day following the last treatment.

[b]Vehicle used was phosphate-buffered saline containing 0.5% heat-inactivated syngeneic mouse serum as a carrier. One unit of Roche rIL-2 is equivalent to one unit of the Biological Modifiers Program IL-2 standard.

Attempts were made to improve the efficacy of rIL-2. Initially, we sought to increase efficacy by the standard methods of increasing the dose, frequency, and/or duration of rIL-2 administration. In both the Lewis lung and colon 38 model systems, the antitumor effect was enhanced somewhat by increasing the frequency of rIL-2 administration (data not shown). However, it became clear from these and other studies that efficacy could not be increased sufficiently to offset the increased risk of toxicity (see Pathogenesis of Toxicity). We therefore evaluated the possibility of increasing efficacy without increasing toxicity by using rIL-2 in combination with α-interferon (IFN), a combination that had been found to be successful in other model systems.[2]

These studies were facilitated by use of a genetically engineered IFN-α A/D hybrid of the human IFN-α A and IFN-α D subtypes. This hybrid molecule has activity in mice unlike that of the parent molecules.[3] A representative experiment testing the efficacy of combination cytokine therapy in the Lewis lung model is shown in Table 15-3. Increased efficacy is shown in the combination of 10,000 units of rIL-2 and 30,000 units of IFN. With this combination, the inhibition of the

Table 15-2. IL-2 Inhibits Growth of Colon 38 Adenocarcinoma in Mice[a]

Treatment[b]	Tumor Weight (g) Mean ± SEM	% Inhibition
Untreated	1.73 ± 0.08	—
Vehicle	1.97 ± 0.57	0
50,000 units	1.02 ± 0.13	48
100,000 units	0.61 ± 0.10	69

[a]Three-tenths mL of a 30% tumor suspension (from in vivo passage) was inoculated sc into BDF$_1$ mice and IL-2 was administered ip once daily, 5 days a week for 3 weeks beginning on the day of tumor transplant. Tumors were excised and weighed on the day following the last treatment.

[b]See Table 15-1.

Table 15-3. IL-2 in Combination with IFN-alpha A/D Results in Enhanced Efficacy Against Spontaneous Pulmonary Metastases of Lewis Lung Carcinoma in Mice[a]

Treatment[b]		Tumor Weight (g) Mean ± SEM (% Inhibition)		Spontaneous Pulmonary Metastases (% Inhibition)	
IL-2	IFN				
Untreated		5.34 ± 0.45	—	16.1 ± 4.9	—
Vehicle		6.42 ± 5.6	(0)	19.0 ± 5.6	(0)
10,000	—	7.45 ± 0.51	(−16)	10.1 ± 0.5	(47)
—	30,000	5.84 ± 0.86	(9)	6.8 ± 2.4	(64)
10,000	30,000	4.65 ± 0.60	(28)	1.8 ± 0.5	(91)

[a]See Table 15-1.

[b]See Table 15-1. Recombinant IFN-α A/D was administered in terms of antiviral units as measured against the α/β mouse reference standard adopted by the NIH (G-002-904-511). IFN was injected ip 3 times a week (M,W,F).

primary tumor and marked reduction of metastases were greater than that achieved by either agent alone and were equivalent to that produced by 300,000 units of rIL-2 alone (compare to Table 15-1). Enhanced potency of combined rIL-2 and IFN therapy has also been observed with colon 38 tumors in mice (data not shown).

The ability of combination rIL-2 and IFN therapy to induce regression of established tumors was evaluated next. The onset of treatment was delayed until 14 days after tumor transplant in the colon 38 model. At this time, the tumors were established and were growing actively, having reached a weight of 0.25–0.5 g. Typical data from one of these experiments are shown in Table 15-4. Clearly, a marked increase in efficacy was observed in mice receiving the combined therapy as opposed to those receiving a single agent. While inhibition of tumor growth was enhanced by combined cytokine therapy as seen on day 22, efficacy improved even further in the ensuing weeks as evidenced by tumor regression and survival of all animals in the combination group on day 43.

Table 15-4. IL-2 in Combination with IFN-alpha A/D Induces the Regression of Established Colon 38 Adenocarcinomas in Mice[a]

Treatment[b]		Tumor Volume (mm³) Mean ± SEM (n)			
IL-2	IFN	Day 22		Day 43	
Untreated		1070 ± 140	(10)	7450 ± 1526	(4)
Vehicle		1078 ± 86	(9)	7349 ± 940	(3)
250,000	—	1134 ± 195	(10)	2665 ± 282	(8)
—	250,000	991 ± 238	(10)	4365 ± 1134	(5)
250,000	250,000	616 ± 83	(10)	163 ± 41	(10)

[a]Tumors were implanted as described in Table 15-1. Treatment was initiated 14 days later as described in Table 15-3 except that duration of treatment was for 4 weeks (days 14–42). Tumors were measured by calipers and volume was calculated according to the formula (4/3)r³.

[b]See Table 15-1.

Clinical Evaluation of IL-2

Recombinant IL-2 was first used in humans in 1984. Clinical trials expanded dramatically during 1985, with a majority of studies being performed by Rosenberg and colleagues at the Surgery Branch of the National Cancer Institute (NCI).[4] In this study, rIL-2 was given either as a single agent or as a form of adoptive immunotherapy. Basically, the adoptive therapy consisted of removing the patients' mononuclear cells, stimulating the cells in culture with rIL-2, reinfusing the patient with the cells, and maintaining the patient on rIL-2. Patients with several types of solid tumors were treated, but responses were marked in renal cell cancer and malignant melanoma. Several dramatic tumor regressions occurred in both types of tumors, with objective response rates (complete and partial) approaching 20% in patients with malignant melanoma. Infusion of LAK cells was associated with higher frequencies of complete tumor regression (5–10%). In a selected group of patients with renal cell cancer, response rates of 30–35% were achieved with combined rIL-2 and LAK cell therapy; 10–15% of responses were complete and these tumor regressions appeared to be durable in the majority of patients.[5]

Six centers were chosen to duplicate Rosenberg's study of rIL-2 combined with LAK cells; results in patients with malignant melanoma were virtually identical to those obtained previously. However, only a 16% response rate, with 5% complete responders, was obtained for patients with renal cell cancer. When parameters that could affect tumor responses to rIL-2 therapy were examined, it was noted that three parameters were important prognostic factors in predicting tumor responses for patients with renal cell cancer: absence of the primary tumor, no lesion greater than 100 cm[3], and minimal hepatic involvement.[4–6]

Administration of rIL-2 by the Rosenberg–NCI regimen is associated with a high frequency of severe toxicities, including vascular leak syndrome (VLS), manifested by peripheral and pulmonary edema, pleural effusions, and ascites. Other side effects that have been observed in humans receiving rIL-2 include fever, hypotension, nausea or vomiting, diarrhea, rash, hyperbilirubinemia, elevated hepatic transaminases, hypoalbumininemia, azotemia, anemia, thrombocytopenia, eosinophilia, and changes in mental status. Since immune activation by rIL-2 appears to be dose dependent, efficacious and toxic doses of rIL-2 are difficult to separate; the NCI treatment regimen requires intensive care unit monitoring.[4–6]

Other ways of administering rIL-2 safely and effectively have been explored. West and colleagues[7] have treated cancer patients with rIL-2 given as a continuous intravenous (iv) infusion with LAK cells and have observed a number of partial tumor regressions in patients with renal cell cancer and malignant melanoma. Continuous infusion regimens for rIL-2 have also been developed by Sondel and Fefer. Sondel[8] treated patients with a 3×10^6 U m^{-2} day^{-1} rIL-2 by continuous iv infusion for 4 days per week, for four consecutive weeks. Three- to tenfold enhancement of peripheral blood lymphocyte numbers, as well as the number of lymphocytes expressing T-cell activation markers, natural killer cell phenotype, and IL-2 receptors were observed. Peripheral blood LAK cell activity increased 250- to 500-fold after 1 month of therapy. Twenty percent of patients with renal cell cancer experienced partial regressions without infusion of exogenously stimulated lymphocytes (LAK cells).

Fefer and colleagues[9] compared the immunostimulatory potential of continuously infused rIL-2 with the bolus administration of this drug. Patients receiving rIL-2 by continuous infusion demonstrated significantly greater enhancement of lymphocyte numbers, natural killer (NK) cells, activated T cells, and LAK activity than patients receiving bolus administration.

At equivalent doses the spectrum of toxic drug reactions is similar with continuous iv and bolus iv administration of rIL-2. However, these reactions are generally more severe with continuously infused rIL-2. This observation correlates with the greater immune stimulation that occurs with this method of providing rIL-2 and suggests that efficacy (immune induction) and toxicity of rIL-2 are closely linked.

Certain tumors can be highly infiltrated with lymphocytes that may be specific for mediating immune attack on autologous cancer cells. Because of the potential high specificity and activity of the immune cells, two groups led by Kradin[10] and Rosenberg[11] have developed methods for expanding these tumor infiltrating lymphocytes (TIL) to greater than 10^{11} cells. These cells are reinfused into donor patients along with rIL-2 and appear to mediate tumor regression in certain patients with malignant melanoma.

Combinations of cytokines are currently being evaluated for their ability to act synergistically to mediate tumor regression. So far, promising results have been observed in phase-I studies with rIL-2 and IFN-α treatment of patients with renal cell cancer and melanoma. Toxicities have been similar in type and severity to those seen with each agent independently. Several complete responses have occurred in patients with both types of cancer. These trials have recently entered phase II.

In summary, rIL-2 is a potent immunostimulatory protein that is capable of mediating a large number of potential antitumor responses. Present and future goals are to optimize the various ways of combining this type of powerful immune modulation with other forms of antitumor therapies, including cytokines, cytotoxic drugs, monoclonal antibodies, and tumor-specific vaccines.

Pathogenesis of Toxicity

As described above, the clinical use of rIL-2 has been complicated by the serious side effects that may result from its administration.[4,5,7] Many of the toxicities associated with high-dose rIL-2 therapy in humans have also been observed in IL-2-treated rodents. Rosenberg and co-workers reported that repetitive administration of high doses of rIL-2 resulted in hepatotoxicity in rats[12] and the development of VLS in mice.[13] In a more extensive examination of the toxicity of rIL-2 in mice, we found that mice given human rIL-2 at doses $\geq 2 \times 10^6$ units kg^{-1} ip twice each day for ≥ 4 days developed VLS (pulmonary edema, pleural effusions, and ascites), elevated hepatic transaminases, azotemia, hypoalbuminemia, thrombocytopenia, and mild eosinophilia.[14,15] In addition, hyperbilirubinemia and anemia were occasionally seen. Hence, the spectrum of toxicities resulting from the administration of high doses of rIL-2 to mice was very similar to the toxic effects of rIL-2 observed in man. The mouse thus appeared to be a suitable species for studying the mechanism by which these toxicities develop.

The possibility that some of the toxic effects of rIL-2 were mediated by rIL-2-activated lymphocytes was suggested by the presence of activated lymphocytes at the sites of tissue damage. Marked lymphoid cell infiltration of pulmonary and hepatic vasculature was present in mice suffering from rIL-2 toxicity, and the pleural and ascitic fluids also contained high numbers of mononuclear cells.[14,15] Hepatocyte necrosis of the single-cell type was present and usually associated with adjacent lymphocytes. Mononuclear cells isolated from the pleural fluids and livers of these mice were 74–98% Thy 1$^+$, 55–83% asialo GM$_1$$^+$, 29–45% Lyt-2$^+$, and <10% L3T4$^+$. Morphologically, the predominant cell type was a large granular lymphocyte with abundant cytoplasm, large nucleus, and azurophilic cytoplasmic granules. Pleural and hepatic lymphoid cells from mice suffering from rIL-2 toxicity possessed potent LAK-like activity: their ability to lyse NK-resistant P815 mastocytoma cells was 10- to 100-fold higher on a per cell basis than splenocytes from the same animals. This LAK-like activity was mediated by Thy 1$^+$, asialo GM$_1$$^+$ cells. A correlation was found between the dose level, duration, and frequency of dosing with rIL-2 required to induce pleural effusions and hepatotoxicity and the dosage regimens required to produce LAK-like cells in the pleural cavities and livers, respectively, of rIL-2-treated mice.

The observations described raised the possibility that LAK-like cells might play a role in the pathogenesis of rIL-2 toxicity. Stronger evidence in support of this hypothesis came from experiments in which mice receiving toxic doses of rIL-2 were treated with anti-asialo GM$_1$ (anti-ASGM-1).[14,15] The administration of anti-ASGM-1 abolished or greatly reduced the severity of rIL-2-induced VLS and acute hepatotoxicity (Figure 15-1) and significantly prolonged the survival of the mice.[14] Administration of anti-ASGM-1 to mice receiving toxic doses of rIL-2 also resulted in a marked reduction in the LAK-like cytolytic activity of their pleural and liver lymphoid cells (Figure 15-1) and a corresponding reduction in the percentage of ASGM-1$^+$ cells in pulmonary and hepatic lymphoid infiltrates.[14,15] It is thus tempting to speculate that ASGM-1$^+$ LAK cells play a central role in the pathogenesis of VLS and acute hepatotoxicity in mice given toxic doses of rIL-2.

Utilizing ASGM-1 allowed us to determine the relative role of ASGM-1$^+$ cells in the efficacy and toxicity of rIL-2 in the colon 38 tumor model[15] described above. In this model, tumor regression appeared to be mediated by Lyt 2$^+$ (CD8$^+$) T cells rather than by ASGM-1$^+$ LAK cells. Indeed, the use of anti-ASGM-1 in addition to rIL-2 led to improved antitumor efficacy in that it permitted the use of a twice-daily rIL-2 dosing regimen which in the absence of anti-ASGM-1 treatment was lethal (Table 15-5).

Taken together, these results suggest strongly that ASGM-1$^+$ lymphoid cells, and quite possibly cells of the NK–LAK lineage, which constitute a subset of ASGM-1$^+$ cells, play a central role in the pathogenesis of some of the toxic effects of rIL-2, including VLS. Additional evidence supporting this hypothesis has been provided by Ettinghausen et al.[16] These investigators found that VLS could be

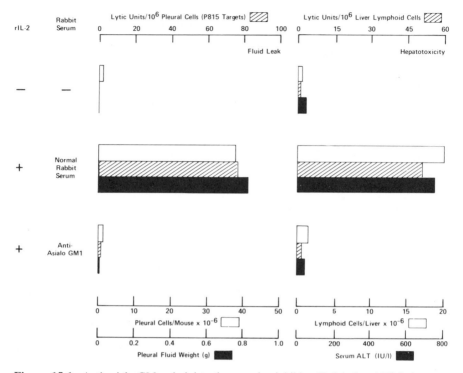

Figure 15-1. Anti-asialo GM$_1$ administration to mice inhibits rIL-2-induced VLS, hepato-toxicity, and generation of LAK-like cytolytic effectors. B6D2F$_1$ mice were given vehicle or 6×10^5 units rIL-2 ip twice daily for 7 days. Some mice also received rabbit anti-ASGM-1 (Wako) or normal rabbit serum, 0.4 mL of a 1 : 5 dilution in phosphate-buffered saline iv on days 2, 5, and 7 of rIL-2 treatment. Administration of anti-ASGM-1 abolished VLS as monitored by measurement of pleural fluid weight, hepatotoxicity as monitored by measurement of serum alanine aminotransferase, and the induction of LAK-like cytolytic effectors. These parameters were all assessed 16 h after the last dose of rIL-2.

induced by adoptive transfer of in vitro-generated ASGM-1$^+$ LAK cells to irradiated mice receiving rIL-2 at a dose that by itself did not cause VLS. The mechanism by which ASGM-1$^+$ cells cause or contribute to damage of normal tissues is unclear. The ASGM-1$^+$ LAK cells may cause direct lytic injury to endothelial cells and hepatocytes. Alternatively, tissue damage may be mediated directly or indirectly by cytokines or enzymes released from ASGM-1$^+$ cells. It is unclear whether rIL-2-activated ASGM-1$^+$ cells are both necessary and sufficient for the induction of toxicity, or whether there are additional requirements for other cell types or the production of soluble mediators whose actions may be blocked without interfering with the antitumor action of LAK cells. In some murine tumor models ASGM-1$^+$ LAK cells were found to be responsible for mediating the antitumor effects of rIL-2, while in other murine tumor models Lyt-2$^+$ T cells were the predominant effectors.[17] It is unknown which, if either, of these two types of effectors mediates the antitumor effects of rIL-2 in human cancer patients. If a class or classes of human

Table 15-5. Effect of Anti-Asialo GM_1 on Antitumor Efficacy and Toxicity of rIL-2 in Colon 38 Tumor-Bearing Mice

Treatment[a]	Tumor Size (mm^3) (N)[b]		Histopathology (Day 31)[c]	
	Day 15	Day 31	Lung Edema	Liver Necrosis
PBS 1× a day + IgG	419 ± 63 (10)	2884 ± 511 (5)	0	0
PBS 1× a day + anti-ASGM-1	278 ± 44 (10)	2570 ± 377 (5)	0	0
5 × 10^5 U rIL-2 2× a day + IgG	310 ± 46 (10)	Lethal (0)	4[d]	3
5 × 10^5 U rIL-2 2× a day + anti-ASGM-1	277 ± 56 (10)	308 ± 90 (8)[e]	0	1
1 × 10^6 U rIL-2 1× a day + IgG	297 ± 54 (10)	947 ± 134 (9)	0	0
1 × 10^6 U rIL-2 1× a day + anti-ASGM-1	326 ± 63 (10)	919 ± 171 (8)	0	0

[a]Mice bearing subcutaneous colon 38 tumors for 14 days (10 mice per group) were given ip injections of rIL-2 or of vehicle (phosphate-buffered saline with 1% normal mouse serum, denoted PBS) the indicated frequency 5 days a week for 3 weeks. On the second day of treatment in each week mice were injected ip with 1 mg normal rabbit IgG or rabbit anti-ASGM-1 gammaglobulin.

[b]Mean tumor volume ± 1 SEM. The numbers in parentheses refer to the number of mice surviving in each group on the indicated day from initiation of treatment. Note that the "day 31" measurements were made 10 days after therapy was terminated.

[c]Histopathology changes graded on the following scale: 0 = none, 1 = very slight, 2 = minor, 3 = moderate, 4 = severe.

[d]Histopathology in this group performed on mice that died following 5 days of rIL-2 treatment (day 19 of tumor growth).

[e]One mouse in this group died of an injection accident (hepatic laceration). The second death appeared to result from rIL-2 toxicity, and this mouse displayed histopathological changes similar to those seen in mice receiving rIL-2 daily plus normal IgG.

tumors could be identified for which $CD8^+$ T cells are the primary mediators of rIL-2-induced tumor regression, elimination of NK–LAK cells in patients suffering from such tumors may make the use of more aggressive rIL-2 dosing regimens possible. This, in turn, may result in improved antitumor efficacy, analogous to the results in the murine colon 38 tumor model shown in Table 15-5. Further advances in our understanding of how the therapeutic and toxic effects of rIL-2 are mediated should permit the development of more successful approaches to the clinical use of rIL-2 as an immunotherapeutic agent.

Approaches to the Identification of IL-2/IL-2 Receptor Antagonists

Introduction

Monoclonal antibodies prepared against IL-2 and the p55 component of the IL-2 receptor have been used to demonstrate the role of this lymphokine–receptor system in in vitro and in vivo immune responses. In vitro, anti-p55 antibodies inhibit the binding of IL-2 to the high-affinity receptor complex and inhibit the proliferative signals resulting from this interaction.[18,19] In vivo, monoclonal antibodies to the

IL-2 receptor have been shown to suppress delayed-type hypersensitivity responses[20,21] and both local[22,23] and systemic[24] graft-versus-host reactions in rodents. Likewise, monoclonal anti-IL-2 receptor antibodies have been shown to prevent or reverse allograft rejection[25-27] and to ameliorate autoimmune disease in rodent models of diabetes mellitis[28,29] and lupus nephritis.[29] Mechanistic studies have suggested that the immunosuppressive effects of the anti-IL-2 receptor antibodies in these in vivo experiments were primarily due to the elimination of IL-2 receptor-bearing cells.[21,30] Taken together these studies indicate that IL-2 receptor-bearing cells represent appropriate targets for immunosuppressive therapy and provide a strong rationale for the development of small organic compounds to inhibit the interaction of IL-2 with its receptor.

IL-2 Receptor

The initial step in IL-2 action is its binding to specific membrane-bound receptors. The first demonstration of specific IL-2 receptors was achieved with the use of [^{35}S]methionine-labeled IL-2.[31] Specific binding sites were found on mitogen- or lectin-activated T cells and certain T-cell lines. This study suggested a single type of binding site for IL-2 (having an apparent dissociation constant of 10^{-11} mol L^{-1}) and the presence of a few thousand receptors on activated T cells. Additional experiments uncovered a more numerous, second class of IL-2 binding site having a low affinity for IL-2.[32] While the precise relationship between the low- and high-affinity forms of the IL-2 receptor have not been completely characterized at the molecular level, the current hypothesis is that the IL-2 receptor is made up of two subunits, a 70-kd and a 55-kd glycoprotein.[33-35] These studies suggest that the 70- and 55-kd proteins bind IL-2 with an intermediate ($K_d = 10^{-9}$ mol L^{-1}) and low ($K_d = 10^{-8}$ mol L^{-1}) affinity, respectively, and that association of these two subunits produces a high ($K_d = 10^{-11}$ mol L^{-1}) affinity form of the receptor. Cloning of the cDNA encoding the 55-kd subunit[36,37] and transfection into non-T cell lines[38] confirms that this protein possesses low affinity for IL-2 and is incapable of mediating a proliferative response in transfected cells. Full characterization of the 70-kd subunit has not yet been achieved and is an area of much intensive study.

Crystallography

X-Ray crystallography is unique in its ability to provide a view of the three-dimensional structure of an entire protein at atomic resolution. The crystallography aspect of our program is aimed at determining the regions of IL-2 and the p55 IL-2 receptor that come into contact with each other and what, if any, structural changes occur upon complex formation. The answers will be derived from analyzing the three-dimensional structures of IL-2, IL-2 receptor, and the IL-2–IL-2 receptor complex. Structural analysis of mutant forms of rIL-2 by themselves and in complex with IL-2 receptor will also provide detailed information on the nature of the interaction between IL-2 and IL-2 receptor (eg, strength and specificity).

Recombinant interleukin-2 has been crystallized in a number of different space groups in triclinic,[39] monoclinic,[40] orthorhombic, and hexagonal[41] (unpublished results) crystal systems and the three-dimensional structure has been determined at 3 Å resolution in the laboratory of David McKay.[42] The latter studies indicate that rIL-2 is composed of six helical segments that include, respectively, residues 11–19 (helix A), 33–56 (helix B and B′), 66–78 (helix D), 83–101 (helix E), and 107–113 and 117–133 (helix F). The helical segment formed by residues 33–54 is interrupted by Pro[47] and may function as two helical segments. The helices formed by residues 33–46, 66–78, 83–101, and 117–133 form an antiparallel α-helical bundle that may be the structural support for helices 11–19, 47–56 and 107–113 to bind the IL-2 receptor.[42]

So far, the IL-2 receptor has not crystallized under any set of conditions but the complex between rIL-2 and the soluble p55 receptor crystallizes readily—again, like IL-2, in a number of forms[40,43] (unpublished results). Analysis of these crystals by SDS PAGE and immunoblot using anti-IL-2 and anti-IL-2 receptor antibodies has shown that the crystals are indeed composed of both rIL-2 and the receptor (data not shown). Unfortunately, crystal forms obtained so far do not diffract well. Several approaches have been taken to improving this situation by reducing the observed microheterogeneity of the IL-2 and IL-2 receptor preparations through additional purification, truncation of the receptor, and removal or limitation of the amount of carbohydrate on the receptor. These efforts have allowed the growth of crystals with an improved diffraction limit of 4–4.5 Å[43] (unpublished results) but more needs to be done to increase the limit to at least 3 Å.

Assuming that the diffraction limit of the complex crystals can be improved to 3 Å or better or that new and better crystal forms can be grown, we will have an unambiguous image of the interactions between rIL-2 and its p55 receptor. Furthermore, we may be able to draw strong inferences of what parts of IL-2 and the p55 receptor interact with the p70 IL-2 receptor. Once the p70 IL-2 receptor has been purified, then we will attempt to crystallize the IL-2–p70 binary complex and the IL-2–p70–p55 ternary complex in order to understand the interactions that generate the low-, medium-, and high-affinity IL-2–IL-2 receptor complexes completely.

Identification of IL-2 Binding Domains

Monoclonal Antibody Mapping

Through analysis of IL-2 structure, insight can be gained into the regions involved in IL-2 action to aid in rational design of IL-2 antagonists. Two approaches for mapping the sites have been through the use of monoclonal antibodies and site-specific mutagenesis. The first approach is aimed at determining the relative functional domains of IL-2 which interact with the p55 and p70 receptor subunits. Monoclonal antibodies were developed against native rIL-2 and their epitopes were determined by binding to synthetic IL-2 peptides and to rIL-2 analogs. The antibodies were tested for their ability to inhibit IL-2-induced proliferation of mouse cytotoxic T cells (CTLL)[44] and to inhibit ^{125}I-human IL-2 binding to mouse CTLL cells and human peripheral blood lymphocyte blast cells.[45] The epitopes of 75 antibodies were correlated with their effect on these two IL-2 assays. Table 15-6 summarizes the results and lists prototype antibodies for each epitope. The antibodies were classified as inhibitory if an excess of antibody to IL-2 inhibited each assay greater than 50%. Most antibodies were tested at concentrations ranging from 1.2 mg mL^{-1} to 0.005 mg mL^{-1} (approx. 10^6- to 500-fold molar excess, respectively).

Antibodies that bind the 1–12 or 9–19 amino acid regions are inhibitory in both assays if their affinities are 4×10^7 M^{-1} or greater (Table 15-6). The second major neutralizing region was determined to be the amino acid sequence 42–56 (Table 15-6). Initially, the epitopes of many antibodies that did not inhibit IL-2 receptor ~~ding or bioactivity were localized to this same epitope. This contradiction was ~~~~~~ ~~ the affini~~~ of these noninhibitory antibodies were determined to be

Table 15-6. Comparison of Antibody Epitopes and Effect on IL-2 Activity

Mab	Epitope[a]	Inhibition of IL-2 Assays[b]		Affinity[c] (M^{-1})
		Bioassay[d]	Receptor Binding[e]	
Neutralizing				
5B1	1–12	+	+	1.2×10^9
7B1	9–19	+	+	1.7×10^8
5B3	1–19	+	+	4.4×10^8
8A6	1–19	+	+	1.6×10^8
1D4	1–19	+	+	4.3×10^7
5A5	21–123	+	+	3.5×10^7
13D2	42–56	+	+	5.2×10^7
17B4	42–56	+	±	1.45×10^8
10B6	40–70	+	±	4.5×10^8
13A6	41–56	+	+	3.6×10^7
Nonneutralizing				
17A1	21–123	–	–	1.1×10^9
3D5	71–87	–	–	2.9×10^8
12B5	66–78	–	–	1.2×10^9
9A2	78–87	–	–	1×10^9
4A4	107–116	–	–	4.2×10^7
3C1	1–12	–	ND	1.1×10^7
1A4	42–56	±	±	1.6×10^7
15C6	42–56	–	–	7.3×10^5
31A4	41–56	–	±	2.8×10^6
7C2	36–56	±	–	7.2×10^6

[a]Determined by binding to synthetic IL-2 peptides and/or to recombinant IL-2 analogs.

[b]Antibodies that reduced rIL-2 induced proliferation or ^{125}I-IL-2 binding by greater than 50% at 1.2 mg mL^{-1} were classified as neutralizing (+). If the inhibition was less than 10%, the antibodies were classified as nonneutralizing (–).

[c]Affinity constants for each antibody were determined by a published method.

[d]Inhibition of IL-2 bioactivity was determined by a microassay with an IL-2-dependent cloned murine cytotoxic T-cell line (CTLL).[44]

[e]Inhibition of binding of ^{125}I-IL-2 to target cells by antibodies was determined as described[45] with minor modifications.

less than 2×10^7 M^{-1}. The antibodies that did inhibit rIL-2 bioactivity at concentrations of 1.2 mg mL^{-1} had affinities of 3.6×10^7 M^{-1} or greater (Table 15-6).

Our data are consistent with previously published results, which indicated that a polyclonal rabbit antibody specific for the amino acid sequence 8–27 and a monoclonal antibody specific for residues 33—54 block IL-2 bioactivity and rIL-2 binding to the high-affinity receptor.[46]

Antibodies that bind to amino acid sequences 71–87, 66–78, 78–87, and 107–116 of the IL-2 molecule do not inhibit rIL-2 bioactivity or ^{125}I-IL-2 binding to the high-affinity receptor when tested at 1.2 mg mL^{-1} (Table 15-6). The affinities of these nonneutralizing antibodies are in the range of 4.2×10^7 to 1.2×10^9 M^{-1}, which is equivalent to affinities of the neutralizing antibodies. We conclude that the regions recognized by the nonneutralizing antibodies are distant from those which interact with the high-affinity IL-2 receptor.

Antibodies specific for sequences 23–41, 87–105, and 116–133 were not identified among the 75 antibodies tested. These regions may be buried within the IL-2 molecule.

The proximity of the individual epitopes within the IL-2 molecule have been elucidated by determining whether or not two monoclonal antibodies can bind to IL-2 simultaneously. The results demonstrate that antibodies can bind simultaneously to sequences 1–12 and 41–55 and to 1–12 and 107–121 (data not shown). These data suggest that the two neutralizing epitopes (1–19 and 41–55) and the N terminus and C terminus of rIL-2 are widely separated or that rIL-2 is flexible enough to accommodate the binding of two large proteins to adjacent structures. The spatial separation of the N-terminal and internal 38–54 sequences has also been shown by Kuo and Robb.[46]

The epitope competition assay was modified to determine whether the purified recombinant p55 subunit of the IL-2 receptor and the neutralizing antibodies could simultaneously bind to IL-2.[47] The data demonstrated that the antibodies specific for the N-terminal epitopes (1–12 and 9–19) did not interfere with rIL-2 binding to the p55 protein, whereas antibodies specific for the internal 41–56 epitope could not bind rIL-2 bound to the p55 protein. In addition, an antibody that is specific for residues 107–116 could not bind rIL-2 bound to p55 protein. From these data, we predict that the N-terminal region of IL-2, in particular residues 9–19, will interact with the p70 subunit of the high affinity IL-2 receptor, whereas the internal segment composed of residues 41–56 will bind to the p55 subunit. In support of this prediction are the following results: (a) The IL-2 mutant in which Asp^{20} is changed to Lys binds the p55 protein but does not compete for the high-affinity IL-2 receptor[45] (see below). (b) Polyclonal rabbit antibodies specific for residues 8–27 have been shown to inhibit binding of ^{125}I-IL-2 to cells that predominately express only the p70 subunit of the IL-2 receptor.[48] (c) A monoclonal antibody specific for residues 33–54 blocks ^{125}I-IL-2 binding to both the p55 and the p70 subunits,[48] suggesting that residues in this internal region may interact with both subunits.

Within the context of the three-dimensional structure of rIL-2 reported by Brandhuber et al.,[42] our data support the suggestion that the 11–19 helix binds the p70 subunit and that helix 47–56 binds the p55 subunit of the IL-2 receptor. The

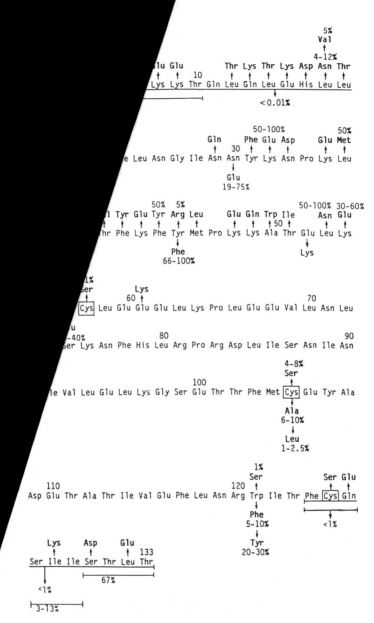

Figure 15-2. Localization and residual bioactivity of site-specific mutations in the rIL-2 protein. The amino acid sequence of mature IL-2 is shown. Amino acid substitutions are shown in boldface, the cysteine residues are boxed, and amino acid deletions are underlined. The percentage residual activity is indicated above or below each mutation. If the bioactivity was equivalent to 100% wildtype activity, no percentage activity is given.

334

data also support
receptor subur
both the p7
gest th
for

n
awa
tor co

Site-Spec

We have also
stitutions and de
quired for receptor
gene was performed t
richia coli expression pl
od of Morinaga et al.[49] Th
protein under the control o
oligonucleotide was designed
deletion. In addition, most of t
endonuclease cleavage site to mon
sequence at the correct location in th

Based on preliminary data, we chose
by site-specific mutagenesis. These region
the N terminus (residues 1–20); region II,
region III, the cysteine residues (58, 105, and
(residues 121–133). To date, over 80 different m
each mutation, rIL-2 analog proteins were produc
bioactivity on murine CTLL cells.[45,50] Selected ana
ability to compete for binding to the human high-affinity
low-affinity p55 subunit, and the intermediate-affinity p7

Results from these structure–function studies (Figure 15-2,
that the integrity of at least three regions of the IL-2 molecule
for substantial activity: the N-terminal 20 amino acids (region I),
amino acids (region IV), and two of the three cysteine residues
region I, deletion of the first 10 amino acids had no significant effect
(Figure 15-2). However, deletion of the first 20 amino acids abolished
bioactivity (<0.01%). Sequential substitutions of the residues in this re
vealed that Leu[17] and Asp[20] were crucial for activity. Competitive binding
(Table 15-7) showed that substitutions of Leu[17] resulted in loss of ability to com
for binding in all three receptor assays. However, substitution of Lys for Asp
produced an analog that failed to bind to the p55–p70 and p70 receptors but was

Table 15-7. Bioactivity Versus Competitive Binding of rIL-2 Analogs

Analog	Bioactivity[a,b]		% Competitive Binding[a]		
	Units mg^{-1}	%	p55–p70[c]	p55[d]	p70[e]
Purified					
Wildtype	2×10^7	100	100	100	100
Asp^{20} to Lys	2.7×10^4	0.135	0.115,0.30	100	0.14,0.2
Trp^{121} to Ser	3×10^4	0.15	0.08	<0.26	0.39
Cys^{58} to Ser	2.7×10^4	0.135	0.1	<0.26	1.03,1.3
Leu^{17} to Asn	3×10^5	1.6	0.39	1	1.2,1.54
Crude					
Asp^{20} to Asn	ND	37.5	0.316	100	
Delete Phe^{124}–Gln^{126}	ND	<0.002	<0.001	19–34.5	<10
Delete Phe^{124}	ND	<0.13	<0.1	27	
Delete Ser^{127}–Ile^{129}	ND	19–37.5	5–24	25–50	ND
Delete Ala^1–Asp^{20}	ND	<1	<1	<10	ND
Leu^{17} to Val	ND	5	2	<10	ND
Leu^{56} to Met	ND	37.5	20	30–37	26,28
Gln^{57} to Glu	ND	33–50	38–42	12.5–16	ND

[a]The percentage bioactivity and competitive binding were calculated from IC$_{50}$ values as described previously.[50]
[b]Measured on murine CTLL cells.
[c]Measured on activated human PBLs.
[d]Measured on purified immobilized human p55.
[e]Measured on human YT cells.

able to compete 100% for binding to p55. A more conservative substitution of Asn at position 20 resulted in a partial loss of bioactivity (to 37.5%), but, as expected, this analog was also fully capable of binding to p55.

In region IV (the *C* terminus), deletion of the last 10 residues eliminated all bioactivity (<1%). Smaller deletions localized the essential region to residues 124–126. Because substitution of Cys^{125} and Gln^{126} did not affect bioactivity, we have focused on Phe^{124} as the crucial residue. Deletion of Phe^{124} resulted in an analog that had no detectable bioactivity (<0.002%) and could not bind to p55–p70 or p70 (Table 15-7). However, like Lys^{20}, this analog retained substantial binding to p55 (27%). A second residue in region IV, Trp^{121}, also appears to be necessary for bioactivity. However, like the substitutions at Leu^{17}, substitution of Ser for Trp^{121} resulted in an analog that had diminished ability to compete for binding in all three receptor assays.

Our results suggest that Leu^{17}, Asp^{20}, Trp^{121}, and Phe^{124} are essential residues for IL-2 bioactivity. From the competitive binding data, we can conclude that Asp^{20} and the region near Phe^{124} form part of the binding site on IL-2 for p70 interaction but are not necessary for p55 binding. A carboxylic acid at position 20 is crucial for full activity. In contrast, because such analogs as Asn^{17} and Ser^{121} had low bioactivities, which correlated with low activities in all three receptor binding assays, mutations at these positions may have generated proteins with abnormal conformations or altered stabilities that were unable to interact with either subunit or with the high-affinity receptor complex. Therefore, Leu^{17} and Trp^{121} may play a role in maintaining the conformation of IL-2, rather than participating directly in binding to either p55 or p70.

To assess the effects of specific substitutions on overall protein conformation, circular dichroism (CD) analysis was performed on selected analog proteins purified to homogeneity (Figure 15-3). The Lys[20] analog produced a CD profile identical to that of the wildtype protein (Figure 15-3A), showing that its conformation had not been grossly altered. The CD spectra of wild-type and Lys[20] proteins indicated that both samples had a high degree of α-helical content (~70%), in agreement with a previous report describing CD results obtained with a refolded rIL-2 analog.[51] In contrast, both Ser[121] and Asn[17] analogs exhibited CD spectra different from that of wildtype rIL-2 (Figure 15-3B). The α-helical content of each analog was reduced at least 50% compared to the wildtype protein (compare ellipticities between 200 nm and 250 nm), suggesting that the conformation of these proteins was severely altered. These altered CD spectra are similar to the spectra obtained with rIL-2 which was partially unfolded in 8 mol L^{-1} urea.[51]

Site-specific mutagenesis of region III, the cysteine residues, clearly indicated that the cysteines at positions 58 and 105 must be maintained for rIL-2 bioactivity, while a substitution of Cys[125] had no effect (Figure 15-2). Our results are consistent with data reported by others[52-54] and suggest that an essential disulfide bond must form between Cys[58] and Cys[105] to yield a biologically active protein. The integrity of an intramolecular bond between these two residues is also necessary for full activity in the natural IL-2 molecule (Robb, 1984). The location of this disulfide bond has been confirmed by direct sequence analysis.[55] Competitive binding assays with purified Ser[58] protein indicate that, as expected, the modified protein was unable to bind to the high affinity receptor complex or its two subunits (Table 15-7).

Attention has been focused on the internal region II (residues 21–65) as an important domain based upon epitope analysis of neutralizing monoclonal antibodies (see previous section). However, we have substituted the majority of the residues on this region with no apparent affect on bioactivity. Alteration of Leu[56] or Gln[57] does cause a modest diminution of activity (Figure 15-2). Because these residues are neighbors of Cys[58], substitutions near this cysteine may have an indirect effect on the conformation of the protein by disrupting the formation of the intramolecular disulfide bond.

The conclusions we have drawn from site-specific mutagenesis can be related to the three-dimensional structure of IL-2[42] (see Crystallography). Our identification of Asp[20] as the contact residue for p70 orients the first α-helical bundle (the A helix) as interacting with this subunit of the IL-2 receptor. Leu[17] is also located in the A helix and may be crucial for maintaining the conformation of this helix. Trp[121] and Phe[124] are located in the F helix, which is proposed to act as part of a structural scaffold. The side chains of both these residues are on the internal face of this helix and are in close proximity to Phe[42] in the B' helix; all three side chains appear to interact with each other (D. McKay, personal communication). This scaffolding model is supported by the observed loss of activity when Phe[42]Phe[44] are substituted with AlaAla (<1% residual bioactivity). At present, our data do not implicate any

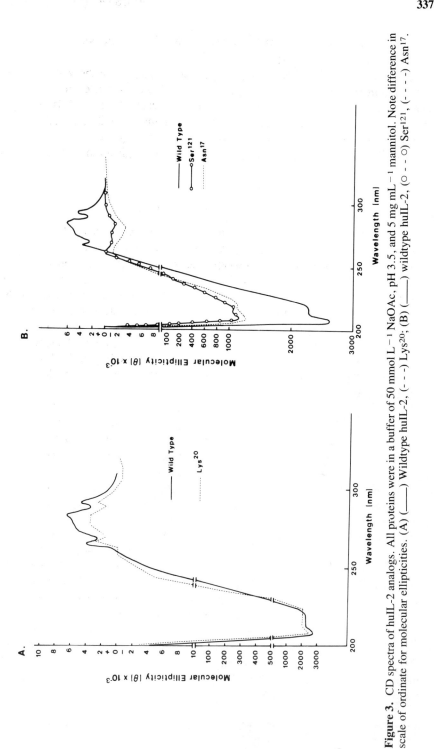

Figure 3. CD spectra of huIL-2 analogs. All proteins were in a buffer of 50 mmol L⁻¹ NaOAc, pH 3.5, and 5 mg mL⁻¹ mannitol. Note difference in scale of ordinate for molecular ellipticities. (A) (———) Wildtype huIL-2, (- - -) Lys[20]; (B) (———) wildtype huIL-2, (○ - - ○) Ser[121], (- - -) Asn[17].

of the residues of the B' helix as important for p55 binding, but we cannot rule out the E helix as the binding region.

Further mutagenesis of rIL-2 will be necessary to determine the validity of the model and to strengthen our conclusions on the function of the relevant residues on bioactivity and receptor interactions. An additional result of this work is the availability of novel analogs of IL-2 that preferentially interact with the p55 protein. Because these analogs allow us to determine the consequences of p55 binding versus p70 binding on lymphoid cells, we can assign biological functions directly to the IL-2 receptor and its individual subunits.

Identification of Novel Organic Antagonists

Complementary to structure–function studies that are directed toward IL-2 antagonist design, another strategy, namely the screening of synthetic compounds, natural products, etc., in the IL-2 radioreceptor assay, is being used to identify IL-2 antagonists. A novel screen has been developed[47] based on the use of a genetically engineered, soluble form of the p55 subunit of the IL-2 receptor. This assay can be carried out either by immobilization of the soluble IL-2 receptor protein directly on 96-well polystyrene plates or by use of a nonneutralizing anti-IL-2 receptor antibody designated 7G7/B6.[56,57] Binding of rIL-2 to the immobilized soluble receptor (ISRA) is determined by use of an rIL-2–biotin adduct. The bound rIL-2–biotin is subsequently detected with horseradish peroxidase-conjugated streptavidin by absorbance at 405 nm.

Binding of rIL-2–biotin to the soluble receptor is shown in Figure 15-4. Plates were coated with the rIL-2 receptor protein and binding of rIL-2–biotin as a function of its concentration was measured. Inhibition of rIL-2–biotin binding by unmodified rIL-2 or 2A3,[58] a neutralizing anti-IL-2 receptor antibody, is also shown. As expected, both IL-2 and 2A3 are able to inhibit the rIL-2–biotin binding to the receptor, thus shifting the dose response. This and a number of other experiments were performed in order to validate the soluble receptor assay for screening of IL-2 antagonists.[59,60]

The IL-2 ISRA was automated using the Hewlett-Packard Microassay System (MAS) which consists of a computer-controlled robot arm integrated with specialized devices for processing a 96-well enzyme immunoassay. The robot transfers test samples from a master plate to a p55-coated plate using a 16-channel pipettor. The master plate, a 96-well tissue culture plate, contains 40 test samples and standards in duplicate. The samples are diversified and include microbial and botanical plant extracts, peptides, antibodies, rIL-2 analogs, and synthetic organic compounds. IL-2–biotin is dispensed to each well and incubated for 2 h. The plates are washed with a wash-dispensing manifold followed by the addition of horseradish peroxidase-conjugated streptavidin. After 2 h, wells are washed, substrate is added, and optical densities are measured in an ELISA reader. Data are stored and processed with an IBM-AT computer. Using this robotic system, we can evaluate 400 test samples in three independent receptor assays during a 14-h time period. No

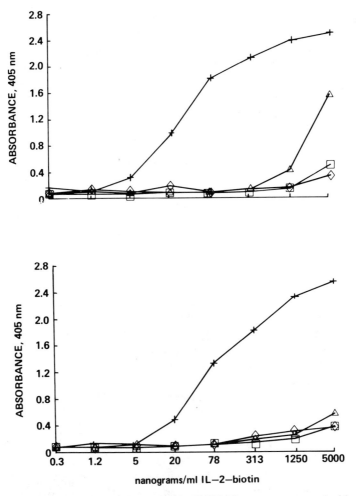

Figure 15-4. Specific IL-2 binding in the ISRA. ELISA plates were saturated with soluble p55 either indirectly on 7G7/B6-coated plates (upper) or directly using affinity-purified receptor alone (lower). IL-2–biotin was serially diluted and added to triplicate wells containing diluting buffer (+), 50 ug mL^{-1} IL-2 ($\triangle$), or 10 ug mL^{-1} 2A3 ($\Diamond$). The IL-2–biotin was also added to wells containing no receptor ($\square$). Bound IL-2-biotin was detected with horseradish peroxidase-conjugated streptavidin by absorbance at 405 nm.

human intervention is required after the initial setup of the receptor-coated plates and the drug master plates.

Samples that are reproducibly active in the solid phase p55 IL-2 receptor assay are subsequently tested in other receptor assays. These include the ability of the test sample to inhibit binding of radioiodinated IL-2 to cells and cell membranes possessing high- and low-affinity receptors. In this way, agents that act upon both the p55 and p70 components of the IL-2 receptor are identified. Agents that demonstrate good activity in the radioreceptor assays are then tested in other IL-2-dependent in vitro and in vivo systems. A chemical synthetic program is initiated upon identification of a structure exhibiting the desired activities.

The IL-2 radioreceptor screening assay is viewed as complementary to the structure–function studies. Structural leads identified in the receptor screen aid in the computer-assisted drug modeling efforts. In turn, advances in characterization of the IL-2 and the IL-2 receptor protein, in particular, lead to an improved, "smarter" screen for identifying new IL-2 antagonists.

Summary

Interleukin-2 as well as a variety of other cytokines have been identified as proteins that modulate the proliferation and activity of the immune and hematopoietic cell systems. Because of their activities, several are being evaluated clinically as therapeutic agents in cancer and other diseases. Interleukin-2 is of particular interest because of the key role it plays in the regulation of the immune response, both the antigen-specific cellular and antibody responses, and the antigen-independent natural killer and LAK responses. Clinical evaluation of rIL-2 in cancer was initiated after demonstration of its efficacy in inducing regression of several mouse tumors. It was uncertain then and it remains unclear how IL-2 mediates tumor shrinkage. Therefore, in the case of a natural product with a very important role in a complex regulatory network, continued preclinical study and careful clinical research should be aggressively pursued to assist in determining how such agents can be used therapeutically in the future.

Our studies, and those of others that we have outlined here, have revealed that the clinical efficacy of rIL-2 is difficult to separate from its toxicity. The efficacy of rIL-2 is apparently manifested through the activation of both antigen-specific and -nonspecific cells of the immune system. Recombinant IL-2 has been used clinically as a single agent and also in conjunction with a novel form of cellular immunotherapy—TIL and LAK therapy. Results to date indicate that rIL-2 therapy with and without concomitant cellular therapy has anticancer potential. However, significant toxicity has been observed with rIL-2 therapy. This toxicity is now being investigated and a better understanding of its mechanism is developing; it is hoped that this information will lead to better ways of reducing high-level toxicity in clinical settings.

Interleukin-2 has also been found to have the potential to combine synergistically with other agents to more effectively treat cancers in experimental animal models. Combined administration of rIL-2 and IFN-α have clear antitumor and antimetastatic activity in murine models, and the promise of this combination is being born out in early clinical studies of rIL-2 combined with human IFN-α-2A (Roferon A). It is encouraging that the combination is effective in animal models where the two agents alone have only marginal activity. Interferon-α and rIL-2 have demonstrated single-agent activity in humans in only a few tumor types to date, and it is possible that this combination may expand the class of indications for their use. Interleukin-2 is an immune enhancer and is therefore thought to act indirectly in cancer via activation of the immune system against tumor cells. Interferon-α also has effects on the immune system but is believed to have its principal clinical effect through direct action on the tumor, perhaps by increasing expression of class I histocompatability or tumor antigens or by direct cytostatic (lytic) activity. Further studies in animal models and in clinical research will yield a better understanding of how these agents work together in cancer therapy and will help to provide more rational clinical use of this promising combination. Studies with other combinations involving rIL-2 are also currently being tested, including IL-2 plus chemotherapy and IL-2 plus other lymphokines, monoclonal antibodies, and tumor vaccines. A general conclusion for rIL-2 and for other natural regulatory proteins with multiple activities is that it will take a large investment of effort and time to fully realize their clinical potential. We believe this effort is worthwhile, however, because of the potent activity that such agents manifest in the appropriate experimental and clinical setting.

The initial focus of biotechnology was on the elaboration of recombinant forms of rare natural regulatory proteins for clinical evaluation as drugs. This was the case for IL-2 and it was only after the gene was cloned, was expressed, and clinical testing was at hand that research was initiated toward development of antagonists of its action. The strategy in this case is that blocking IL-2 action is theoretically an effective means to suppress an immune response. Potential indications for its use would be in prevention of transplant rejection or in autoimmune diseases. Our strategy is based on the hypothesis that receptor blockade is an appropriate target for therapeutic intervention. The extracellular site is pharmacologically accessible and the interaction of IL-2 and its receptor is highly specific; therefore the drugs resulting can be highly specific in their action. Further, highly specific blocking agents can be developed through molecular biology that would interfere with ligand–receptor interactions. As described, significant progress has been made in elucidating the structure of IL-2. Progress on the receptor lags somewhat and has been focused mainly on the p55 subunit because the p70 subunit has not yet been cloned. Our plan is to determine the detailed three-dimensional structure of these proteins, both alone and in their functionally interacting state. Our structural and synthetic chemists will then possess information needed to design small organic compounds that modulate this interaction and that can be evaluated clinically as immunosuppressive agents. One question that will have to be addressed is whether we can design agents that can effectively block the formation of the functional high-affinity complex that these proteins establish in vivo.

We have also used the rIL-2 and receptor proteins to implement automated, high-flux screens for receptor blocking agents from among a large category of synthetic organic compounds and natural products. Our strategy is to take advantage of the diverse spectrum of structures that nature has generated as a potential source for a lead structure for our chemistry effort. This endeavor is closely interrelated with the structure–function analysis, described previously. Indeed, we see each of these approaches as being facilitative if not essential to the progress of the other. Together, we believe that our research on IL-2 should lead to the development of novel pharmaceutical agents useful in diseases that include cancer, transplant rejection, and autoimmune disorders.

References

1. Hinuma S, Naruo K, Ootsu T, Houkan T, Shiho O, Tsukamoto K. *Immunology*. 1987;60:173.

2. Brunda MJ, Bellantoni D, Sulich V. *Int J Cancer*. 1987;40:365.

3. Rehberg E, Kelder B, Hoal EG, Pestka S. *J Biol Chem*. 1982;257:11,497.

4. Rosenberg SA, Lotze MT, Muul LM, Leitman S, Chang AE, Ettinghausen SE, Matory WL, Skibber JM, Shiloni E, Vetto JT, Seipp CA, Simpson C, Reichert CM. *New Engl J Med*. 1985;313:1485.

5. Rosenberg SA, Lotze MT, Muul LM, Chang AE, Avis FP, Leitman S, Linehan WM, Robertson CN, Lee RE, Rubin JT, Seipp CA, Simpson CG, White DE. *New Engl J Med*. 1987;316:889.

6. Fisher RI, Coltman CA, Doroshaw JH, Rayner AA, Hawkins MJ, Wiernik P, McMannis JD, Weiss AR, Margolin K, Parkinson DR, Gemlo BT, Hoth DF, Paietta E. *Ann Int Med*. 1988;108:518.

7. West, WH, Tauer KW, Yannelli JR, Marshal GD, Orr DW, Thurman GB, Oldham RK. *New Engl J Med*. 1987;316:898.

8. Sondel PM, Kohler PC, Hank JA, Moore KH, Rosenthal NS, Sosman JA, Bechhofer R, Storer B. *Cancer Res*. 1988;48:2561.

9. Thompson JA, Lee DJ, Lindgren CG, Benz LA, Collins C, Levitt D, Fefer A. *J Clin Oncol*. 1988;6:669.

10. Kradin RL, Boyle LA, Preffer FI, Callahan RJ, Barlai-Kovach M, Strauss HW, Dubinett S, Kurnick JT. *Cancer Immunol Immunother*. 1987;24:76.

11. Topalian SL, Solomon D, Avis FP, Chang AE, Freerksen DL, Linehan WM, Lotze MT, Robertson CW, Seipp C, Simon P, Simpson CG, Rosenberg SA. *J Clin Oncol*. 1988;6:839.

12. Matory YL, Chang AE, Lipford EH III, Braziel R, Hyatt CL, McDonald HD, Rosenberg SA. *J Biol Resp Mod*. 1985;4:377.

13. Rosenstein M, Ettinghausen SE, Rosenberg SA. *J Immunol*. 1986;137:1735.

14. Gately MK, Anderson TD, Hayes TJ. *J Immunol*. 1988;141:189.

15. Anderson TD, Hayes TJ, Gately MK, Bontempo JM, Stern LL, Truitt GA. *Lab Invest*. 1988;59:598.

16. Ettinghausen SE, Puri RK, Rosenberg SA. *J Natl Cancer Inst*. 1988;80:177.

17. Muul JJ, Yang JC, Lafreniere R, Shu S, Rosenberg SA. *J Immunol*. 1987;139:285.

18. Malek TR, Ortega G, Takway JP, Chan C, Shevach EM. *J Immunol*. 1984;133:1976.

19. Osawa H, Diamantstein T. *J Immunol*. 1983;30:1983.

20. Kelley VE, Naor D, Tarcic N, Gaulton GN, Strom TB. *J Immunol*. 1986;137:2111.

21. Kelley VE, Gaulton GN, Strom TB. *J Immunol*. 1987;138:2771.

22. Volk, H-D, Brocke S, Osawa H, Diamanstein T. *Eur J Immunol*. 1986;16:1309.

23. Volk H-D, Brocke S, Osawa, H, Diamantstein T. *Clin Exp Immunol*. 1986;66:126.

24. Ferrara JLM, Marion A, McIntyre JF, Murphy GF, Burakoff SJ, *J Immunol*. 1986;137:1874.

25. Kirkman RL, Barrett LV, Gaulton GN, Kelley VE, Ythier A, Strom TB. *J Exp Med*. 1985;162:358.

26. Granstein RD, Goulston C, Gaulton GN. *J Immunol*. 1986;136:898.

27. Kupiec-Weglinski JW, Diamantsten T, Tilney NL, Strom TB. *Proc Natl Acad Sci (USA)*. 1986;83:262A.

28. Hahn HJ, Lucke S, Kloting I, Volk H-D, Baehr RV, Dianmantstein T. *Eur J Immunol*. 1987;17:1075.

29. Kelley VE, Gaulton GN, Hattori M, Ikegami H, Eisenborth G, Strom TB. *J Immunol*. 1988;140:59.

30. Mousaki A, Volk HD, Osawa H, Diamantstein T. *Eur J Immunol*. 1987;17:335.

31. Robb RJ, Munck A, Smith KA. *J Exp Med*. 1981;154:1455.

32. Robb RJ, Greene WC, Rusk AM. *J Exp Med*. 1984;160:1126.

33. Dukovich M, Wano Y, Thuy LB, Katz P, Cullen BR, Kehr JH, Greene WC. *Nature (London)*. 1987;327:518.

34. Sharon M, Klausner RD, Cullen BR, Chizzonite R, Leonard WJ. *Science*. 1986;234:859.

35. Smith KA. *Immunol Today*. 1988;9:36.

36. Leonard WJ, Crabtree G, Rudikoff S, Pumphrey J, Robb RJ, Kronke M, Svetlik PB, Peffer NJ, Waldmann TA, Greene WC. *Nature (London)*. 1984;311:626.

37. Nikaido T, Shimizu NI, Sabe H, Teshigawara K, Maeda M, Uchiyama T, Yodoi J, Honjo T. *Nature (London)*. 1984;311:631.

38. Greene WC, Robb RJ, Svetlik PB, Rusk CM, Depper JM, Leonard WJ. *Proc Natl Acad Sci (USA)*. 1986;83:3992.

39. Brandhuber BJ, Boone T, Kenney WC, McKay DB. *J Biol Chem*. 1987;262:12,306.

40. Stura EA, Wilson IA. Personal communication. 1988.

41. Sano C, Ishikawa K, Nagashima W, Tsuji T, Kawakita T, Fukuhara K, Mitsui Y, Iitaka Y. *J Biol Chem*. 1987;262:4769.

42. Brandhuber BJ, Boone T, Kenney WC, McKay DB. *Science*. 1987;238:1707.

43. Lambert G, Stura EA, Smart J, Wilson IA. "Abstracts of Papers," Annual Meeting of the American Crystallographic Association, Philadelphia, PA; June 26–July 1, 1988: Paper No. PJ4.

44. Stern AS, Pan Y-CE, Urdal DL, Mochizuki DY, DeChiara S, Blacher R, Wideman J, Gillis S. *Proc Natl Acad Sci (USA)*. 1984;81:871.

45. Ju G, Collins L, Kaffka KL, Tsien W-H, Chizzonite R, Crowl R, Bhatt R, Kilian PL. *J Biol Chem*. 1987;262:5723.

46. Kuo L-M, Robb RJ. *J Immunol*. 1986;137:1538.

47. Hakimi J, Seals C, Anderson LE, Podlaski FJ, Lin P, Danho W, Jenson JC, Perkins A, Donadio PE, Familletti PC, Pan Y-CE, Tsien W-H, Chizzonite RA, Casabo L, Nelson DL, Cullen BR. *J Biol Chem*. 1987;262:17,336.

48. Robb RJ, Rusk CM, Yodoi J, Greene WC. *Proc Natl Acad Sci (USA)*. 1987;84:2002.

49. Morinaga Y, Franceschini T, Inouye S, Inouye M. *Bio/Technology*. 1984;636.

50. Collins L, Tsien W-H, Seals C, Hakimi J, Weber D, Bailon P, Hoskings J, Greene WC, Toome V, Ju G. *Proc Natl Acad Sci (USA)*. 1988; 85:7709.

51. Arakawa T, Boone T, Davis JM, Kenney W. *Biochemistry*. 1986;25:8274.

52. Wang A, Lu S-D, Mark DF. *Science*. 1984;224:1431.

53. Liang S-M, Thatcher DR, Liang C-M, Allet B. *J Biol Chem*. 1986;261:334.

54. Liang S-M, Lee N, Zoon KC, Manishewitz JF, Chollet A, Liang C-M, Quinnan GV. *J Biol Chem*. 1988;263:4768.

55. Robb RJ, Kutny RM, Panico M, Morris HR, Chowdhry V. *Proc Natl Acad Sci (USA)*. 1984;81:6486.

56. Rubin LA, Kurman CC, Biddison WE, Goldman ND, Nelson DL. *Hybridoma*. 1985;4:91.

57. Rubin LA, Kurman CC, Fritz ME, Biddison WE, Boutin B, Yarchoan R, Nelson DL. *J Immunol*. 1985;135:3172.

58. Urdal DL, March CJ, Gillis S, Larsen A, Dower SK. *Proc Natl Acad Sci (USA)*. 1984;81:6481.

59. Hakimi J, Seals C, Anderson L, Danho W. *FASEB J*. 1988;2:A1251.

60. Hakimi J, Cullen B, Chizzonitte RA, Ju G, Bailon P, Tsien W-H, Schuman M, Liu, CM. In Biology of Actinomycetes, *1988 Proceedings of the 7th International Symposium Biol. Actinomycetes*. Japan Scientific Societies Press; 1988:189–194.

CHAPTER 16

Present Possibilities to Evaluate the Immunomodulatory Properties of Some Immunoregulatory Drugs

Jozef Rovenský and Jan Pekárek

State Institute for Control of Drugs, Bratislava, Czechoslovakia Institute of Sera and Vaccines, Prague, Czechoslovakia

Dušan Mlynarčík

Faculty of Pharmacy Comenius University, Bratislava, Czechoslovakia

Evžen Kasafírek

Research Institute for Pharmacy and Biochemistry, Prague, Czechoslovakia

Vladimír Lackovič

Virological Institute Slovak Academy of Sciences, Bratislava, Czechoslovakia

Věra Hříbalová

Institute of Hygiene and Epidemiology, Prague, Czechoslovakia

Milan Buc

Faculty of Medicine Comenius University, Bratislava, Czechoslovakia

At present the use of immunomodulatory drugs both to treat and to prevent some diseases has been increasing. The number of immunodeficient patients is growing constantly because of excessive stress, toxic factors, and administration of drugs that may adversely influence the human immunological system. Where genetic factors are concerned, the situation is even more complicated, since it is necessary to administer immunomodulatory drugs by means of a substitution in cases of inborn or genetically determined defects.

The immunological system comprises an array of many complex reactions that are mostly coordinated; however, in some instances these reactions may compete. The immunological system is a very intricate network that is composed of many individual parts. This system is therefore very sensitive to any intervention. Because of its complexity, any disturbance to the system can cause clinical manifestations of immunodeficiency. This is very important since a presenting clinical syndrome may be the result of several possible disturbances, each of which can have a very different mechanism. The phenomenon of immunodeficiency may result from many factors, for example, (1) the absence of some cell types or certain factors, (2) the inability of these cells to respond to the impulses that ought to activate them, or (3) their inability to release some regulatory or cooperating substances. The same clinical picture may be caused by a surplus of suppressoric factors, which neutralize the inductive part of the immune response. A further conceivable cause of the presenting syndrome is the failure of mutual cooperation and balance among the individual parts of the immune system. For therapeutic purposes it is very important to discriminate among these etiologies. A successful treatment leading to the normalization of the immune function must intervene only in the damaged part of the immune system. If this principle is not closely observed even a well-meant stimulation could activate undesired parts of the immune system. For example, with antitumor immunity it is necessary to prevent stimulation of the suppressor mechanism, which very often is the cause of the progression of the tumor because it may block the part of the immunity response responsible for the elimination or destruction of the tumor cells. It is therefore necessary to employ only such drugs or procedures as will influence solely the damaged part of the immune system and ensure its correct function.

To secure the success of such therapy it is necessary to examine the effects of the individual immunomodulatory drugs on each part or reaction of the immune system and, for therapy, to use only such drugs as have selective effects on definite individual parts of the immune system and at the very least are not able to cause its deregulation. Unfortunately many of these methods represent only a very rough indicator of the effect of a given drug on a respective immune reaction.

For a reliable evaluation of an individual drug, it is therefore necessary to use a whole battery of methods that can ensure verification of its effect on the designated part of the immune system.

Some studies along these lines have been performed using these drugs in vitro and in vivo or both. For instance, specific laboratory animals or some particular animal model is useful in certain diseases. According to our experience, use of human peripheral blood leukocytes is very appropriate for some in vitro tests. In animal model systems, it becomes possible to use either normal, healthy, non-influenced animals or animals whose immune potential has been damaged by some intervention, eg, by x-irradiation or cytostatic drugs administration.

Therefore, we shall present a short survey of some methods that are used in laboratories to screen immunomodulatory drugs, together with the results obtained with certain drugs that we have examined.

Methods

The Lymphocyte Transformation Test (LTT)

This test evaluates the effect of immunomodulatory drugs on the blast transformation of lymphocytes as initiated by various mitogens. Various mitogens selectively stimulate particular T-cell subpopulations. For example, phytohemaglutinin (PHA) stimulates chiefly T_H cells, and concanavalin A stimulates mostly T_S lymphocytes. Thus, it becomes possible to follow up the effects of immunomodulatory drugs on the respective T-lymphocyte subpopulations.

The Active E Rosette Assay

This test is also suitable for following up on the immunomodulatory properties of various drugs. Wybran et al.[1] have shown that human blood T cells bear receptors for metenkephalin (Met-Enk) and morphine. The method for detecting such receptors is based on an assay of rosettes formed by sheep red blood cells and lymphocytes. This test, termed the active T-rosette assay, identifies only T lymphocytes and is technically performed under conditions suboptimal for rosetting, ie, a temperature of 37°C and low ratio of sheep red blood cells to lymphocytes.[2] The enkephalin and its analogs are cultivated for 1 hour at 37°C in various concentrations. The cells are washed and then their capacity to form active rosette is tested (see Table 16-1).

Recovery Assay of T Lymphocytes

This test is used to assess immunological activity of dialyzable leukocyte extract (DLE) and thymosine[3-5]; it has been adapted for assessing the immunomodulatory activities of other drugs such as, in our case, the enkephalins. Peripheral blood lymphocytes lose the receptor for sheep red blood cells (SRBC) after cultivation in trypsin and do not form E-rosettes or keep their vitality. By recultivation at 37°C E-receptor recovery can be made to occur gradually. Trypsinized peripheral blood

Table 16-1. The Effect of Various Analogs of Enkephalins on Active E Rosettes

Concentration[a] (μg mL^{-1})	Analogs (%)				
	I	II	III	IV	Standard
Control	41.50 ±2.28	41.50 ±2.90	43.62 ±2.28	41.50 ±2.28	41.50 ±2.28
1	45.28 ±5.05	48.52 ±8.38	53.27 ±8.63	48.20 ±9.18	40.70 ±8.05
10	43.43 ±4.91	42.48 ±4.27	65.03[b] ±2.66	49.92[b] ±2.27	40.48 ±1.27
100	49.93[b] ±4.81	46.15 ±4.31	52.07 ±7.01	50.43 ±7.46	45.22 ±2.02

[a] 4×10^6 lymphocytes in 1 mL.
[b] $P < 0.05$.

Table 16-2. The Effect of Enkephalins on the Rosette-Forming Ability of Trypsinized MN Cells after 3-h Time Intervals

	Analogs $\bar{x}$				Standard $\bar{x}$
	I	II	III	IV	
Medium	15.5	17.1	24.0	20.3	21.9
Enkephalins	22.1[a]	26.7[b]	35.2[a]	23.6	24.2
Enkephalins + Naloxone	21.2[b]	24.41[b]	24.7[a]	N.D.	24.9

[a]$P < 0.001$; concentration of analog: 100 μg mL^{-1}; 4×10^6 mL^{-1} lymphocytes.
[b]$P < 0.01$.

lymphocytes were cultivated with various concentrations of enkephalins for 3 hours at 37°C. Their effect on the recovery of the receptor for E on T lymphocytes was followed (see Table 16-2).

Assay of Theophylline-Sensitive and Theophylline-Resistant E Rosettes

The principle of this test consists in the fact that treatment of T-lymphocytes with theophylline, a phosphodiesterase inhibitor, results in an increased accumulation of cAMP inside the cells and inhibits the ability of T suppressor cells to form rosettes with SRBC, without influencing the rosetting ability of the remaining T cells.[5-7] The test is performed by cultivating an aliquot of peripheral blood lymphocytes for 2 hours at 37°C in 1 mL control medium. Another aliquot is also incubated in the same way except that 1 mmol theophylline is added to the medium. The cells are washed, resuspended in a control medium, and then mixed with SRBC at a 50:1 ratio of erythrocytes to lymphocytes. The cells are then tested for their capacity to form E rosettes. A third sample is usually incubated for 2 hours with immunomodulators and theophylline (see Table 16-4).

Table 16-3. Response of Lymphocytes to Concanavalin A in the Presence of Analogs of Enkephalins

Concentration[a] (μg mL^{-1})	Analogs				Standard
	I	II	III	IV	
Control	63.12	77.70	86.47	63.12	64.60
	±38.7	±33.3	±34.7	±38.7	±12.4
10	61.67	61.10[a]	92.00	64.35	66.78
	±39.19	±22.2	±36.51	±40.1	±21.22
50	53.50	56.18	62.67	56.19	70.94
	±30.2	±27.65	±16.86	±35.3	±20.45
100	49.95	45.55[a]	47.13[a]	50.49	57.53
	±34.50	±23.83	±19.9	±35.6	±21.59

[a]$P < 0.05$.

Table 16-4. The Influence of Various Analogs of Enkephalins on Theophylline Resistance and Theophylline Sensitivity in T Lymphocytes

	Analogs (%)				
	I	II	III	IV	Standard
Theophylline-resistant T cells	50.5	55.3	58.0	42.87	48.5
Theophylline-sensitive T cells	5.5	4.4	0	11.86	5.0
Control without theophylline	56.4	59.5	57.7	54.7	53.5
Control with theophylline	50.5	52.3	45.5	50.4	48.5
Control theophylline sensitive	5.9	7.2	12.2	4.35	5.0

[a]Concentration of analog: 100 μg mL^{-1}; 4 $\times$ 10^6 mL^{-1} lymphocytes.

Natural Killer Cell Activity Test

Wybran described the stimulatory effect of enkephalin on human natural killer (NK) cell activity. This system is mediated by NK cells, which appear to be mainly large lymphocytes containing azurophilic granules.[2,8] The NK cells are able to kill a variety of malignant cells without prior sensitization. The Ficoll-Hypaque technique is used to separate mononuclear cells from the peripheral blood of normal blood donors. The cell suspension is depleted of adherent cells by inoculating it in RPMI-1640 medium for 40 min at 37°C in plastic Petri dishes. The K-562 strain of erythroleukemia cells is used as target cells for the detection of NK-cell cytolytic activity (Table 16-5). The K-562 cells (approx. 2 $\times$ 10^6) are labeled with 100 μCi of Na^{51}CrO$_4$ (Zentralinstitut für Kernforschung, Dresden, GDR).

The ratio of effector cells and 50 μL of target cells (K-562) with 50 μL of RPMI-1640 medium (in controls) or enkephalin preparations (0.005–10 μg), partially purified preparation of human leukocyte interferon are tested. The chromium release cytotoxicity test is performed according to Lotzová et al.[9]

The Polyclonal Activation Test

Lymphocytes of peripheral blood are cultivated with PWM for 7 days. Activation of T lymphocytes manifests via blast cell transformation and the stimulation of B lymphocytes to form antibodies. Polyclonal activation of B-lymphocytes is realized by factors released from the activated T_H cells. The T and B cells act cooperatively to cause differentiation of B cells into antibody-forming plasma cells. Impairment of this system results in the failure of B-lymphocyte differentiation and their inability to form antibodies. Helper T lymphocytes are responsible for this phenomenon. Any impairment of the function of T_H cells reflects the inability of B cells to form antibodies, ie, immunoglobulins. This test is an indicator of the impairment of cooperation between the T_H lymphocytes and B cells. This test also can be used to screen immunomodulatory drugs. An example of the use of this test to examine Isoprinosine and commercial preparations of Transfer factor SEVAC is given in Table 16-6.

Table 16-5. The Influence of Analogs of Enkephalins on NKC Activity

Compound	Amount[a]	% Cytotoxicity	Index
Control (basal activity)		64.2	1.00
Interferon		69.3	1.07
Analog I	5	67.2	1.04
	0.5	66.4	1.03
	0.05	64.1	0.99
	0.005	63.3	0.98
Analog II	5	73.2	1.14
	0.5	67.9	1.05
	0.05	64.1	0.99
	0.005	63.9	0.99
Analog III	5	72.2	1.12
	0.5	75.1	1.16
	0.05	69.0	1.07
	0.005	63.9	0.99
Analog IV	5	70.9	1.10
	0.5	67.3	1.04
	0.05	64.5	1.0
	0.005	64.7	1.0
Standard	5	70.5	1.09
	0.5	65.0	1.01
	0.05	63.9	0.99
	0.005	64.3	1.0

[a]μg per 0.2 mL.

Estimation of Adjuvant Activity

The ability of a substance to induce a cell-mediated immunity response was assessed by an animal model, experimental allergic encephalitis (EAE).[10] Albino guinea pigs, weighing 250 g, when injected with 0.4 mg of encephalitigenic fraction together with a substance possessing an adjuvant activity, manifest the clinical signs of EAE. The cells reportedly responsible for initiating EAE are the T_H lymphocytes.[11] Substances able to activate T_H lymphocytes in the comitogenic test

Table 16-6. The effect of Isoprinosine and Transfer Factor SEVAC on Polyclonal Activation[a]

	Cultured with:					
	∅	PWM	TF[b]	TF + PWM	ISO[c]	ISO + PWM
IgM	33.14	401.85	166.3	2232	11.4	2468.5
IgA	105.96	517.0	162.2	3157.0	200.0	4702.6
IgG	146	387.5	240.0	785.5	283	1133.82

[a]The results represent the average of the tests performed on lymphocytes from 10 individual patients.

[b]TF = Transfer factor SEVAC; the amount tested corresponded to the amount of biologically active substance contained in the original 2×10^6 peripheral blood leukocytes.

[c]ISO = isoprinsine; tested in the amount of 100 μg mL^{-1}.

have been shown to have simultaneous ability to induce the EAE in guinea pigs when injected together with the encephalitogenic fraction.[12] In the comitogenic test, newborn guinea pig thymocytes are cultivated with different doses of the substances tested in the presence of PHA, 25 μg mL^{-1}, 10.10^6 cells. Blastogenic activity was measured on the third day by the incorporation of [^{3}H]thymidine. Substances having adjuvant activity stimulated PHA-induced blast cell transformation (Tables 16-7 and 16-8).

Characterization of Enkephalins

Opiate peptides have multiple effects, influencing the central nervous system as analgesics, the endocrine system, or immunity as immunomodulatory substances.[9,13-15] Among these endogenous optiates the dominant are enkephalins. Positions 2 and 5 of the enkephalin molecule are important functional groups for biological activity. Whereas in position 2 the D configuration of hydrophobic amino

Table 16-7. The Correlation Between Comitogenic and EAE-Provoking Activity of MDP and Its Synthetic Analogs and Derivatives

	PHA	Con A	Comit. EAE
A. PEPTIDES WITHOUT SUGAR COMPONENT			
Dipeptide	−	−	−
L-Ala–D-iGln			
Tetrapeptide	−	−	−
L-Ala–D-iGln–L-Lys–D-Ala–NH$_2$			
Hexapeptide	−	−	−
L-Ala–D-iGln–L-Lys–D-Ala–(L-Ala)$_2$–OMe			
Nonapeptide	−	−	−
L-Ala–D-iGln–L-Lys(Ac)–D-Ala(Gly)$_5$–NH$_2$			
Octadecapeptide	−	−	−
L-Ala–D-iGln–L-Lys(Ac)–D-Ala–(L-Ala)$_2$			
L-Ala–D-iGln–L-Lys–D-Ala–(L-Ala)$_2$			
L-Ala–D-iGln–L-Lys–D-Ala–(L-Ala)$_2$–OMe			
B. CORRESPONDING MURAMYL PEPTIDES			
Muramyl dipeptide (MDP)	+	+	+
MurNac–L-Ala–D-iGln			
Muramyl tetrapeptide	+	+	+
MurNac–L-Ala–D-iGln–L-Lys(Ac)–D-Ala-NH$_2$			
Muramyl hexapeptide	+	+	+
MurNac–L-Ala–D-iGln–L-Lys–D-Ala–(L-Ala)$_2$–OMe			
Muramyl nonapeptide	+	+	+
MurNac–L-Ala–D-iGln–L-Lys(Ac)–D-Ala–(Gly)$_5$–NH$_2$			
Muramyl octadecapeptide	+	+	+
MurNac–L-Ala–D-iGln–L-Lys(Ac)–D-Ala–(L-Ala)$_2$			
MurNac–L-Ala–D-iGln–L-Lys–D-Ala–(L-Ala)$_2$			
MurNac–L-Ala–D-iGln–L-Lys–D-Ala–(L-Ala)$_2$–OMe			
C. MURAMYL DIPEPTIDE DERIVATIVES			
MurNac–L-A$_2$bu–D-iGln	−	−	−
norMurNac–L-Abu–D-iGln	+	+	+

Table 16-8. Comitogenic and EAE-Provoking Activity of Some Immunomodulators[a]

	PHA	Con A	Comit. EAE
MDP	+	+	+
LPS	−	−	−
Ei	+	+	−
DLE	−	+	−

[a]MDP, muramyl dipeptide; LPS, lipopolysaccharide; Ei, Ei factor isolated from *Listenia monocytogenes*; DLE, dialyzable leukocytes extract.

acids seems to be the optimum one, position 5 has not been unequivocally determined so far. Besides highly active analogs containing methioninol sulfoxide or prolinamide, or less active analogs containing norleucine, this position has been substituted with a great variety of different amino acids.[16-22]

We have attempted to extend this group by a series of analogs substituted with methionin-like amino acids. For this purpose, we have synthesized and tested the biological activity of enkephalin analogs altered in position 5 and optionally also in position 2. Alterations in position 5 were produced by means of alkycysteine derivatives, ie, S-methylcysteine (a), S-ethylcysteine (b), S-isopropylcysteine (c), S-propylcysteine (d), and methionide (e). Alteration in position 2 was carried out with D-alanine. In this way, we have synthesized enkephalin analogs of the general formula:

1   2   3   4   5
Tyr-D-Ala-Gly-Phe-X

in which the structures of the substituents X at position 5 are:

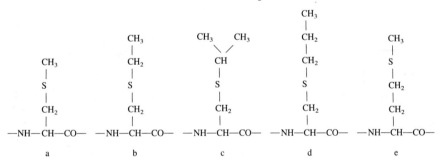

a   b   c   d   e

Unless noted otherwise, all amino acids with the exception of glycine were L-configuration. The analogs are as follows:

		X
I	a Cys (Me)	S-Methylcysteine
II	b Cys (Et)	S-Ethylcysteine
III	c Cys (i-Pr)	S-Isopropylcysteine
IV	d Cys (Pr)	S-Propylcysteine
Standard	e Met	Methionine

The aim of the study was to evaluate the influence of various enkephalin analogs on T lymphocytes and NK-cell reactions.

The enkephalin analogs were synthetized by fragment condensation in solution, similarly to methione-enkephalin synthesis.[25,26]

Analysis of the Results

A significant difference in the formation of active E rosettes was found with analog III, which had a stimulatory effect. Analogs I and IV had a milder activity, and analog II was without any effect (Table 16-1).

In the recovery assay analog III increased the E-rosette-forming capacity of trypsinized cells. This ability could be reversed by naloxone, a specific inhibitor of opiate activity (Table 16-2).

Neither of the tested analogs had an effect on PHA-induced proliferation. On the other hand, a marked effect on proliferation induced by Con A was found with analogs II and III (Table 16-3). These results correspond with the results of a further test, wherein the effect of these preparations was followed on theophylline-sensitive E-rosette cells. Here, analogs II and III also had an inhibitory effect on theophylline-sensitive T cells, which are though to be suppressor cells; on the other hand, analog IV had a stimulatory effect on theophylline-sensitive cells (Table 16-4).

Finally, the effect of the respective analogs on NK cell activity was assessed. It was found that almost all substances tested had a stimulatory effect, which in some cases (II, III, and IV) was even higher than that of interferon, tested in tandem (Table 16-5).

In accordance with some other authors these analogs had a stimulatory effect on NK cell activity. In our experiments analogs II, III, and IV had an especially significant effect, which was even greater than that of interferon. Neither of the substances tested influenced PHA-induced proliferation, as had been also shown by Wybran.[8] On the other hand, a pronounced effect was found with two of our analogs, II and III, on the Con A-induced proliferation. Concanavalin A mainly influences suppressor cells. For this reason, we tried these substances were used in another test (the theophylline-resistant and -sensitive E-rosette test), where analogs II and III also had an inhibitory activity on the suppressor cells. A pronounced stimulatory effect on the suppressor cells was found with substance IV. Higher stimulating activity of analog IV in comparison with other analogs is probably due to its different steric structure, which corresponds less to the receptor structure.

Because of the selective effect of some of our analogs on the respective T-cell subpopulations, these analogs are very promising for the future treatment of diseases that are characterized by immunological disturbance.

Conclusions

To check certain immunomodulatory drugs precisely it is necessary to examine them by various immunological tests which also include animal models and represent particular reactions of the immunological response. It is of great importance to know the effect of every substance on the particular immunological reaction appropriate to each part of the immune system. The immune system represents a fine network of different reactions influencing each other. When the immune system is impaired or its coordination is disturbed, it is necessary to repair only the impaired part, as any ill-considered intervention can cause a deeper disturbance. The treatment itself must be carried out by a clinical immunologist who can apply the immunomodulatory drugs as the means of treatment. Thus to start the treatment aimed at the normalization of the function of the immune system, the physician must know precisely the function and the ability of the immunomodulatory drug. In addition to the positive effect of the drug he has to also know its eventual adverse reaction on other parts of the immune system. Therefore, a good knowledge of the effect of each individual immunomodulatory drug on the particular part of the immune system is a necessary prerequisite for its therapeutical application. In the near future immunologists are expected to be able to define exactly the precise mechanisms of the impairment of the immune system of the individual patient, for example, the absence of certain factors, failure of certain functions, failure in production of lymphokines, or lack of T_H cells, or on the other hand, the excess of suppressor activity. Then it will be most important to have at our disposal such drugs as can influence selectively only that particular part of the immune system. If this requirement is met, the treatment of every defect of immunity will depend on the erudition of the physician. It is obvious that the first step toward this aim is a deep knowledge of the effect of a particular immunomodulatory drug. This type of research requires the introduction of many testing systems and this is the aim of most immunologists at present. It is also possible to solve this problem by application of some seemingly nontraditional systems. For the assessment of the effect of the drugs on the state of cell-mediated immunity, the recovery assay is used. This test proves to be valuable in two modifications. On the one hand, the recovery test can be performed on lymphocytes of immunodeficient persons, who are supposed to have defect in the recovery of the E receptors, and also on lymphocytes of normal persons, where the receptors are deprived by trypsinization. In the above mentioned experiments the latter modification was used to evaluate drugs with known effects eg, Levamisole, DLE, thymosine, on cell-mediated immunity. As it is evident from this chapter, this modification proved to be useful also for testing the effect of enkephalins and their analogs. The other test that uses human lymphocytes is the test of polyclonal activation by PWM. Patients with T_H lymphocyte defects are not able to respond to the polyclonal impulse of PWM by increased production of immunoglobulins. This fact is used to evaluate the ability of immunomodulatory drugs to restore normal T_H lymphocyte function. Incubation of the patient's lymphocytes with DLE, isoprinosine, etc, has led to a normal polyclonal activation of PWM response. This test has also another advantage as it can be used to indicate the most specific therapy. We have stated that drugs that are able to restore normal function of a patient's T_H lymphocytes in vitro are also effective in vivo.

To evaluate adjuvant activity, the comitogenic activity test was used. This test is based on the ability of some drugs with adjuvant activity (MDP and its derivatives) to stimulate the blast transformation of guinea pig thymocytes evoked by some mitogens (PHA, Con A). The results obtained in this test were compared with an in vivo method, the EAE model. The drug that could evoke EAE when injected together with encephalitogen worked also in the comitogen test.

Evaluation of the immunomodulatory effect of drugs may be performed by various methods. The number of tests described and their diversity enable us to evaluate this biological activity using different models. In this Chapter, we have described and discussed only some of the ways in which the immunomodulatory activity of a new chemical compound can be assessed.

References

1. Wybran J, Appelboom T, Famaey JP, Govaerts AJ. *Immunol.* 1979;123:1068.

2. Wybran J. *Fed Proc.* 1985;92:44.

3. Holt JLP, Rovenský J, Cebecauer L. "Abstracts of Lectures." British Society for Immunology Meeting, London; April 21–23, 1976: p. 33.

4. Schroder I, Rovenský J. *J Allergol Immunopathol.* 1982;10:171.

5. Rovenský J, Goldstein AL, Holt PJL, Miština T. *Čas. Lék. Čes.* 1981;120:761.

6. Limatibul S, Shore A, Dosch MH, Gelfand EW. *Clin Immunol Immunopathol.* 1978;10:65.

7. Shore A, Dosch MH, Gelfand EW. *Nature (London).* 1978;247:586.

8. Wybran J. In Guillemin R, Cohn M, Melneclub T, eds. *Neural Modulation of Immunity.* New York: Raven Press Inc; 1985:157–161.

9. Lotzová E, McCredie KB, Marounz JA, Dicke KA, Freireich EJ. *Transplant Proc.* 1979;11:1390.

10. Pekárek J, Rotta J, Rýc M, Zaoral M, Straka R, Ježek J. In Zaoral M, Havlas Z, Mikeš O, Procházka Ž, eds. *Synthetic Immunomodulators and Vaccines.* Třeboň: 1985:129–140.

11. Swanborg RH. *J Immunol.* 1983;1503.

12. Iribe H, Koga T. *Cell Immunol.* 1984;88:9.

13. Simon EJ, Hiller JM. *Ann Rev Pharmacol Toxicol.* 1978;18:371.

14. Pfeifer A, Herz A. *Hormone Metabol Res.* 1984;16:386.

15. Faith RE, Liang HJ, Murgo AJ, Plotnikof NP. *Clin Immunobiol Immunopathol.* 1984;31:412.

16. Roemer D, Buescher HH, Hill RC, Pless J, Bauer W, Cardinaux F, Closse A, Hauser D, Huguenin R. *Nature (London).* 1977;268:547.

17. Bajusz S, Ronai AZ, Szekely JI, Graf L, Dunai-Kovacs Z, Berzetéi I. *FEBS Lett.* 1977;76:91.

18. Day AR, Luján M, Dowey WL, Harris LS, Redding JA, Freer RJ. *Res Commun Chem Pathol Pharmacol.* 1976;14:597.

19. Chang JK, Fong BTW, Pert A, Pert CB. *Life Sci.* 1976;18:1473.

20. Beddell CR, Clarck RB, Hardy GW, Lowe LA, Ubatuba FB, Vane JR, Wilkinson FRS, Wilkinson S. *Proc R Soc London B.* 1977;198:249.

21. Adler MW. *Life Sci.* 1980;26:497.

22. Dutta AS, Gormley JJ, Hayward CF, Morley JS, Shaw JS, Stacey GJ, Turnbull MT. *Life Sci.* 1977;21:559.

23. Audiger Y, Gout R, Mazarguil H, Cros J. *Eur J Pharmacol.* 1980;64:187.

24. Schiller PW, Maziak LA, Lemieux C, Nguyen TMD. *Int J Peptide Protein Res.* 1986;28:493.

25. Losse G, Wehrstedt KD. *J Prakt Chem.* 1978;320:96.

26. Voelter W, Altenburg A. *Justus Liebigs Ann Chem.* 1983;1641.

Index